Liver Transplantation

Editor

DAVID GOLDBERG

CLINICS IN
LIVER DISEASE

www.liver.theclinics.com

Consulting Editor
NORMAN GITLIN

February 2021 • Volume 25 • Number 1

ELSEVIER

1600 John F. Kennedy Boulevard • Suite 1800 • Philadelphia, Pennsylvania, 19103-2899

http://www.theclinics.com

CLINICS IN LIVER DISEASE Volume 25, Number 1
February 2021 ISSN 1089-3261, ISBN-13: 978-0-323-79192-2

Editor: Kerry Holland
Developmental Editor: Donald Mumford

Clinics in Liver Disease (ISSN 1089-3261) is published quarterly by Elsevier Inc., 360 Park Avenue South, New York, NY 10010-1710. Months of issue are February, May, August, and November. Business and Editorial Offices: 1600 John F. Kennedy Blvd., Ste. 1800, Philadelphia, PA 19103-2899. Customer Service Office: 3251 Riverport Lane, Maryland Heights, MO 63043. Periodicals postage paid at New York, NY and additional mailing offices. Subscription prices are $319.00 per year (U.S. individuals), $100.00 per year (U.S. student/resident), $752.00 per year (U.S. institutions), $409.00 per year (international individuals), $200.00 per year (international student/resident), $790.00 per year (international instituitions), $371.00 per year (Canadian individuals), $100.00 per year (Canadian student/resident), and $790.00 per year (Canadian institutions). Foreign air speed delivery is included in all *Clinics* subscription prices. All prices are subject to change without notice. **POSTMASTER:** Send address changes to *Clinics in Liver Disease*, Elsevier Health Sciences Division, Subscription Customer Service, 3251 Riverport Lane, Maryland Heights, MO 63043. **Customer Service: Telephone: 1-800-654-2452 (U.S. and Canada); 314-447-8871 (outside U.S. and Canada). Fax: 314-447-8029. E-mail: journalscustomer service-usa@elsevier.com (for print support); journalsonlinesupport-usa@elsevier.com (for online support).**

Reprints. For copies of 100 or more of articles in this publication, please contact the Commercial Reprints Department, Elsevier Inc., 360 Park Avenue South, New York, NY 10010-1710. Tel.: 212-633-3874; Fax: 212-633-3820; E-mail: reprints@elsevier.com.

Clinics in Liver Disease is covered in *MEDLINE/PubMed (Index Medicus)*, Science Citation Index Expanded, Journal Citation Reports/Science Edition, and Current Contents/Clinical Medicine.

Contributors

CONSULTING EDITOR

NORMAN GITLIN, MD, FRCP (LONDON), FRCPE (EDINBURGH), FAASLD, FACP, FACG
Head of Hepatology, Southern California Liver Centers, San Clemente, California

EDITOR

DAVID GOLDBERG, MD, MSCE
Associate Professor of Medicine, University of Miami Miller School of Medicine, Miami, Florida

AUTHORS

BLESSING AGHAULOR, MD, MPH
Division of Gastroenterology and Hepatology, Department of Medicine, Northwestern University Feinberg School of Medicine, Chicago, Illinois

DAVID D. AUFHAUSER Jr. MD
Fellow, Division of Transplantation, Department of Surgery, University of Wisconsin-Madison School of Medicine and Public Health, Madison, Wisconsin

KHURRAM BARI, MD, MS
Associate Professor, Division of Gastroenterology and Hepatology, University of Cincinnati, Cincinnati, Ohio

KALYAN RAM BHAMIDIMARRI, MD, MPH
Chief of Hepatology, Division of Digestive Health and Liver Diseases, University of Miami Miller School of Medicine, Miami, Florida

DANIELLE BRANDMAN, MD, MAS
Associate Professor of Clinical Medicine, Department of Medicine, Division of Gastroenterology, University of California San Francisco, San Francisco, California

ANDRES F. CARRION, MD
Associate Professor of Clinical Medicine, Division of Digestive Health and Liver Diseases, University of Miami Miller School of Medicine, Miami, Florida

CLAUDIA COTTONE, MD
Department of Internal Medicine at Northwestern Medicine McHenry Hospital, Rosalind Franklin University of Medicine and Science, McHenry, Illinois

KRISTOPHER P. CROOME, MD, MS
Department of Transplant, Mayo Clinic Florida, Jacksonville, Florida

C. KRISTIAN ENESTVEDT, MD
Associate Professor of Surgery, Division of Abdominal Organ Transplantation and HPB Surgery, School of Medicine, Oregon Health & Science University, Portland, Oregon

DAVID P. FOLEY, MD
Professor and Chair, Division of Transplantation, Department of Surgery, University of Wisconsin-Madison School of Medicine and Public Health, Madison, Wisconsin

SWAYTHA GANESH, MD
Medical Director, Living Donor Liver Transplantation Program, Department of Medicine, University of Pittsburgh Medical Center, Center for Liver Diseases, Pittsburgh, Pennsylvania

CLAIRE R. HARRINGTON, MD
Department of Medicine, Northwestern University Feinberg School of Medicine, Chicago, Illinois

JESSICA HAUSE, MD
Division of Gastroenterology and Hepatology, Department of Medicine, University of Wisconsin-Madison School of Medicine and Public Health, Madison, Wisconsin

ABHINAV HUMAR, MD
Chief, Division of Abdominal Transplantation Surgery and Clinical Director, Thomas E. Starzl Transplantation Institute, Thomas E. Starzl Professor in Transplantation Surgery, University of Pittsburgh Medical Center, UPMC Montefiore, Pittsburgh, Pennsylvania

NAUDIA JONASSAINT, MD, MHS
Medical Director, Division of Gastroenterology, Hepatology, and Nutrition, Vice Chair for Diversity and Inclusion, Department of Medicine, University of Pittsburgh Medical Center, Center for Liver Diseases, Pittsburgh, Pennsylvania

ALLISON KWONG, MD
Division of Gastroenterology and Hepatology, Stanford University, Stanford, California

JOSH LEVITSKY, MD
Comprehensive Transplant Center, Division of Gastroenterology and Hepatology, Northwestern University Feinberg School of Medicine, Chicago, Illinois

ERIC F. MARTIN, MD
Assistant Professor of Clinical Medicine, Medical Director of Living Donor Liver Transplant, Division of Digestive Health and Liver Disease, University of Miami Miller School of Medicine, Miami Transplant Institute, Miami, Florida

PAUL MARTIN, MD, FRCP, FRCPI
Professor of Medicine, Chief, Division of Digestive Health and Liver Diseases, University of Miami Miller School of Medicine, Miami, Florida

NEIL MEHTA, MD
Division of Gastroenterology, University of California San Francisco, San Francisco, California

AKSHATA MOGHE, MD, PhD
Advanced/Transplant Hepatology Fellow, Division of Gastroenterology, Hepatology and Nutrition, Department of Medicine, University of Pittsburgh Medical Center, Pittsburgh, Pennsylvania

MICHELE MOLINARI, MD, MSc
Associate Professor, Department of Surgery, University of Pittsburgh Medical Center, UPMC Montefiore, Pittsburgh, Pennsylvania

NATHALIE A. PENA POLANCO, MD
Division of Digestive Health and Liver Diseases, University of Miami Miller School of Medicine, Miami, Florida

JOHN P. RICE, MD
Associate Professor of Medicine, Division of Gastroenterology and Hepatology, Department of Medicine, University of Wisconsin-Madison School of Medicine and Public Health, Madison, Wisconsin

YEDIDYA SAIMAN, MD, PhD
Division of Gastroenterology and Hepatology, University of Pennsylvania Perelman School of Medicine, Philadelphia, Pennsylvania

MARINA SERPER, MD, MS
Division of Gastroenterology and Hepatology, University of Pennsylvania Perelman School of Medicine, Department of Medicine, Corporal Michael J Crescenz VA Medical Center, Philadelphia, Pennsylvania

PRATIMA SHARMA, MD, MS
Associate Professor, Division of Gastroenterology and Hepatology, Michigan Medicine, University of Michigan, Ann Arbor, Michigan

C. BURCIN TANER, MD
Department of Transplant, Mayo Clinic Florida, Jacksonville, Florida

LISA B. VANWAGNER, MD, MSc, FAST, FAHA
Division of Gastroenterology and Hepatology, Department of Medicine and Division of Epidemiology, Department of Preventive Medicine, Northwestern University Feinberg School of Medicine, Chicago, Illinois

ROSS VYHMEISTER, MD
Gastroenterology Fellow, Department of Medicine, Oregon Health & Science University, Portland, Oregon

GUANG-YU YANG, MD, PhD
Department of Pathology, Northwestern University Feinberg School of Medicine, Chicago, Illinois

Contents

Obesity Management of Liver Transplant Waitlist Candidates and Recipients   1

Danielle Brandman

>Obesity is increasing in prevalence in liver transplant candidates and recipients. The rise in liver transplantation for nonalcoholic steatohepatitis reflects this increase. Management of obesity in liver transplant candidates can be challenging due to the presence of decompensated cirrhosis and sarcopenia. Obesity may increase peritransplant morbidity but does not have an impact on long-term post-transplant survival. Bariatric surgery may be a feasible option in select patients before, during, or after liver transplantation. Use of weight loss drugs and/or endoscopic therapies for obesity management ultimately may play a role in liver transplant patients, but more research is needed to determine safety.

Expanding the Limits of Liver Transplantation for Hepatocellular Carcinoma: Is There a Limit?   19

Allison Kwong and Neil Mehta

>Liver transplantation is a treatment option for hepatocellular carcinoma within Milan criteria. With careful selection practices, patients with larger tumors can do well with successful downstaging followed by liver transplantation and should not be excluded based on tumor size or number alone. When considering expanded criteria for hepatocellular carcinoma, however, survival outcomes after liver transplantation should be comparable with patients without hepatocellular carcinoma. Surrogate measures of tumor biology, such as α-fetoprotein, other biomarkers, and dynamic tumor behavior including response to locoregional therapy can aid in risk stratification of patients before liver transplantation.

Frailty and Sarcopenia in Patients Pre– and Post–Liver Transplant   35

Yedidya Saiman and Marina Serper

>Greater than half of patients with decompensated liver disease suffer from frailty and/or sarcopenia, which can lead to increased pre– and post–liver transplant morbidity and mortality. Although frailty and sarcopenia can impact patients with end-stage liver disease in similar ways, they are unique clinical entities with differing underlying etiologies. Early assessment and identification of frailty and sarcopenia in patients is critical to guide clinical decision-making regarding transplantation and to implement nutritional and exercise-based treatment regiments. Nonetheless, accurate diagnosis and, in particular, predicting patients that will develop frailty and/or sarcopenia remains challenging, and the success of clinical interventions is limited.

Therefore, the care of LT candidates on the waiting list must be centered on anticipation and prompt intervention for these complications.

Akshata Moghe, Swaytha Ganesh, Abhinav Humar, Michele Molinari, and Naudia Jonassaint

There is an acute shortage of deceased donor organs for liver transplantation in the United States. Nearly a third of patients either die or become too sick for transplant while on the transplant waitlist. Living donor liver transplantation (LDLT) bridges the gap between demand and supply of organs for liver transplantation. This article reviews current living donor selection criteria, and avenues for expansion of criteria with novel surgical techniques and ongoing outcomes research. Ways in which institutions can establish and expand LDLT programs using the Living Donor Champion model are discussed. Efforts to expand recipient indications for LDLT are described.

Ross Vyhmeister and C. Kristian Enestvedt

Hepatitis C virus has historically been the leading indication for liver transplant, followed by nonalcoholic steatohepatitis (NASH) and alcoholic liver disease. Severe alcoholic hepatitis has become a growing indication for liver transplant, and overall alcohol use rates continue to increase in the United States. Rates of obesity and NASH in the United States continue to increase and are expected to place increasing demand on liver transplant infrastructure. In the current absence of robust pharmacologic therapy for NASH, the use of bariatric procedures and surgeries is being explored, as are other innovative approaches to curtail this upward trend.

Blessing Aghaulor and Lisa B. VanWagner

Cardiovascular disease complications are the leading cause of early (short-term) mortality among liver transplant recipients. The increasingly older candidate pool has multiple comorbidities necessitating cardiac and pulmonary vascular disease risk stratification of patients for optimal allocation of scarce donor livers. Arrhythmias, heart failure, stroke, and coronary artery disease are common pretransplant cardiovascular comorbidities and contribute to cardiovascular complications after liver transplant. Valvular heart disease and portopulmonary hypertension present intraoperative challenges during liver transplant surgery. The Cardiovascular Risk in Orthotopic Liver Transplantation score estimates the risk of cardiovascular complications in liver transplant candidates within the first year after transplant.

Machine perfusion (MP) has emerged as a promising preservation technique to reduce the risks associated with transplant of high risk (steatotic, elderly, and donation after circulatory death) hepatic allografts. Multiple strategies for MP are under investigation. MP facilitates assessment of organ viability and enables liver-directed therapy before transplant. Clinical trials suggest MP may improve the use of hepatic allografts, mitigate ischemia-reperfusion injury, and reduce the incidences of early allograft dysfunction, biliary complications, and ischemic cholangiopathy. As MP sees more widespread use outside of trial settings, more investigation will be needed to establish optimal application of this technology.

Despite record-breaking numbers of liver transplants (LTs) performed in the United States in each of the last 7 years, many patients remain on the wait list as the demand for LT continues to exceed the supply of available donors. The emergence of highly effective and well-tolerated direct-acting antiviral therapy has transformed the clinical course and management of hepatitis C virus (HCV) in both the pretransplant and posttransplant setting. Historically, donor livers infected with HCV were either transplanted into patients already infected with HCV or discarded.

Increased life expectancy and advances in the care of chronic liver disease has increased the number of elderly patients needing liver transplant. Organ donation policies prioritize transplant to the sickest. There is an ongoing debate with regard to balancing the principles of equity and utility. Several hospitals have adopted center-specific policies and there has been an increased trend of transplant in elderly patients since 2002. Appropriate patient selection and long-term outcomes in the setting of limited organ availability pose several challenges. This article reviews the data and discusses the pros and cons of transplants in the elderly.

Liver transplant for severe alcohol-associated hepatitis remains a controversial practice despite evidence for a substantial survival benefit compared with medical therapy and posttransplant alcohol relapse rates comparable with previously published studies in alcohol-associated cirrhosis. The controversy stems in part from concern regarding patient selection practices, lack of long-term follow-up data, and the potential negative public perception of the practice affecting organ donation. Despite these concerns, it seems that early liver transplant for alcohol-associated hepatitis is increasingly being offered to selected patients across the United States and the world.

CLINICS IN LIVER DISEASE

SERIES OF RELATED INTEREST

Gastroenterology Clinics of North America
www.gastro.theclinics.com
Gastrointestinal Endoscopy Clinics of North America
www.giendo.theclinics.com

THE CLINICS ARE AVAILABLE ONLINE!
Access your subscription at:
www.theclinics.com

CLINICS IN LIVER DISEASE

FORTHCOMING ISSUES

May 2021
Complications of Cirrhosis
Andres Cardenas and Thomas Reiberger, editors

August 2021
Alcoholic Hepatitis
Paul Kwo, editor

November 2021
Challenging Issues in the Management of Chronic Hepatitis B Virus
Mitchell Shiffman, editor

RECENT ISSUES

November 2020
Hepatocellular Carcinoma: Moving into The 21st Century
Catherine Frenette, editor

August 2020
Consultations in Liver Disease
Steven L. Flamm, Editor

May 2020
Hepatic Encephalopathy
Vinod K. Rustgi, Editor

SERIES OF RELATED INTEREST

Gastroenterology Clinics of North America
www.gastro.theclinics.com
Gastrointestinal Endoscopy Clinics of North America
www.giendo.theclinics.com

THE CLINICS ARE AVAILABLE ONLINE!

Access your subscription at:
www.theclinics.com

Preface

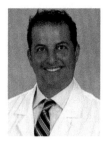

David Goldberg, MD, MSCE
Editor

Despite advances in the care of patients with chronic liver disease, notably the revolution of direct-acting antivirals to treat hepatitis C, the need for lifesaving liver transplants remains. The number of liver transplants performed increases every year, yet the demand continues to outstrip the supply. Despite this, the landscape of liver transplantation has been rapidly changing, with respect to expansions of the donor pool, aging of the recipient population, and changing diagnoses leading to liver transplantation.

In a short period of time, hepatitis C has no longer become the leading indication for liver transplantation. At the same time, there has been a growth in several populations of transplant recipients: (1) younger patients with acute alcoholic hepatitis; (2) older, obese patients with nonalcoholic steatohepatitis; and (3) patients with hepatocellular carcinoma exceeding traditional transplant criteria. Each of these patient populations has required a frameshift in our pretransplant risk assessment (eg, psychosocial evaluation of patients with alcoholic hepatitis and pretransplant cardiovascular assessment in patients with nonalcoholic steatohepatitis), and our posttransplant management (eg, immunosuppression, obesity, cardiovascular disease). Furthermore, we have had to deal with the complexities of transplanting these unique patient populations, including an increasing prevalence of obesity, as well as frailty and sarcopenia in our end-stage liver disease patients awaiting a transplant.

Despite increases in deceased organ donation, the supply of available organs falls well short of the demand, which has led the transplant community to continue to innovate in the field of organ donation and utilization. Two areas in which we have seen a growth have been (1) donation after circulatory death donors; and (2) living donor liver transplantation. Each of these offers the potential to help meet the organ supply-demand gap. Advances in technology, namely machine perfusion, have raised our hopes

Dr Goldberg has received research funding support, paid to his institution, from Merck, Gilead, and AbbVie, and has done consulting for Pfizer for creation of unbranded educational content.

Clin Liver Dis 25 (2021) xiii–xiv
https://doi.org/10.1016/j.cld.2020.09.002
1089-3261/21/© 2020 Published by Elsevier Inc.

that we can continue to improve utilization of donor organs to help save more lives through liver transplantation.

We hope that this special issue of *Clinics in Liver Disease* focused on liver transplantation will be of use to the broad group of health care providers caring for patients with end-stage liver disease as well as liver transplant recipients. In the future, we hope that we will continue to improve our ability to care for our patients with end-stage liver disease, and for those who require a transplant, to have enough organs to perform a life-saving transplant that will provide long-term survival to all those who are in need.

David Goldberg, MD, MSCE
University of Miami
Miller School of Medicine
1120 NW 14th Street, Room 807
Miami, FL 33136, USA

E-mail address:
dsgoldberg@med.miami.edu

Obesity Management of Liver Transplant Waitlist Candidates and Recipients

Danielle Brandman, MD, MAS

KEYWORDS

- Obesity • Liver transplantation • NAFLD • Bariatric surgery

KEY POINTS

- Obesity prevalence is increasing in liver transplant candidates and recipients, which increases waitlist mortality and post-transplant morbidity but ultimately results in good long-term post-transplant survival in those who receive a transplant.
- Frailty and sarcopenia are common in patients with obesity and cirrhosis, so these factors must be considered when providing dietary counseling.
- Sleeve gastrectomy performed prior to or during liver transplantation at an experienced center may improve candidates' suitability for transplant and resolve metabolic syndrome comorbidities.

OBESITY, LIVER DISEASE, AND IMPACT ON LIVER TRANSPLANT CANDIDACY

The prevalence of obesity has drastically increased over time, with 13% of the world's population affected as of 2016[1] and many countries affected more deeply, such as the United States, with an obesity prevalence of 42.4% as of 2018.[2] The presence of obesity increases the risk of morbidity and mortality related to diabetes and cardiovascular disease.[3] The increased incidence and prevalence of nonalcoholic fatty liver disease (NAFLD) have paralleled the obesity epidemic, with 20% of the world population and 30% of the US population likely to have NAFLD.[4] The increase in NAFLD has resulted in rising rates of decompensated cirrhosis and hepatocellular carcinoma (HCC) due to nonalcoholic steatohepatitis (NASH). Consequently, NASH has become the second most common indication for liver transplantation in the United States[5] and is rapidly rising in other countries as well.[6,7] Because NASH patients commonly are affected by obesity, the management of these patients to insure excellent outcomes before and after liver transplantation warrants close attention. The prevalence of obesity also has risen in liver transplant candidates with other underlying liver disease,

Department of Medicine, Division of Gastroenterology, University of California San Francisco, 513 Parnassus Avenue, Box 0538, Room S357, San Francisco, CA 94143, USA
E-mail address: Danielle.brandman@ucsf.edu

Clin Liver Dis 25 (2021) 1–18
https://doi.org/10.1016/j.cld.2020.08.001
1089-3261/21/© 2020 Elsevier Inc. All rights reserved.

liver.theclinics.com

with 17% of all US liver transplant candidates having a body mass index (BMI) greater than 35 kg/m^2 as of 2018 and approximately 25% with BMI greater than 30 kg/m^2.[8]

Obese patients are at increased risk for hepatic decompensation, acute-on-chronic liver failure, and liver-related death.[9–11] Obesity, in combination with diabetes and hypertension, appears to increase the risk of HCC substantially.[12–14] Patients with HCC in the setting of NASH may have higher risk histology seen on explant at the time of liver transplantation, but obesity alone does not appear to independently have an impact on HCC histology in liver transplant recipients.[15] The high rates of decompensation and HCC in obese patients illustrates a clear need for liver transplantation in this patient population.

Current guidelines from the American Association for the Study of Liver Disease and American Society of Transplantation recognize the potential impact of severe obesity on post-transplant outcomes, and, as such, have given a recommendation that the presence of class III obesity (**Table 1** lists obesity classes) is a relative contraindication to liver transplantation, but this is a weak recommendation with only moderate-quality evidence and does not incorporate data published after development of these recommendations showing good long-term outcomes in obese liver transplant recipients.[16] Dietary counseling is recommended for liver transplant candidates with class I obesity and higher.[16] European guidelines do not offer a specific cutoff BMI at which patients may not be offered liver transplant but do recommend that those with class II obesity or greater should be managed by a multidisciplinary team that does include a dietician.[17]

Historically, patients with obesity tend to fare poorly on the liver transplant waiting list.[18,19] The most recent analysis of United Network for Organ Sharing (UNOS) data has shown that patients with BMI greater than or equal to 35 kg/m^2 have a 1.07-fold to 1.27-fold greater risk of waitlist dropout than patients with BMI 25 kg/m^2 to 29.9 kg/m^2.[18] Whether this is due to a direct higher risk of mortality in obese patients is unclear. One factor contributing to poorer waitlist outcomes is decreased rates of acceptance of organs for waitlisted patients who are obese.[20,21] Smaller proportions of obese patients also make it to the waiting list, with many programs imposing BMI cutoffs to determine candidacy for transplant,[22] with as many as 19% of centers not performing transplants on patients with class III obesity.[21]

OBESITY AND LIVER TRANSPLANT OUTCOMES

The perception of patients with high BMI being suboptimal candidates for liver transplantation has been deeply rooted in data from the general surgery literature,[23] other solid organ literature,[24] and previously supported by single-center and pre–Model of End-Stage Liver Disease (MELD) era studies reporting poor post-transplant outcomes in this patient population.[25–28] Obese liver transplant candidates may not be viewed as favorably as nonobese candidates, due to concerns about more complex surgery,[29] prolonged recovery, and post-transplant hospital stay,[30] higher rates of wound

Table 1 Classification of obesity severity	
BMI class	Body Mass Index (kg/m^2)
Class I	30–34.99
Class II	35–39.99
Class III	$\geq$40

complications,[30-36] more frequent pulmonary complications,[36,37] and increased risk of major cardiovascular events.[38] A meta-analysis that included 132,126 liver transplant recipients observed a higher risk of death at 30 days post-transplant in comparison with normal weight and overweight patients. This study, however, included a relatively small proportion of patients who had undergone liver transplantation in the modern era; therefore, the results may not be reflective of current outcomes.[39] More modern data in liver transplant recipients have helped reshape the narrative surrounding the impact of obesity on post–liver transplant outcomes. A more recent meta-analysis identifies the importance of year of publication as a factor influencing post-transplant outcomes, with earlier studies more likely to report poorer outcomes in obese liver transplant recipients.[40] Several large, multicenter studies have reported similar survival after liver transplantation in obese patients versus nonobese patients[41,42] and receive good survival benefit from transplant.[43] No standard criteria exist to select the ideal transplant candidate with obesity, although it is likely that those selected represent a fitter group, thereby accounting for their good outcomes. Recent data from European registries, however, report class III obesity as associated with a 1.35-fold greater risk of post-transplant death in comparison with normal-weight recipients.[44] The discordant results may be accounted for by US programs having more experience in the management of obese patients, because severe obesity is more common in the United States.

Few data exist regarding liver transplant recipients with BMI greater than or equal to 50 kg/m^2, because these patients rarely are accepted for liver transplant listing and eventually undergo transplant. Evaluation of 123 liver transplant recipients (out of 104,250) with BMI in this range showed high rates of mortality (10%) at 30 days. The short-term survival was markedly better in patients with lower BMI (99.2%), with the difference in long-term survival persisting although differences were less pronounced (66% vs 74%, respectively, at 5 years).[45] The observed shorter survival in obese liver transplant recipients in part may be accounted for by higher degrees of visceral fat, which are associated with increased risk of diabetes.[46]

Diabetes prior to liver transplantation is a known risk factor for decreased long-term survival after liver transplantation, particularly if sustained post-transplant.[47] Because many patients with obesity also are affected by diabetes, the impact of increasing prevalence of these comorbid conditions on post-transplant survival warrants attention. A large multicenter study showed no difference in survival on the basis of BMI alone, although the concomitant presence of diabetes plus obesity was associated with worse 5-year survival (66%) than in patients with diabetes who were not obese (80%), without diabetes but were obese (90%), and without diabetes or obesity (88%).[48] Similar findings also were reported in UNOS-based studies and a large meta-analysis.[49-51]

New-onset diabetes post-transplant is more common in patients with NASH as their indication for transplant; given that the majority of NASH recipients are obese, there is good reason for concern about the potential for increased risk of morbidity and mortality in this population.[52] Despite concerns about patients with NASH cirrhosis being at higher risk for death after liver transplantation, large, multicenter studies thus far have reported similar long-term post-transplant survival for NASH versus non-NASH recipients.[44,53,54] In a recent US study, liver transplant recipients with NASH cirrhosis had better survival if they were obese.[55] This may suggest either that patients with NASH who have lower BMI at the time of transplant are malnourished or that the obese NASH recipients are highly selected as better candidates at the outset. Increased risk of post-transplant cardiovascular events in NASH recipients may be accounted for by higher prevalence of cardiac risk factors and older age rather than obesity alone.[56]

STRATEGIES FOR OBESITY MANAGEMENT IN LIVER TRANSPLANT CANDIDATES: LIFESTYLE MODIFICATION

Before recommendations for weight loss are provided, it is critical to accurately assess the nutritional status of patients with decompensated cirrhosis, because malnutrition and sarcopenia are common.[57–59] Frailty appears to compound the risk of death on the liver transplant waiting list, with a large multicenter study demonstrating that frail candidates with class I obesity have a 1.7-fold increased risk of waitlist mortality compared with nonobese candidates, and those with class II to class III obesity having a 3.2-fold increased risk.[59] In nonfrail patients, the risk of waitlist mortality was similar between all 3 BMI categories, suggesting that frailty may be a particularly ominous sign in obese liver transplant candidates that warrants close attention. Sarcopenia in these patients likely is contributing to frailty in these patients, because sarcopenia is common in patients with NASH cirrhosis and/or obesity.[60–62] Given the known association of frailty and waitlist mortality,[63] efforts, such as exercise and prehabilitation, to improve this parameter should be promoted to try to mitigate the deleterious effect of frailty.[64,65]

Additionally, it can be difficult to accurately determine a patient's true BMI, because up to 20% of patients with ascites may have BMI overestimated.[41] Promotion of weight loss in patients with decompensated cirrhosis should be done with caution, given concern for worsening preexisting sarcopenia if patients eat a diet that restricts calories and/or protein too aggressively, because further muscle loss may increase mortality.[66] Currently, no specific guidelines exist for promotion of weight loss in patients with decompensated cirrhosis, although avoidance of higher caloric intake in these patients along with high protein requirements is recommended.[67,68] Structured weight loss programs have been used in patients with advanced liver disease. For example, the Mayo Clinic obesity protocol takes a multidisciplinary approach to patients listed for liver transplantation with BMI greater than 35 kg/m^2, utilizing dietary and exercise counseling, a food diary, and weekly weight assessment[69]; the success rate of this protocol in patients who have not undergone transplant has not been reported.

Weight loss through dietary changes is safe in patients with compensated cirrhosis and may improve severity of portal hypertension.[70] Exercise, particularly if administered through a supervised physical exercise program, may aid in successful weight loss efforts and also contribute to reductions in portal pressures.[71]

STRATEGIES FOR OBESITY MANAGEMENT IN LIVER TRANSPLANT CANDIDATES: PHARMACOTHERAPY

Few drugs are approved for the purpose of weight management, and little is known about the safety or effectiveness of these drugs in patients with advanced liver disease. Herbal weight loss supplements should be avoided due to the risk of liver failure with several of these agents.[72] Prescription weight loss drugs may be safe, but few data on safety in patients with cirrhosis are available. Orlistat impairs absorption of dietary fats through inhibition of gastric and pancreatic lipase. This drug has minimal systemic absorption but has been associated with cases of severe liver injury and liver failure.[73] Lorcaserin, a selective 5-HT_{2C} receptor agonist that resulted in a 4.5% to 5.8% body weight change in its registration trials, has similar pharmacokinetics in patients with mild to moderate impairments in hepatic function (Child-Pugh class A–B), suggesting that dose adjustments of this drug may not be necessary in patients with liver disease.[74] One case report of a patient with Child-Pugh class B8 and MELD of 15 described reduction in BMI from 50.3 kg/m^2 to 40.7 kg/m^2 over a 9-month period with use of lorcaserin, which also was accompanied by improvement in MELD score to 11.[75] Phentermine/

topiramate yielded 7.8% to 10.9% body weight reduction in their registration trials. Concern about adverse cardiac or neurologic effects of lorcaserin and phentermine/topiramate has been raised and resulted in withdrawal of approval of these drugs in Europe.[76,77] Other drugs, such as bupropion/naltrexone and liraglutide, appear to have favorable safety profiles, but again the data in patients with cirrhosis are lacking. Additional studies are needed to garner adequate data to consider use of prescription weight loss drugs in patients with end-stage liver disease and likely require collaborative care delivered by an obesity specialist and hepatologist if used.

STRATEGIES FOR OBESITY MANAGEMENT IN LIVER TRANSPLANT CANDIDATES: BARIATRIC SURGERY PRIOR TO TRANSPLANT

The effectiveness of bariatric surgery in producing durable loss of excess body weight and improvement in metabolic syndrome comorbidities in patients with severe obesity is well established in the general population,[78,79] although few data exist regarding how this may translate to improvement in mortality.[80,81] Bariatric surgery is more effective than standard medical therapy for improving control and inducing remission of diabetes in patients with class I obesity,[82] with both Roux-en-Y gastric bypass (RYGB) and sleeve gastrectomy having a similar impact.[83] Several societies now recommend laparoscopic bariatric surgery for patients with class I obesity and diabetes and/or hypertension that is suboptimally controlled with medication, class II obesity with comorbidities, and/or class III obesity.[84,85] The 2 most common bariatric surgical procedures, RYGB and sleeve gastrectomy, have similar results with regard to percentage of excess body weight loss (EBWL),[86] although sleeve gastrectomy has lower rates of complications.[87] Gastric banding had been appealing due to less complex surgery and the potential to adjust the band depending on weight loss or symptoms, but typically it yields lower EBWL[78,86] and has higher long-term complication rates.[88] Bariatric surgical procedures that are emerging, such as laparoscopic greater curvature plication, 1 anastomosis gastric bypass, and 1 anastomosis duodenal switch, have few long-term data on outcomes and insufficient data for patients with cirrhosis.[89–91]

Obesity refractory to medical management in a patient with advanced liver disease poses a particular challenge for transplant programs, because many patients may be too sick to tolerate bariatric surgery when presenting with hepatic decompensation. Bariatric surgery may be performed successfully in carefully selected patients with cirrhosis. The weight loss afforded by surgery can help facilitate transplant candidacy for patients who otherwise might be declined for transplant on the basis of weight.

The benefits of sleeve gastrectomy in liver transplant candidates include less technically complex surgery, preservation of access to the biliary tree, and fewer concerns about impaired absorption of immunosuppressant drugs after transplant.[92–94] Sleeve gastrectomy has been identified as a cost-effective management strategy in patients with compensated NASH cirrhosis who were overweight or obese (all classes), with quality-adjusted life-year benefit of $10,274 in moderate obesity and $6563 in severe obesity.[95] Several small retrospective cohort studies have reported good outcomes of bariatric surgery (majority having sleeve gastrectomy) in patients with cirrhosis with and without portal hypertension.[96–98] The largest series that included 32 liver transplant candidates with Child-Pugh class A and B cirrhosis underwent laparoscopic sleeve gastrectomy at a high-volume liver transplant center, which helped to facilitate active listing for transplant and ultimately liver transplantation in 14 of these patients.[99] The complication rate in this cohort (3%) was comparable to that observed in the general sleeve gastrectomy population.

Although favorable results have been reported for sleeve gastrectomy, caution must be exercised when considering bariatric surgery in patients with advanced liver disease. Analysis of a population-based study that included patients who underwent bariatric surgery from the Nationwide Inpatient Sample (NIS) between 1998 and 2007 demonstrated that those with decompensated cirrhosis had higher postoperative mortality than patients with compensated cirrhosis or who did not have cirrhosis (16.3% vs 0.9% vs 0.3%, respectively).[100] Of particular concern was the unacceptably high in-hospital mortality (41%) of patients with decompensated cirrhosis who had bariatric surgery at low volume bariatric surgery centers. An updated analysis of the NIS from 2012 to 2015 shows higher risk of inpatient mortality, greater need for surgical revision, and more wound complications after bariatric surgery in patients with chronic liver disease (encompassed International Classification of Diseases, Ninth Revision, codes for patients with and without cirrhosis), although no data are provided on presence of hepatic decompensation preoperatively.[101]

Limited experience with biliopancreatic diversion with or without duodenal switch in patients with cirrhosis is available,[102] so this procedure should be avoided because of concern for risk of rapidly progressive liver disease,[103–105] difficulty in accessing the biliary tree after liver transplantation, and higher risk of protein-calorie malnutrition.[90]

Patients who have had bariatric surgery long before liver transplantation may represent unique challenges, and a suggested approach to obesity management in these patients is provided (**Fig. 1**). A single-center study comparing patients who had had

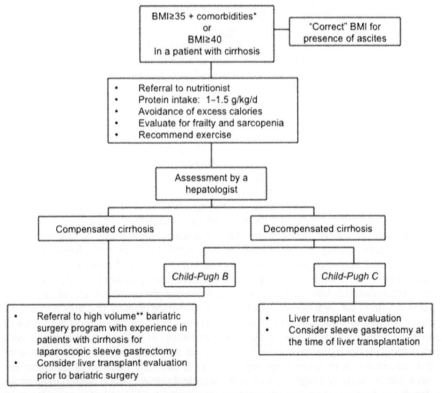

Fig. 1. Algorithm to manage class II and class III obesity in patients with cirrhosis. *Comorbidities: diabetes, hypertension, hyperlipidemia, sleep apnea, osteoarthritis, or any other comorbidity expected to improve with weight loss. **>100 per year.

prior bariatric surgery (most commonly RYGB) to age-matched controls reported higher prevalence of malnutrition as assessed by the subjective global assessment in the patients with prior bariatric surgery (64% vs 39%, respectively).[106] Although the bariatric surgery candidates had similar BMI and severity of liver disease, once listed for transplant, the bariatric surgery patients were less likely to undergo transplant, although those transplanted had similar outcomes after transplant.[106] In this cohort, patients who had RYGB were more likely to be delisted or die on the waiting list than patients who had other types of bariatric surgery (44% vs 17%, respectively). This study likely was underpowered to adequately assess factors that contributed to these differences in pretransplant outcome, although it suggested that RYGB should be avoided in patients who may require liver transplantation in the future. Another single-center study, however, that did not evaluate waitlist outcomes demonstrated similar survival at 1-year and 2-year post-transplant in patients who had had prior bariatric surgery (again, most commonly RYGB).[107]

STRATEGIES FOR OBESITY MANAGEMENT IN LIVER TRANSPLANT CANDIDATES: BARIATRIC SURGERY AT THE TIME OF TRANSPLANT

Patients who have Child-Pugh class C cirrhosis and severe obesity are too sick and too late into their liver disease course to be able to access bariatric surgery prior to liver transplantation. In this select group of patients, the option for simultaneous sleeve gastrectomy and liver transplant is appealing. Using a structured weight management protocol, liver transplant candidates at a large US transplant center with listing BMI greater than or equal to 35 kg/m^2 who were unable to lose enough weight to bring their BMI to less than 35 kg/m^2 underwent simultaneous sleeve gastrectomy (SG) and liver transplantation.[108] The weight loss in patients who had sleeve gastrectomy at the time of transplant had sustained weight loss 3 years after transplant, whereas the patients who had liver transplant alone regained most of the weight lost prior to transplant,[108] with the transplant–sleeve gastrectomy patients having significantly lower BMI 3 years post-transplant (30.9 vs 38.5, respectively), and survival similar between groups. This improvement in post-transplant weight was reflected in numerically lower prevalence of metabolic syndrome as a whole and its individual comorbidities, with the lack of statistically significant differences likely due to lack of power. All but 1 patient had a MELD score of at least 26 and BMI ranging from 40 to 61 at the time of transplant, and only 1 patient had a complication directly attributable to bariatric surgery (leak from gastric staple line). The Mayo experience suggests that sleeve gastrectomy at the time of liver transplantation may be a viable option for obesity management even in high MELD patients. Limited experience at other centers with similar results has been reported in small case series[109,110] but does warrant further study to confirm results can be replicated. Additionally, widespread use of this practice may be limited by potential lack of insurance reimbursement for the combined procedure.

OBESITY AND WEIGHT GAIN AFTER LIVER TRANSPLANTATION

Weight gain after liver transplantation is common,[111,112] due to increased appetite with improvement in oral intake, immunosuppression, genetic factors,[113] preexisting obesity,[112] and potentially addiction transfer in patients who had prior substance use problems.[114] The majority of weight gained post-transplant occurs within the first 2 years to 3 years,[112,115–120] with new-onset obesity occurring in up to 26% of patients.[120] Increased weight and obesity may carry greater risk of development of the metabolic syndrome,[121] thereby increasing the likelihood of cardiovascular morbidity and mortality.[122,123] An analysis of UNOS data observed better 5-year survival in patients who gained rather than lost weight (90% vs 77%, respectively)[115]; although the investigators did an excellent job controlling for confounding variables, such as HCC and hepatitis C recurrence, it is possible that unmeasured confounders may explain some of this association. Management of obesity and other metabolic syndrome comorbidities in liver transplant recipients can be challenging and may be managed best primarily by primary care providers, although barriers to optimal management in this complex patient population are common.[124] Patel and colleagues[111] demonstrated with single-center data that, despite receiving office-based weight loss counseling from hepatologists, 38% of patients were able to lose some weight, although only 11% had sustained weight loss over a 48-week period. The success of the counseling provided, however, may have been limited by the low frequency of contact (every 6 months), because prior studies have demonstrated that likelihood of successful weight loss is greater with more frequent contact.[125]

Modern immunosuppression regimens contain medications that may influence onset and severity of metabolic syndrome comorbidities. Nonetheless, several studies failed to demonstrate a relationship between specific immunosuppression type and weight gain or BMI after liver transplantation,[126–128] so no recommendation regarding optimal immunosuppressant regimens to prevent weight gain can be made.

Recurrence of NAFLD after liver transplantation is almost universal, and de novo NAFLD increasingly is recognized.[129–137] Graft loss due to recurrent or de novo NAFLD rarely has been reported, but with more patients with NAFLD being listed for liver transplantation at younger ages,[138] it is possible that this phenomenon may become more common. Because patients with recurrent or de novo NAFLD after liver transplantation may have higher rates of metabolic syndrome and poorer survival,[129] it will be important to identify any factors that can mitigate poorer survival. Any structured weight loss intervention is likely to provide benefit for NAFLD management[139] so should be promoted in liver transplant recipients with NAFLD after transplant.

BARIATRIC SURGERY AFTER LIVER TRANSPLANTATION

Because many patients may not have had the opportunity to have bariatric surgery prior to transplantation or they gain substantial weight after transplantation, a surgery may need to be considered. Several small studies have now described outcomes of bariatric surgery after liver transplantation, with the vast majority of the studies performing sleeve gastrectomy at least 2 years post-transplant.[140–147] Bariatric surgery has yielded good weight loss in liver transplant recipients but has been associated with relatively high rates of complications, particularly in earlier series utilizing open gastric bypass.[141] Sleeve gastrectomy generally has been better tolerated, although complications related to poor wound healing and need for reoperation does warrant some caution.[141,142,145]

ENDOSCOPIC MANAGEMENT OF OBESITY IN LIVER TRANSPLANT CANDIDATES AND RECIPIENTS

Minimally invasive and endoscopic procedures are appealing to consider in patients with cirrhosis because most are nonsurgical, although they generally yield smaller degrees of weight loss (10%–15% EBWL) compared with the classic surgical procedures and are not covered by insurance.[85]

The intragastric balloon mediates weight loss through effects on gastric emptying and accommodation and neurohormonal mediation of satiety largely due to reduced ghrelin levels.[148] Weight loss achieved with this intervention reaches 13.2% total body weight loss at 6 months,[149] but regaining weight after balloon removal is common.[150] This suggests that the balloon may have a potential role in weight management, particularly to help patients initiate successful weight loss, but that additional longer-term measures are needed to promoted sustained weight loss. The procedure appears to be safe, with serious adverse events occurring rarely and less severe complications of nausea and vomiting typically being transient problems.

Only 1 study to date has reported experience with intragastric balloon placement in patients with decompensated cirrhosis (7 of 8 included with Child-Pugh score of at least 8) awaiting liver transplantation.[151] In this study, a majority of patients had substantial reduction in weight sufficient to proceed with liver transplantation, although the complications of vomiting and/or esophageal or gastric erosions is concerning. Because only 1 of these patients had significant ascites, it is not known whether the intragastric balloon would be safe and effective in the presence of refractory ascites, because such patients already experience nausea, vomiting, and/ or early satiety commonly.[152] The safety of this device in the setting of varices is not known.

Other procedures and devices, such as gastric stimulators, other endoscopically implanted devices or materials (eg, transpyloric shuttle and hyaluronic acid injection), endoluminal gastric restrictive procedures, derivative procedures (eg, bypass liners and duodenal mucosal resurfacing), or transluminal therapy (eg, endoscopic aspiration therapy) all show potential promise in adding tools to the bariatric surgeon's or endoscopist's armamentarium in the future.[153] It is not known whether these procedures will be considered safe in patients with advanced liver disease and/or liver transplant recipients. Devices, such as the duodenal-jejunal bypass liner and gastro-duodenojejunal sleeve, are likely to make access to the biliary tree more challenging for liver transplant recipients with biliary complications. Another consideration is the risk of reduced immunosuppressant absorption with these devices in liver transplant recipients. These endoscopic therapies for weight management may someday play a role in obesity management in liver transplant candidates and recipients, but the safety needs further study before they are widely adopted.

CLINICS CARE POINTS

- Liver transplant candidates with obesity are at high risk of hepatic decompensation, indicating high need for liver transplantation. Because they have post-transplant outcomes similar to their normal-weight counterparts, BMI alone should not be viewed as a contraindication for liver transplantation.
- Weight management in patients with decompensated cirrhosis is challenging and requires coordinated multidisciplinary care.
- Sarcopenia and decompensated cirrhosis can worsen if calories and protein are restricted. Dietary counseling in these patients should be provided by nutritionists with expertise in the management of patients with liver disease.
- Bariatric surgery should be considered early in patients with cirrhosis, ideally prior to hepatic decompensation. Sleeve gastrectomy can be performed at centers with experience with patients with cirrhosis, and liver transplant evaluation may be considered concurrently.
- Weight loss drugs and endoscopic management for obesity in cirrhosis require further study before widespread adoption is implemented.

DISCLOSURE

The author has no disclosures relevant to this work.

REFERENCES

1. Organization WH. WHO fact sheet: obesity and overweight 2020. Available at: https://www.who.int/news-room/fact-sheets/detail/obesity-and-overweight. Accessed April 10, 2020.
2. Hales CMCM, Fryar CD, Ogden CL. Prevalence of obesity and severe obesity among adults: United States, 2017-2018. NCHS Data Brief 2020;360:7.
3. Collaborators GBDO, Afshin A, Forouzanfar MH, et al. Health effects of overweight and obesity in 195 countries over 25 years. N Engl J Med 2017; 377(1):13–27.
4. Vernon G, Baranova A, Younossi ZM. Systematic review: the epidemiology and natural history of non-alcoholic fatty liver disease and non-alcoholic steatohepatitis in adults. Aliment Pharmacol Ther 2011;34(3):274–85.
5. Noureddin M, Vipani A, Bresee C, et al. NASH leading cause of liver transplant in women: updated analysis of indications for liver transplant and ethnic and gender variances. Am J Gastroenterol 2018;113(11):1649–59.
6. Calzadilla-Bertot L, Jeffrey GP, Jacques B, et al. Increasing incidence of nonalcoholic steatohepatitis as an indication for liver transplantation in Australia and New Zealand. Liver Transpl 2019;25(1):25–34.
7. Holmer M, Melum E, Isoniemi H, et al. Nonalcoholic fatty liver disease is an increasing indication for liver transplantation in the Nordic countries. Liver Int 2018;38(11):2082–90.
8. Kwong A, Kim WR, Lake JR, et al. OPTN/SRTR 2018 annual data report: liver. Am J Transplant 2020;20(Suppl s1):193–299.
9. Everhart JE, Lok AS, Kim HY, et al. Weight-related effects on disease progression in the hepatitis C antiviral long-term treatment against cirrhosis trial. Gastroenterology 2009;137(2):549–57.
10. Berzigotti A, Garcia-Tsao G, Bosch J, et al. Obesity is an independent risk factor for clinical decompensation in patients with cirrhosis. Hepatology 2011;54(2): 555–61.
11. Sundaram V, Jalan R, Ahn JC, et al. Class III obesity is a risk factor for the development of acute-on-chronic liver failure in patients with decompensated cirrhosis. J Hepatol 2018;69(3):617–25.
12. Kanwal F, Kramer JR, Li L, et al. Effect of metabolic traits on the risk of cirrhosis and hepatocellular cancer in nonalcoholic fatty liver disease. Hepatology 2020; 71(3):808–19.
13. Welzel TM, Graubard BI, Zeuzem S, et al. Metabolic syndrome increases the risk of primary liver cancer in the United States: a study in the SEER-Medicare database. Hepatology 2011;54(2):463–71.
14. Yang JD, Ahmed F, Mara KC, et al. Diabetes is associated with increased risk of hepatocellular carcinoma in patients with cirrhosis from nonalcoholic fatty liver disease. Hepatology 2020;71(3):907–16.
15. Lewin SM, Mehta N, Kelley RK, et al. Liver transplantation recipients with nonalcoholic steatohepatitis have lower risk hepatocellular carcinoma. Liver Transpl 2017;23(8):1015–22.
16. Martin P, DiMartini A, Feng S, et al. Evaluation for liver transplantation in adults: 2013 practice guideline by the American association for the study of liver diseases and the American society of transplantation. Hepatology 2014;59(3): 1144–65.
17. European Association for the Study of the Liver. Electronic address eee. EASL clinical practice guidelines: liver transplantation. J Hepatol 2016;64(2):433–85.

18. Kardashian AA, Dodge JL, Roberts J, et al. Weighing the risks: morbid obesity and diabetes are associated with increased risk of death on the liver transplant waiting list. Liver Int 2018;38(3):553–63.

19. Aguilar M, Liu B, Holt EW, et al. Impact of obesity and diabetes on waitlist survival, probability of liver transplantation and post-transplant survival among chronic hepatitis C virus patients. Liver Int 2016;36(8):1167–75.

20. Ravaioli M, Grande G, Di Gioia P, et al. Risk avoidance and liver transplantation: a single-center experience in a national network. Ann Surg 2016;264(5):778–86.

21. Segev DL, Thompson RE, Locke JE, et al. Prolonged waiting times for liver transplantation in obese patients. Ann Surg 2008;248(5):863–70.

22. Halegoua-De Marzio DL, Wong SY, Fenkel JM, et al. Listing practices for morbidly obese patients at liver transplantation centers in the United States. Exp Clin Transplant 2016;14(6):646–9.

23. Choban PS, Flancbaum L. The impact of obesity on surgical outcomes: a review. J Am Coll Surg 1997;185(6):593–603.

24. Hoogeveen EK, Aalten J, Rothman KJ, et al. Effect of obesity on the outcome of kidney transplantation: a 20-year follow-up. Transplantation 2011;91(8):869–74.

25. Nair S, Verma S, Thuluvath PJ. Obesity and its effect on survival in patients undergoing orthotopic liver transplantation in the United States. Hepatology 2002; 35(1):105–9.

26. Dick AA, Spitzer AL, Seifert CF, et al. Liver transplantation at the extremes of the body mass index. Liver Transpl 2009;15(8):968–77.

27. Molina Raya A, Garcia Navarro A, San Miguel Mendez C, et al. Influence of obesity on liver transplantation outcomes. Transplant Proc 2016;48(7):2503–5.

28. Conzen KD, Vachharajani N, Collins KM, et al. Morbid obesity in liver transplant recipients adversely affects longterm graft and patient survival in a single-institution analysis. HPB (Oxford) 2015;17(3):251–7.

29. Ayala R, Grande S, Bustelos R, et al. Obesity is an independent risk factor for pre-transplant portal vein thrombosis in liver recipients. BMC Gastroenterol 2012;12:114.

30. Hakeem AR, Cockbain AJ, Raza SS, et al. Increased morbidity in overweight and obese liver transplant recipients: a single-center experience of 1325 patients from the United Kingdom. Liver Transpl 2013;19(5):551–62.

31. LaMattina JC, Foley DP, Fernandez LA, et al. Complications associated with liver transplantation in the obese recipient. Clin Transplant 2012;26(6):910–8.

32. Singhal A, Wilson GC, Wima K, et al. Impact of recipient morbid obesity on outcomes after liver transplantation. Transpl Int 2015;28(2):148–55.

33. Diaz-Nieto R, Lykoudis PM, Davidson BR. Recipient body mass index and infectious complications following liver transplantation. HPB (Oxford) 2019;21(8): 1032–8.

34. Dare AJ, Plank LD, Phillips AR, et al. Additive effect of pretransplant obesity, diabetes, and cardiovascular risk factors on outcomes after liver transplantation. Liver Transpl 2014;20(3):281–90.

35. Schaeffer DF, Yoshida EM, Buczkowski AK, et al. Surgical morbidity in severely obese liver transplant recipients - a single Canadian Centre Experience. Ann Hepatol 2009;8(1):38–40.

36. Nair S, Cohen DB, Cohen MP, et al. Postoperative morbidity, mortality, costs, and long-term survival in severely obese patients undergoing orthotopic liver transplantation. Am J Gastroenterol 2001;96(3):842–5.

37. Febrero B, Ramirez P, Espinosa F, et al. Risk of respiratory complications in obese liver transplant patients: a study of 343 patients. Transplant Proc 2015; 47(8):2385–7.
38. D'Avola D, Cuervas-Mons V, Marti J, et al. Cardiovascular morbidity and mortality after liver transplantation: the protective role of mycophenolate mofetil. Liver Transpl 2017;23(4):498–509.
39. Barone M, Viggiani MT, Losurdo G, et al. Systematic review with meta-analysis: post-operative complications and mortality risk in liver transplant candidates with obesity. Aliment Pharmacol Ther 2017;46(3):236–45.
40. Beckmann S, Drent G, Ruppar T, et al. Body weight parameters are related to morbidity and mortality after liver transplantation: a systematic review and meta-analysis. Transplantation 2019;103(11):2287–303.
41. Leonard J, Heimbach JK, Malinchoc M, et al. The impact of obesity on long-term outcomes in liver transplant recipients-results of the NIDDK liver transplant database. Am J Transplant 2008;8(3):667–72.
42. Perez-Protto SE, Quintini C, Reynolds LF, et al. Comparable graft and patient survival in lean and obese liver transplant recipients. Liver Transpl 2013;19(8): 907–15.
43. Pelletier SJ, Schaubel DE, Wei G, et al. Effect of body mass index on the survival benefit of liver transplantation. Liver Transpl 2007;13(12):1678–83.
44. Haldar D, Kern B, Hodson J, et al. Outcomes of liver transplantation for non-alcoholic steatohepatitis: a European Liver Transplant Registry study. J Hepatol 2019;71(2):313–22.
45. Alvarez J, Mei X, Daily M, et al. Tipping the scales: liver transplant outcomes of the super obese. J Gastrointest Surg 2016;20(9):1628–35.
46. Terjimanian MN, Harbaugh CM, Hussain A, et al. Abdominal adiposity, body composition and survival after liver transplantation. Clin Transplant 2016;30(3): 289–94.
47. Roccaro GA, Goldberg DS, Hwang WT, et al. Sustained posttransplantation diabetes is associated with long-term major cardiovascular events following liver transplantation. Am J Transplant 2018;18(1):207–15.
48. Adams LA, Arauz O, Angus PW, et al. Additive impact of pre-liver transplant metabolic factors on survival post-liver transplant. J Gastroenterol Hepatol 2016;31(5):1016–24.
49. Wong RJ, Cheung R, Perumpail RB, et al. Diabetes mellitus, and not obesity, is associated with lower survival following liver transplantation. Dig Dis Sci 2015; 60(4):1036–44.
50. Younossi ZM, Stepanova M, Saab S, et al. The impact of type 2 diabetes and obesity on the long-term outcomes of more than 85 000 liver transplant recipients in the US. Aliment Pharmacol Ther 2014;40(6):686–94.
51. Saab S, Lalezari D, Pruthi P, et al. The impact of obesity on patient survival in liver transplant recipients: a meta-analysis. Liver Int 2015;35(1):164–70.
52. Stepanova M, Henry L, Garg R, et al. Risk of de novo post-transplant type 2 diabetes in patients undergoing liver transplant for non-alcoholic steatohepatitis. BMC Gastroenterol 2015;15:175.
53. Henson JB, Wilder JM, Kappus MR, et al. Transplant outcomes in older patients with nonalcoholic steatohepatitis compared to alcohol-related liver disease and hepatitis C. Transplantation. 2020;104(6):e164–73.
54. Thuluvath PJ, Hanish S, Savva Y. Liver transplantation in cryptogenic cirrhosis: outcome comparisons between NASH, alcoholic, and AIH cirrhosis. Transplantation 2018;102(4):656–63.

55. Satapathy SK, Jiang Y, Agbim U, et al. Posttransplant outcome of lean compared with obese nonalcoholic steatohepatitis in the United States: the obesity paradox. Liver Transpl 2020;26(1):68–79.
56. VanWagner LB, Lapin B, Skaro AI, et al. Impact of renal impairment on cardiovascular disease mortality after liver transplantation for nonalcoholic steatohepatitis cirrhosis. Liver Int 2015;35(12):2575–83.
57. van Vugt JL, Levolger S, de Bruin RW, et al. Systematic review and meta-analysis of the impact of computed tomography-assessed skeletal muscle mass on outcome in patients awaiting or undergoing liver transplantation. Am J Transplant 2016;16(8):2277–92.
58. Paternostro R, Lampichler K, Bardach C, et al. The value of different CT-based methods for diagnosing low muscle mass and predicting mortality in patients with cirrhosis. Liver Int 2019;39(12):2374–85.
59. Haugen CE, McAdams-DeMarco M, Verna EC, et al. Association between liver transplant wait-list mortality and frailty based on body mass index. JAMA Surg 2020;154(12):1103–9.
60. Carias S, Castellanos AL, Vilchez V, et al. Nonalcoholic steatohepatitis is strongly associated with sarcopenic obesity in patients with cirrhosis undergoing liver transplant evaluation. J Gastroenterol Hepatol 2016;31(3):628–33.
61. Cruz RJ Jr, Dew MA, Myaskovsky L, et al. Objective radiologic assessment of body composition in patients with end-stage liver disease: going beyond the BMI. Transplantation 2013;95(4):617–22.
62. Berzigotti A, Saran U, Dufour JF. Physical activity and liver diseases. Hepatology 2016;63(3):1026–40.
63. Lai JC, Rahimi RS, Verna EC, et al. Frailty associated with waitlist mortality independent of ascites and hepatic encephalopathy in a multicenter study. Gastroenterology 2019;156(6):1675–82.
64. Lai JC, Sonnenday CJ, Tapper EB, et al. Frailty in liver transplantation: an expert opinion statement from the American Society of Transplantation Liver and Intestinal Community of Practice. Am J Transplant 2019;19(7):1896–906.
65. Tandon P, Ismond KP, Riess K, et al. Exercise in cirrhosis: translating evidence and experience to practice. J Hepatol 2018;69(5):1164–77.
66. Welch N, Dasarathy J, Runkana A, et al. Continued muscle loss increases mortality in cirrhosis: impact of aetiology of liver disease. Liver Int 2020;40(5):1178–88.
67. Medici VMM, Kappus MR. Liver disease. Silver Spring (MD): American Society for Parenteral and Enteral Nutrition; 2017.
68. Plauth M, Bernal W, Dasarathy S, et al. ESPEN guideline on clinical nutrition in liver disease. Clin Nutr 2019;38(2):485–521.
69. Heimbach JK, Watt KD, Poterucha JJ, et al. Combined liver transplantation and gastric sleeve resection for patients with medically complicated obesity and end-stage liver disease. Am J Transplant 2013;13(2):363–8.
70. Berzigotti A, Albillos A, Villanueva C, et al. Effects of an intensive lifestyle intervention program on portal hypertension in patients with cirrhosis and obesity: the SportDiet study. Hepatology 2017;65(4):1293–305.
71. Macias-Rodriguez RU, Ilarraza-Lomeli H, Ruiz-Margain A, et al. Changes in hepatic venous pressure gradient induced by physical exercise in cirrhosis: results of a pilot randomized open clinical trial. Clin Transl Gastroenterol 2016;7(7):e180.

72. Garcia-Cortes M, Robles-Diaz M, Ortega-Alonso A, et al. Hepatotoxicity by dietary supplements: a tabular listing and clinical characteristics. Int J Mol Sci 2016;17(4):537.
73. LiverTox: Clinical and Research Information on Drug-Induced Liver Injury. Orlistat. Available at: https://www.ncbi.nlm.nih.gov/books/NBK547852/?term=orlistat. Accessed2020.
74. Christopher RJ, Morgan ME, Tang Y, et al. Pharmacokinetics and tolerability of lorcaserin in special populations: elderly patients and patients with renal or hepatic impairment. Clin Ther 2017;39(4):837–848 e837.
75. Gutierrez JA, Landaverde C, Wells JT, et al. Lorcaserin use in the management of morbid obesity in a pre-liver transplant patient. Hepatology 2016;64(1):301–2.
76. Colman E, Golden J, Roberts M, et al. The FDA's assessment of two drugs for chronic weight management. N Engl J Med 2012;367(17):1577–9.
77. Siebenhofer A, Jeitler K, Horvath K, et al. Long-term effects of weight-reducing drugs in people with hypertension. Cochrane Database Syst Rev 2016;(3):CD007654.
78. Sjostrom L, Lindroos AK, Peltonen M, et al. Lifestyle, diabetes, and cardiovascular risk factors 10 years after bariatric surgery. N Engl J Med 2004;351(26):2683–93.
79. Buchwald H, Avidor Y, Braunwald E, et al. Bariatric surgery: a systematic review and meta-analysis. JAMA 2004;292(14):1724–37.
80. Sun Y, Liu B, Smith JK, et al. Association of preoperative body weight and weight loss with risk of death after bariatric surgery. JAMA Netw Open 2020;3(5):e204803.
81. Arterburn DE, Olsen MK, Smith VA, et al. Association between bariatric surgery and long-term survival. JAMA 2015;313(1):62–70.
82. Hsu CC, Almulaifi A, Chen JC, et al. Effect of bariatric surgery vs medical treatment on type 2 diabetes in patients with body mass index lower than 35: five-year outcomes. JAMA Surg 2015;150(12):1117–24.
83. Sha Y, Huang X, Ke P, et al. Laparoscopic Roux-en-Y gastric bypass versus sleeve gastrectomy for type 2 diabetes mellitus in nonseverely obese patients: a systematic review and meta-analysis of randomized controlled trials. Obes Surg 2020;30(5):1660–70.
84. Di Lorenzo N, Antoniou SA, Batterham RL, et al. Clinical practice guidelines of the European Association for Endoscopic Surgery (EAES) on bariatric surgery: update 2020 endorsed by IFSO-EC, EASO and ESPCOP. Surg Endosc 2020;34(6):2332–58.
85. Mechanick JI, Apovian C, Brethauer S, et al. Clinical practice guidelines for the perioperative nutrition, metabolic, and nonsurgical support of patients undergoing bariatric procedures - 2019 update: cosponsored by American Association of Clinical Endocrinologists/American College of Endocrinology, The Obesity Society, American Society for Metabolic and Bariatric Surgery, Obesity Medicine Association, and American Society of Anesthesiologists. Obesity (Silver Spring) 2020;28(4):O1–58.
86. Puzziferri N, Roshek TB 3rd, Mayo HG, et al. Long-term follow-up after bariatric surgery: a systematic review. JAMA 2014;312(9):934–42.
87. Young MT, Gebhart A, Phelan MJ, et al. Use and outcomes of laparoscopic sleeve gastrectomy vs laparoscopic gastric bypass: analysis of the American College of Surgeons NSQIP. J Am Coll Surg 2015;220(5):880–5.
88. Himpens J, Cadiere GB, Bazi M, et al. Long-term outcomes of laparoscopic adjustable gastric banding. Arch Surg 2011;146(7):802–7.

89. Abdelbaki TN, Huang CK, Ramos A, et al. Gastric plication for morbid obesity: a systematic review. Obes Surg 2012;22(10):1633–9.
90. O'Brien PE, Hindle A, Brennan L, et al. Long-term outcomes after bariatric surgery: a systematic review and meta-analysis of weight loss at 10 or more years for all bariatric procedures and a single-centre review of 20-year outcomes after adjustable gastric banding. Obes Surg 2019;29(1):3–14.
91. Neichoy BT, Schniederjan B, Cottam DR, et al. Stomach intestinal pylorus-sparing surgery for morbid obesity. JSLS 2018;22(1). e2017.00063.
92. Lin MY, Tavakol MM, Sarin A, et al. Laparoscopic sleeve gastrectomy is safe and efficacious for pretransplant candidates. Surg Obes Relat Dis 2013;9(5):653–8.
93. Diwan TS, Lichvar AB, Leino AD, et al. Pharmacokinetic and pharmacogenetic analysis of immunosuppressive agents after laparoscopic sleeve gastrectomy. Clin Transplant 2017;31(6). https://doi.org/10.1111/ctr.12975.
94. Yemini R, Nesher E, Winkler J, et al. Bariatric surgery in solid organ transplant patients: long-term follow-up results of outcome, safety, and effect on immunosuppression. Am J Transplant 2018;18(11):2772–80.
95. Klebanoff MJ, Corey KE, Samur S, et al. Cost-effectiveness analysis of bariatric surgery for patients with nonalcoholic steatohepatitis cirrhosis. JAMA Netw Open 2019;2(2):e190047.
96. Pestana L, Swain J, Dierkhising R, et al. Bariatric surgery in patients with cirrhosis with and without portal hypertension: a single-center experience. Mayo Clin Proc 2015;90(2):209–15.
97. Dallal RM, Mattar SG, Lord JL, et al. Results of laparoscopic gastric bypass in patients with cirrhosis. Obes Surg 2004;14(1):47–53.
98. Shimizu H, Phuong V, Maia M, et al. Bariatric surgery in patients with liver cirrhosis. Surg Obes Relat Dis 2013;9(1):1–6.
99. Sharpton SR, Terrault NA, Posselt AM. Outcomes of sleeve gastrectomy in obese liver transplant candidates. Liver Transpl 2019;25(4):538–44.
100. Mosko JD, Nguyen GC. Increased perioperative mortality following bariatric surgery among patients with cirrhosis. Clin Gastroenterol Hepatol 2011;9(10): 897–901.
101. Mavilia MG, Wakefield D, Karagozian R. Outcomes of bariatric surgery in chronic liver disease: a national inpatient sample analysis. Obes Surg 2020; 30(3):941–7.
102. Giannini EG, Coppo C, Romana C, et al. Long-term follow-up study of liver-related outcome after bilio-pancreatic diversion in patients with initial, significant liver damage. Dig Dis Sci 2018;63(7):1946–51.
103. Addeo P, Cesaretti M, Anty R, et al. Liver transplantation for bariatric surgery-related liver failure: a systematic review of a rare condition. Surg Obes Relat Dis 2019;15(8):1394–401.
104. Geerts A, Darius T, Chapelle T, et al. The multicenter Belgian survey on liver transplantation for hepatocellular failure after bariatric surgery. Transplant Proc 2010;42(10):4395–8.
105. Castillo J, Fabrega E, Escalante CF, et al. Liver transplantation in a case of steatohepatitis and subacute hepatic failure after biliopancreatic diversion for morbid obesity. Obes Surg 2001;11(5):640–2.
106. Idriss R, Hasse J, Wu T, et al. Impact of prior bariatric surgery on perioperative liver transplant outcomes. Liver Transpl 2019;25(2):217–27.
107. Safwan M, Collins KM, Abouljoud MS, et al. Outcome of liver transplantation in patients with prior bariatric surgery. Liver Transpl 2017;23(11):1415–21.

108. Zamora-Valdes D, Watt KD, Kellogg TA, et al. Long-term outcomes of patients undergoing simultaneous liver transplantation and sleeve gastrectomy. Hepatology 2018;68(2):485–95.

109. Nesher E, Mor E, Shlomai A, et al. Simultaneous liver transplantation and sleeve gastrectomy: prohibitive combination or a necessity? Obes Surg 2017;27(5): 1387–90.

110. Tariciotti L, D'Ugo S, Manzia TM, et al. Combined liver transplantation and sleeve gastrectomy for end-stage liver disease in a bariatric patient: first European case-report. Int J Surg Case Rep 2016;28:38–41.

111. Patel SS, Siddiqui MB, Chadrakumaran A, et al. Office-based weight loss counseling is ineffective in liver transplant recipients. Dig Dis Sci 2020;65(2):639–46.

112. Anastacio LR, Ferreira LG, de Sena Ribeiro H, et al. Body composition and overweight of liver transplant recipients. Transplantation 2011;92(8):947–51.

113. Watt KD, Dierkhising R, Fan C, et al. Investigation of PNPLA3 and IL28B genotypes on diabetes and obesity after liver transplantation: insight into mechanisms of disease. Am J Transplant 2013;13(9):2450–7.

114. Brunault P, Salame E, Jaafari N, et al. Why do liver transplant patients so often become obese? The addiction transfer hypothesis. Med Hypotheses 2015; 85(1):68–75.

115. Martinez-Camacho A, Fortune BE, Gralla J, et al. Early weight changes after liver transplantation significantly impact patient and graft survival. Eur J Gastroenterol Hepatol 2016;28(1):107–15.

116. Everhart JE, Lombardero M, Lake JR, et al. Weight change and obesity after liver transplantation: incidence and risk factors. Liver Transpl Surg 1998;4(4): 285–96.

117. Palmer M, Schaffner F, Thung SN. Excessive weight gain after liver transplantation. Transplantation 1991;51(4):797–800.

118. Stegall MD, Everson G, Schroter G, et al. Metabolic complications after liver transplantation. Diabetes, hypercholesterolemia, hypertension, and obesity. Transplantation 1995;60(9):1057–60.

119. Wawrzynowicz-Syczewska M, Karpinska E, Jurczyk K, et al. Boron-Kaczmarska A. Risk factors and dynamics of weight gain in patients after liver transplantation. Ann Transplant 2009;14(3):45–50.

120. Richards J, Gunson B, Johnson J, et al. Weight gain and obesity after liver transplantation. Transpl Int 2005;18(4):461–6.

121. Kuo HT, Sampaio MS, Ye X, et al. Risk factors for new-onset diabetes mellitus in adult liver transplant recipients, an analysis of the Organ Procurement and Transplant Network/United Network for Organ Sharing database. Transplantation 2010;89(9):1134–40.

122. Laish I, Braun M, Mor E, et al. Metabolic syndrome in liver transplant recipients: prevalence, risk factors, and association with cardiovascular events. Liver Transpl 2011;17(1):15–22.

123. Laryea M, Watt KD, Molinari M, et al. Metabolic syndrome in liver transplant recipients: prevalence and association with major vascular events. Liver Transpl 2007;13(8):1109–14.

124. Heller JC, Prochazka AV, Everson GT, et al. Long-term management after liver transplantation: primary care physician versus hepatologist. Liver Transpl 2009;15(10):1330–5.

125. American College of Cardiology/American Heart Association Task Force on Practice Guidelines OEP. Executive summary: Guidelines (2013) for the management of overweight and obesity in adults: a report of the American College

of Cardiology/American Heart Association Task Force on Practice Guidelines and the Obesity Society published by the Obesity Society and American College of Cardiology/American Heart Association Task Force on Practice Guidelines. Based on a systematic review from the The Obesity Expert Panel, 2013. Obesity (Silver Spring) 2014;22(Suppl 2):S5–39.

126. Ramirez CB, Doria C, Frank AM, et al. Completely steroid-free immunosuppression in liver transplantation: a randomized study. Clin Transplant 2013;27(3):463–71.

127. Bianchi G, Marchesini G, Marzocchi R, et al. Metabolic syndrome in liver transplantation: relation to etiology and immunosuppression. Liver Transpl 2008;14(11):1648–54.

128. Fussner LA, Heimbach JK, Fan C, et al. Cardiovascular disease after liver transplantation: when, what, and who is at risk. Liver Transpl 2015;21(7):889–96.

129. Narayanan P, Mara K, Izzy M, et al. Recurrent or De Novo allograft steatosis and long-term outcomes after liver transplantation. Transplantation 2019;103(1):e14–21.

130. Vallin M, Guillaud O, Boillot O, et al. Recurrent or de novo nonalcoholic fatty liver disease after liver transplantation: natural history based on liver biopsy analysis. Liver Transpl 2014;20(9):1064–71.

131. Kakar S, Dugum M, Cabello R, et al. Incidence of recurrent NASH-related allograft cirrhosis. Dig Dis Sci 2019;64(5):1356–63.

132. Malik SM, Devera ME, Fontes P, et al. Recurrent disease following liver transplantation for nonalcoholic steatohepatitis cirrhosis. Liver Transpl 2009;15(12):1843–51.

133. Yalamanchili K, Saadeh S, Klintmalm GB, et al. Nonalcoholic fatty liver disease after liver transplantation for cryptogenic cirrhosis or nonalcoholic fatty liver disease. Liver Transpl 2010;16(4):431–9.

134. Dureja P, Mellinger J, Agni R, et al. NAFLD recurrence in liver transplant recipients. Transplantation 2011;91(6):684–9.

135. Bhagat V, Mindikoglu AL, Nudo CG, et al. Outcomes of liver transplantation in patients with cirrhosis due to nonalcoholic steatohepatitis versus patients with cirrhosis due to alcoholic liver disease. Liver Transpl 2009;15(12):1814–20.

136. Bhati C, Idowu MO, Sanyal AJ, et al. Long-term outcomes in patients undergoing liver transplantation for nonalcoholic steatohepatitis-related cirrhosis. Transplantation 2017;101(8):1867–74.

137. Contos MJ, Cales W, Sterling RK, et al. Development of nonalcoholic fatty liver disease after orthotopic liver transplantation for cryptogenic cirrhosis. Liver Transpl 2001;7(4):363–73.

138. Shingina A, DeWitt PE, Dodge JL, et al. Future trends in demand for liver transplant: birth cohort effects among patients with NASH and HCC. Transplantation 2019;103(1):140–8.

139. Koutoukidis DA, Astbury NM, Tudor KE, et al. Association of weight loss interventions with changes in biomarkers of nonalcoholic fatty liver disease: a systematic review and meta-analysis. JAMA Intern Med 2019;179(9):1262–71.

140. Butte JM, Devaud N, Jarufe NP, et al. Sleeve gastrectomy as treatment for severe obesity after orthotopic liver transplantation. Obes Surg 2007;17(11):1517–9.

141. Al-Nowaylati AR, Al-Haddad BJ, Dorman RB, et al. Gastric bypass after liver transplantation. Liver Transpl 2013;19(12):1324–9.

142. Lin MY, Tavakol MM, Sarin A, et al. Safety and feasibility of sleeve gastrectomy in morbidly obese patients following liver transplantation. Surg Endosc 2013; 27(1):81–5.
143. Khoraki J, Katz MG, Funk LM, et al. Feasibility and outcomes of laparoscopic sleeve gastrectomy after solid organ transplantation. Surg Obes Relat Dis 2016;12(1):75–83.
144. Elli EF, Gonzalez-Heredia R, Sanchez-Johnsen L, et al. Sleeve gastrectomy surgery in obese patients post-organ transplantation. Surg Obes Relat Dis 2016; 12(3):528–34.
145. Osseis M, Lazzati A, Salloum C, et al. Sleeve gastrectomy after liver transplantation: feasibility and outcomes. Obes Surg 2018;28(1):242–8.
146. Tsamalaidze L, Stauffer JA, Arasi LC, et al. Laparoscopic sleeve gastrectomy for morbid obesity in patients after orthotopic liver transplant: a matched case-control study. Obes Surg 2018;28(2):444–50.
147. Ayloo S, Guss C, Pentakota SR, et al. Minimally invasive sleeve gastrectomy as a surgical treatment for nonalcoholic fatty liver disease in liver transplant recipients. Transplant Proc 2020;52(1):276–83.
148. Bazerbachi F, Vargas EJ, Abu Dayyeh BK. Endoscopic bariatric therapy: a guide to the intragastric balloon. Am J Gastroenterol 2019;114(9):1421–31.
149. Force ABET, Committee AT, Abu Dayyeh BK, et al. ASGE Bariatric Endoscopy Task Force systematic review and meta-analysis assessing the ASGE PIVI thresholds for adopting endoscopic bariatric therapies. Gastrointest Endosc 2015;82(3):425–38.e5.
150. Kotzampassi K, Grosomanidis V, Papakostas P, et al. 500 intragastric balloons: what happens 5 years thereafter? Obes Surg 2012;22(6):896–903.
151. Choudhary NS, Puri R, Saraf N, et al. Intragastric balloon as a novel modality for weight loss in patients with cirrhosis and morbid obesity awaiting liver transplantation. Indian J Gastroenterol 2016;35(2):113–6.
152. Neijenhuis M, Gevers TJG, Atwell TD, et al. Development and validation of a patient-reported outcome measurement for symptom assessment in cirrhotic ascites. Am J Gastroenterol 2018;113(4):567–75.
153. Carrano FM, Peev MP, Saunders JK, et al. The role of minimally invasive and endoscopic technologies in morbid obesity treatment: review and critical appraisal of the current clinical practice. Obes Surg 2020;30(2):736–52.

Expanding the Limits of Liver Transplantation for Hepatocellular Carcinoma
Is There a Limit?

Allison Kwong, MD[a], Neil Mehta, MD[b],*

KEYWORDS

- Hepatocellular carcinoma • Liver transplantation • Organ allocation • Organ utility
- Survival benefit • Survival threshold

KEY POINTS

- Liver transplantation is an established treatment option for hepatocellular carcinoma. Acceptable survival outcomes have been achieved with more liberal tumor size and number criteria beyond conventional Milan criteria.
- When considering expanded criteria for HCC, survival outcomes after LT should be comparable with patients within Milan criteria and those without HCC.
- Surrogate measures of tumor biology, such as α-fetoprotein, other biomarkers, imaging features, and dynamic tumor behavior including response to locoregional therapy can help to risk stratify and select patients appropriate for liver transplantation.

INTRODUCTION

Liver transplantation (LT) is now an established treatment option for early stage hepatocellular carcinoma (HCC) within Milan criteria, defined as a single lesion less than 5 cm or two to three lesions each less than 3 cm.[1] This approach has been successful, leading to excellent post-LT outcomes including low risk of post-LT HCC recurrence and high survival rates.

However, a minority of patients with HCC qualify for these fairly restrictive LT criteria. Over the past two decades, there has been interest in expanding criteria to

Funding: Dr. A. Kwong is supported by the National Institute of Allergy and Infectious Diseases under the award number R25AI147369. The funding agency played no role in the preparation, review, or approval of the article.
[a] Division of Gastroenterology and Hepatology, Stanford University, 420 Broadway Street, 3rd Floor, Redwood City, CA 94063, USA; [b] Division of Gastroenterology, University of California, San Francisco, 513 Parnassus Avenue, S-357, San Francisco, CA 94143, USA
* Corresponding author.
E-mail address: Neil.Mehta@ucsf.edu

Clin Liver Dis 25 (2021) 19–33
https://doi.org/10.1016/j.cld.2020.08.002
1089-3261/21/© 2020 Elsevier Inc. All rights reserved.

liver.theclinics.com

be able to offer this treatment option to a wider population of patients with HCC. This has been explored in diverse cohorts, albeit with variable results. This review addresses whether there are limits to expanding criteria for LT for this indication.

Expanded criteria for LT will have collateral effects on the liver transplant waitlist, including those with HCC within Milan and those without HCC. Considerations include (1) organ utility and a minimum survival threshold, (2) definitions for overall survival and transplant benefit for each of these populations, and (3) optimal risk stratification for post-LT outcomes.

OUTCOMES OF LIVER TRANSPLANTATION

HCC within Milan criteria is established as an appropriate indication for LT and is the standard against which expanded criteria are evaluated. In the United States, patients with HCC meeting prespecified criteria receive LT priority through Model for End-Stage Liver Disease (MELD) exception points, which attempt to approximate the urgency for LT compared with general waitlist population with chronic liver disease. This includes patients with unresectable HCC who are always within conventional Milan criteria, and those who are initially beyond Milan criteria and are successfully "downstaged" to within Milan criteria after locoregional therapy (LRT). The standard downstaging protocol in the United States, that is, United Network for Organ Sharing downstaging (UNOS-DS) criteria, specify an upper limit of one lesion less than or equal to 8 cm, two to three lesions less than or equal to 5 cm, or four to five nodules all less than 3 cm, with total tumor diameter less than or equal to 8 cm, and that HCC must be within Milan criteria after LRT.[2] In 2018, 1571 (20.4%) of liver transplants in the United States were performed for patients with HCC exception points.[3] This proportion has increased steadily since the introduction of MELD HCC exception in 2002. The incidence of HCC is expected to increase with the aging population and greater prevalence of chronic liver disease caused by nonalcoholic steatohepatitis, both known risk factors for HCC.[4]

Organ Utility and the Minimum Survival Threshold for Hepatocellular Carcinoma

Organ allocation systems seek to make the best use of donated organs, currently a limited resource in many countries. Under the guiding principles of equity and justice, the benefit of transplanting patients with HCC should not outweigh the harm for not transplanting patients without HCC. In the context of more liberal or expanded criteria for HCC, this risk-benefit calculation may differ.

Conventionally, the minimum acceptable survival after LT has been recognized to be 50% at 5 years. This benchmark was first proposed in 1999 and is based on expert opinion and clinical judgment rather than objective assessment. In addition, it has not been adjusted to reflect the improvements in post-LT survival since. A Markov model from 2008 suggested that a 5-year survival rate of at least 61% among patients beyond Milan criteria must be achieved to outweigh the harm to others awaiting LT and loss of utility, in terms of quality-adjusted life-years.[4] In areas where patients with HCC draw from the deceased donor pool, it is generally accepted that survival outcomes should be comparable with those without HCC.[5] In the 2018 SRTR Annual Data Report for LT, 3- and 5-year survival was 81.7% and 76.6% for patients with HCC, compared with 81.4% and 76.4% for patients without HCC.[3] Although patients with HCC are generally less frail and have lower MELD at the time of LT, the post-LT mortality risk in the first several years post-transplant is driven by rate of HCC recurrence, which has been estimated to be up to 5.7% at 1 year and 12.8% at 5 years in the modern era.[6]

Current LT survival outcomes in HCC exceed proposed utility thresholds and standard metrics for post-LT survival. However, expanding criteria to allow for greater tumor burden could compromise these outcomes. Particularly in the context of organ shortage, minimum survival threshold for expanded HCC criteria is expected to be comparable with patients within Milan criteria, as well as those without HCC. A Markov model from 2008 suggested that a 5-year survival rate of at least 61% among patients beyond Milan criteria must be achieved toooutweigh the harm to others awaiting LT and loss of utility, in terms of quality-adjusted life-years.[4] In 2009, Mazzaferro and colleagues[7] used a benchmark of 70% 5-year post-LT survival, the outcome expected for patients within Milan criteria, to propose and justify the up-to-seven criteria, a more flexible alternative to the Milan criteria. Thresholds for waitlist mortality or intention-to-treat survival have not been widely considered, although these are arguably relevant to patients and their providers. Intent-to-treat survival considers survival from time of listing, with or without transplantation.

Patients with extensive HCC may have different personal thresholds. For many, LT is the only potentially curative option, and they may be willing to take on much higher risks of post-LT mortality and HCC recurrence for the chance at a cure. However, on a societal level, with ongoing organ shortage and deceased donor organs considered as a shared national resource, a minimum survival threshold at a comparable level with patients without HCC is necessary.

Deceased Donor Availability

Anticipated waiting times may vary widely even within a single organ allocation system. For example, in the United States, waiting times for patients with HCC are influenced by local deceased donor organ availability. Patients with HCC now wait a minimum of 6 months before gaining exception points, and in May 2019, the number of exception points granted was adjusted to a constant based on the local median MELD (median MELD at transplant minus 3). These changes have helped to equalize waiting times in the United States allocation system. Still, waitlist times may differ by geographic area. The risk of waitlist dropout varies as a consequence, and so the risk assessment in these situations may need to consider these geographic variations.[8]

Living Donor Availability

Selection criteria and acceptable survival thresholds may also be different for patients with a living donor option, with regard to acceptable post-LT survival and outcome. Because patients with living donors are not drawing from the deceased donor pool, the survival threshold calculus may change, although this would have to be balanced against the added risk to a potential donor. Transplant centers may accept less-restrictive criteria in these situations, although the post-LT survival rates may be lower. On an individual level, patients and their donors may be willing to accept a higher or lower risk of post-LT recurrence and survival. A threshold of 50% 5-year survival has been previously proposed for patients with HCC undergoing living donor LT (LDLT), an improvement on the 20% survival expected at the time with palliative treatments (LRT).[9] Under the tenet that LT for HCC should have similar expected survival compared with nontumor patients, the recent ILTS Transplant Oncology Consensus Conference proposed elevating this benchmark to 60% 5-year survival after LDLT. Outcomes for LDLT and deceased donor liver transplant (DDLT) for HCC have been comparable in the MELD era.[10–12]

Patients with an available living donor often benefit from a shorter wait time, reducing the risk of waitlist dropout but also allowing less time to assess the dynamics of the tumor biology. Static data, such as PET, may be more useful in these scenarios.

Risk stratification is needed to adequately provide informed consent and counsel the patient and their donor appropriately.

Organ Allocation Policy

Selection criteria for LT should take into account the local availability of donor organs, anticipated wait time, and post-LT outcome. The goal in organ allocation is to minimize waitlist mortality and achieve acceptable post-LT graft and patient survival. A secondary goal, although not explicit, is to maximize transplant benefit.

In the United States, patients with HCC are currently assigned the same amount of exception points and thus similar allocation priority and probability of undergoing LT, regardless of tumor characteristics. The diverse risks of waitlist dropout and post-LT HCC recurrence are currently not well-represented by the current system.

Survival Benefit of Liver Transplantation

The concept of survival benefit in LT considers the expected survival without LT against expected survival after LT, balancing the two-fold risks of waitlist mortality and LT. Considering the heterogeneity of the HCC population, the survival benefit of LT for HCC can be quite variable. In an intention-to-treat analysis, Lai and colleagues[13] demonstrate the largest LT survival benefit for patients with HCC outside Milan criteria, with low α-fetoprotein (AFP) and incomplete response or inability to undergo LRT. In contrast, patients with low LT survival benefit are of two distinct categories: poor radiologic response and high AFP, with too advanced or aggressive malignancy to benefit from LT; and complete radiologic response and low MELD with well-treated tumor and thus greater survival without LT than with LT.

A proportion of patients presenting with HCC tumor burden beyond Milan and UNOS-DS may still benefit greatly from LT, where a higher urgency for LT may mitigate, or justify, the slightly lower yet still excellent post-LT outcomes. For example, a patient with HCC exceeding UNOS-DS criteria with a 9-cm tumor, who is able to achieve reduction in viable tumor to 3 cm and normal AFP after radioembolization has much to gain from LT and should undergo LT before the tumor progresses beyond transplantable criteria. By contrast, a patient with compensated liver disease and a single, well-treated 3-cm tumor without residual or recurrent tumor may be at lower risk for waitlist dropout with no imminent need for LT and may derive a lower transplant benefit.

PUSHING THE ENVELOPE: IS THERE A LIMIT?

There is clearly a limit to LT for HCC. There is general consensus that LT is futile in the context of extrahepatic spread. Macrovascular invasion, such as portal vein tumor thrombosis, has also conventionally been considered a contraindication to LT, although a recent study demonstrated 60% 5-year post-LT survival in a subgroup of patients who achieved complete radiologic regression of the vascular invasion by LRT before LT.[14]

The extent and biology of HCC confined to the liver that will benefit from LT is less well-defined. The combination of tumor size and number has been shown in multiple settings to predict response to LRT and the risk of HCC recurrence, which is the basis for current downstaging protocols that specify upper limits for initial tumor burden (eg, UNOS-DS criteria). Certainly, infiltrative tumors that overtake the entire liver parenchyma are associated with poor prognosis. However, there are tumors that may be large or numerous but still have more favorable tumor biology compared with smaller tumors. This can occur in cases disadvantaged by a delayed diagnosis from overdue screening, or the rare situation of having no underlying liver disease.

Expanding Beyond Milan

Over the past two decades, more liberal selection criteria have been proposed, expanding on the Milan criteria and exploring different cutoffs for combined tumor number and size at the time of LT. These include the UCSF criteria (one lesion up to 6.5 cm, or two to three lesions each <4.5 cm, and total tumor diameter <8 cm), "up-to-seven" criteria (sum of the size of largest tumor [cm] and number of tumors not exceeding 7), Valencia criteria (three tumors each <5 cm, total tumor diameter ≤10 cm), and the extended Toronto criteria (no upper limit on size or number; excluding patients with cancer-related symptoms, extrahepatic disease, vascular invasion, or poorly differentiated tumors).[7,15–17] Caused in part by variable results and ongoing organ shortages in many parts of the world including the United States, further expansion of LT criteria based on tumor number and size has not routinely been adopted.

Downstaging

Downstaging is a pathway by which patients with HCC beyond Milan may be eligible for LT, but only once the tumor burden is reduced to within Milan criteria with LRT. The downstaging approach allows for observation of tumor response and tumor behavior over time, which may in itself serve as a selection tool for patients who will do well after LT.[18] Outcomes for certain LT recipients successfully downstaged using LRT have not been significantly different from those always within Milan, in terms of post-LT survival and HCC recurrence. Post-transplant survival after 3 years in one US-based study was 79.1% for those meeting UNOS-DS criteria and downstaged before LT, compared with 83.2% for those always within Milan ($P = .17$). Patients exceeding UNOS-DS criteria experienced lower 3-year survival at 71.4% ($P = .04$ compared with Milan).[19] HCC recurrence rates at 3 years were 6.9% for Milan, 12.8% for UNOS-DS, and 16.7% for patients exceeding UNOS-DS. In 2017, UNOS implemented a national downstaging protocol (UNOS-DS), by which patients beyond Milan criteria can be eligible for priority LT listing via HCC exception points (one lesion ≤8 cm, two to three lesions <5 cm, or four to five nodules all <3 cm, with total tumor diameter <8 cm) **(Table 1)**.[20] In patients exceeding these UNOS-DS criteria, inferior outcomes related not only to post-LT survival but also waitlist outcomes have been observed, including 80% risk of waitlist dropout after 3 years, 5-year post-LT survival of 50%, and a 5-year intention-to-treat survival of 21.1%.[21] The sum of tumor number and largest tumor diameter and Child-Pugh class B or C were predictors of waitlist dropout. There was escalating risk of waitlist dropout with higher tumor burden, with a 68% probability of successful downstaging in patients where the sum of tumor number and largest tumor diameter was greater than or equal to 8 cm, 47% where it was greater than or equal to 12 cm, and 38% where it was greater than or equal to 14 cm. Based on the observation that the rate of downstaging dropped lower than the threshold of 50% at 1 year combined with the high rate of waitlist dropout even after successful downstaging, the authors propose an upper limit to tumor burden, calculated by the sum of tumor number and largest tumor diameter, of 12 cm.[21]

BEYOND TUMOR SIZE AND NUMBER

Risk estimation of post-LT mortality and HCC recurrence has typically relied on some combination of pre-LT tumor size and number. Although these often do predict

Table 1 **Downstaging protocols in patients with HCC presenting beyond Milan criteria**	
UNOS-DS Protocol	**All Comers Protocol**
Inclusion criteria	

1. HCC exceeding UNOS T2 criteria but meeting one of the following:
   a. Single lesion ≤8 cm
   b. 2 or 3 lesions each ≤5 cm with the sum of the maximal tumor diameters ≤8 cm
   c. 4 or 5 lesions each ≤3 cm with the sum of the maximal tumor diameters ≤8 cm
2. Absence of vascular invasion or extrahepatic disease based on cross-sectional imaging
	1. HCC exceeding UNOS-DS by any of the following:
	   a. HCC tumor number
	   b. HCC tumor size
	   c. Total HCC tumor diameter
	2. Absence of vascular invasion or extrahepatic disease based on cross-sectional imaging

Criteria for successful downstaging: residual tumors within Milan criteria	
Criteria for downstaging failure and exclusion from liver transplant	
1. Progression of tumors beyond inclusion criteria for downstaging based on tumor size and number 2. Any evidence of extrahepatic, lymphatic, or vascular tumor spread	1. Progression of tumor burden beyond Milan criteria after initial successful downstaging 2. Development of any new HCC lesions (not including residual/recurrent disease at previous LRT site) 3. Any evidence of extrahepatic, lymphatic, or vascular tumor spread
Additional guidelines	
Minimum observation period of 3 mo between downstaging and liver transplant	Minimum observation period of 6 mo between downstaging and liver transplant

transplant outcome, they are not completely reliable. Pre-LT imaging and explant characteristics are discordant in up to 15% to 25% of cases.[22,23] Underestimation of true tumor burden on pre-LT imaging compared with explant pathology has been associated with increased risk of post-LT HCC recurrence and death.[23] Setting a limit based solely on tumor size and number can then be arbitrary, ruling in patients with aggressive tumor and ruling out patients who might otherwise benefit from LT. In addition, other variables including dynamic tumor behavior, serum biomarkers, and imaging have been found to predict LT outcome, independent of tumor burden (**Table 2**).

Dynamic Tumor Behavior as an Indicator of Tumor Biology

Radiologic response to LRT remains an essential criterion for downstaging protocols, selecting for patients with more favorable tumor biology and selecting out those with an unacceptably high risk of HCC recurrence and mortality after LT. Dynamic tumor behavior, such as response to LRT and/or tumor progression while awaiting LT, may be an indicator for tumor biology. Tumor progression after LRT is associated with inferior outcomes after LT.[24,25] The observation that patients with HCC outside of Milan criteria who were successfully downstaged achieved similar outcomes to those within Milan after a period of waiting time inspired the "ablate and wait" strategy, which requires a period of observation before LT during which the tumor biology is clarified.[26] In a recent multicenter study, waiting times that were either too short

Table 2
Proposed selection criteria for LT using pretransplant characteristics, and effect on outcome in selected studies

Predictor	Cutoff	5-y RFS (%)	5-y Post-LT Survival (%)	Multivariable Risk Ratio (95% CI)
Tumor number + size				
Yao et al[15] (N = 70)	1 lesion ≤6.5 cm, 2–3 lesions each ≤4.5 cm with total tumor diameter ≤8 cm		75.2	
Silva et al (N = 257) (Valencia)	Up to 3 tumors, each <5 cm, cumulative tumor burden <10 cm	72	62	
	Milan	86	69	
Mazzaferro et al[7] (N = 1556) (up-to-seven)	Sum of size of largest tumor + number of tumors ≤7		71.2	
	Milan		73.3	
Sapisochin et al[17] (N = 605)	No limit	75	68	
	Milan	84	78	
Response to LRT				
Millonig et al[45] (N = 106)	Complete response		85.1	
	Partial response		63.9	
	No response		51.4	
Lai et al[24] (N = 422)	mRECIST progression			OS HR 1.6 (1.0–3.1)
	No progression			RFS HR 3.5 (1.9–6.6)
Yao et al (N = 606)	Downstaging	77.8	90.8	
	Milan	81.0	88.0	
AFP (ng/mL)				
Todo et al[46] (N = 653)	≤200		72.2	OS HR 2.54 (1.66–3.88)
	>1000		34.0	RFS HR 3.44 (2.09–5.66)
Duvoux et al[31] (N = 1033)	≤100	83.3	67.5	RFS HR 1.95 (1.21–1.35)
	100–1000	73.2	51.1	RFS HR 2.57 (1.55–4.28)
	>1000	47.0	39.1	

(continued on next page)

Table 2
(continued)

Predictor	Cutoff	5-y RFS (%)	5-y Post-LT Survival (%)	Multivariable Risk Ratio (95% CI)
Hameed et al[30] (N = 211)	≤1000	52.7		
	>1000	80.3		RFS HR 1.54 (0.36–6.50)
Berry and Ioannou (N = 8659)	0–15		73.9	OS HR 1.02 (0.93–1.12)[a]
	16–65		65.3	OS HR 1.38 (1.23–1.54)
	66–320		60.4	OS HR 1.65 (1.45–1.88)
	>320		52.6	OS HR 2.37 (2.06–2.73)
AFP, slope				
Lai et al[24] (N = 422)	>15 ng/mL/mo			OS HR 3.8 (2.0–6.9)
Vibert et al (N = 153)	≤15 ng/mL/mo	76		RFS HR 5.4 (2.8–10.1)
	>15 ng/mL/mo	54		
Giard et al[34] (N = 336)	>7.5 ng/mL/mo	69.8	59.5	RFS HR 3.0 (1.3–7.2)
	≤7.5 ng/mL/mo	87.4	75.3	
AFP (ng/mL), response to LRT				
Mehta et al[32] (N = 407)	≥1000–101–499	92.8	88.4	RFS HR 0.35 (0.14–0.86)
	≥1000 to ≤100	86.7	67.0	RFS HR 0.14 (0.04–0.43)
	No reduction	65.0	48.8	Reference
AFP-L3%				
Chaiteerakij et al[36] (N = 127)	>35%			Univariate HR 3.2 (1.7–6.1)
Des-gamma-carboxyprothrombin				
Takada and Uemoto47 (N = 136)	≥400 mAU/mL	49	34	Risk ratio, recurrence 5.62 (2.12–14.93)
	<400 mAU/mL	89	81	
Shirabe et al[48] (N = 119)	>300 mAU/mL	48		RFS HR 3.82 (1.58–19.18)
	≤300 mAU/mL	91		
Chaiteerakij et al (N = 127)	≥7.5 ng/mL			Univariate HR 3.5 (1.9–6.7)
Neutrophil/lymphocyte ratio				
Bertuzzo et al[49] (N = 219)	≥5	6.3	14.7	OS HR 4.87 (2.47–9.58)
	<5	89.5	73.2	RFS HR 19.14 (6.95–52.71)

Halazun et al[50] (N = 150)	≥5	25	28	OS HR 6.10 (2.29–16.29)
	<5	75	64	RFS HR 8.42 (2.85–24.88)
Limaye et al[51] (N = 160)	≥5	27	38	OS HR 2.22 (1.10–14.00)
	<5	79	68	RFS HR 67 (11–413)
PET				
Hsu et al[39] (N = 147)	TNR ≥2	29.6		RFS HR 13.52 (4.77–38.29)
	Positive, TNR 1–2	85.0		RFS HR 1.92 (0.52–7.12)
	Negative	84.8		Reference
Kornberg et al[52] (N = 116)	Positive	38.1	46.3	RFS HR 22.88 (6.39–83.01)
	Negative	93.3	88.7	
Ye et al[53] (N = 103)	Positive	21.9	49.9	OS HR 4.57 (1.52–14.72)
	Negative	76.0	76.2	

Abbreviations: CI, confidence interval; HR, hazard ratio; OS, overall survival; RFS, recurrence-free survival; TNR, tumor/nontumor ratio.
[a] Reference group = patients without HCC.
Data from Refs.[7,17,24,30–32,34,36,39,45–53]

(<6 months) or too long (>18 months) before LT resulted in a 60% increased risk of HCC recurrence after LT (16% vs 10%).[27] A shorter waiting time may not allow the tumor to declare its biology, whereas a longer waiting time may give tumors the opportunity to develop more aggressive tumor biology. In October 2015, UNOS implemented a mandatory 6-month waiting period after the initial application to obtain HCC exception points. This policy change equalized the waitlist dropout risk between patients with HCC and patients without HCC and prolonged the overall waiting time for patients with HCC.[28]

Serum Biomarkers and Imaging

To safely expand the limits of LT for HCC, selection criteria need to consider more than simply tumor size, number, and the response to LRT. In the Toronto experience with extended criteria, for which there were no specific limits on tumor number or size, liver biopsy of the largest lesion was performed in all patients exceeding Milan criteria, and those with poorly differentiated tumor were excluded.[17] With these selection criteria, Sapisochin and colleagues[17] demonstrated similar rates of survival at 1, 3, and 5 years compared with those within Milan. However, liver biopsy is not always practical and may lead to procedural complications, and so surrogate noninvasive markers of tumor differentiation would be preferable. Markers of tumor biology, such as novel biomarkers, and imaging have been demonstrated to predict outcomes after LT for HCC, independent of tumor size and number, and will be useful to help risk stratify LT candidates with an initial tumor burden beyond Milan.

Higher AFP levels have been consistently identified as a negative predictor of post-LT outcome, at all stages of HCC, correlating with vascular invasion and tumor differentiation.[6,17,19,29–31] Hameed and colleagues[30] identified AFP greater than 1000 ng/mL as the strongest pretransplant variable predicting vascular invasion, with 5-year survival of 52.7%. The trend of AFP levels also correlates with outcome. Among those with AFP greater than 1000 ng/mL, the reduction of AFP to less than 200 or 500 ng/mL after LRT has been associated with lower post-LT mortality.[32,33] A rise in AFP of more than 7.5 to 15 ng/mL per month also predicts poor outcome.[24,34] In the downstaging population in particular, AFP greater than 100 ng/mL identified a particular subgroup with higher risk of HCC recurrence and death, with 3-year survival of 59.5%, compared with 80.6% among patients with AFP less than 20 ng/mL, and 72.1% among patients with AFP with 20 to 99 ng/mL.[19]

Other serum biomarkers, such as the neutrophil/lymphocyte ratio, AFP-L3, and des-gamma carboxyprothrombin (DCP), and radiographic features including 18F-fluorodeoxyglucose avidity on PET, also predict HCC recurrence and post-LT mortality.[6,35–38] PET positivity, especially with tumor/nontumor ratio greater than two, has been associated with worse tumor differentiation and microvascular invasion and may be advantageous in regions with shorter LT wait times or before LDLT.[39] These markers have been incorporated in some proposed pre-LT risk stratification protocols, such as the Kyoto criteria for LDLT (up to 10 tumors, largest 5 cm, and DCP <400 mAU/mL) and the National Cancer Center Korea (total tumor diameter <10 cm and negative PET scan).[40–42]

Pretransplant Risk Stratification

It is increasingly clear that tumor size and number alone are not the sole determinants of post-LT outcome. If criteria for initial tumor size and number are liberalized, surrogate markers including dynamic tumor behavior, biomarkers, and imaging, will be needed to represent tumor biology and refine the selection conditions for LT.

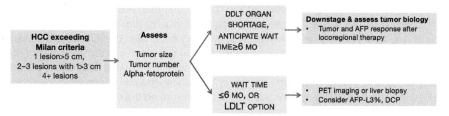

Fig. 1. Proposed evaluation for patients with HCC exceeding Milan criteria.

Combining biomarkers or imaging with tumor number and size may help to more accurately risk stratify this population.

Risk scores incorporating AFP cutoffs or categories improve prediction of post-LT HCC recurrence.[31,35] For example, in the Metroticket 2.0 analysis, the addition of AFP added to number and size of tumors outperformed Milan, UCSF, and up-to-seven criteria in the prediction of 5-year post-LT HCC-specific survival.[43]

Increasing the allowable criteria for tumor size and number may require more stringent limits for other markers of tumor biology to select the patients who will benefit from LT. The Metroticket 2.0 analysis demonstrates that with higher tumor burden, a lower AFP threshold is needed to meet the target of 70% 5-year survival: that is, if sum of number and size of tumors less than or equal to 7 cm (up-to-seven), then AFP should be less than 200 ng/mL; if up-to-five then AFP 200 to 400 ng/mL; and if up-to-four, then AFP 400 to 1000 ng/mL. Using a similar framework combining AFP with tumor burden in an intention-to-treat analysis, Lai and colleagues[44] proposed the following upper limits for successful LT: AFP less than or equal to 20 ng/mL and up-to-12; AFP 21 to 200 and up-to-10; AFP 201 to 500 and up-to-seven; AFP 501 to 1000 and up-to-five. The acceptable survival probability in this study was greater than or equal to 87% from the time of referral, recalibrated from the Metroticket 2.0 analysis.

Expanding HCC criteria in terms of tumor size and burden requires consideration of dynamic tumor behavior and biomarkers to represent tumor biology and differentiation, if liver biopsy is not available. Practical implementation of these risk scores should expect patients with high tumor burden exceeding Milan criteria not only to meet the AFP thresholds described previously, but also demonstrate at least one of the following: response to LRT, low AFP-L3 or DCP, negative PET, or exclusion of poorly differentiated tumor on histology (**Fig. 1**).

Liver allocation policy for DDLT in the United States now considers some of these variables, with recent implementation of a formalized downstaging protocol to ensure response to LRT for patients initially beyond Milan, a 6-month observation time before LT, and an AFP cutoff of 500 ng/mL after LRT in patients with AFP greater than 1000 ng/mL. Further study is needed to identify appropriate biomarker thresholds, the specific utility of specific radiographic features, such as 18F-fluorodeoxyglucose-avidity on PET, and the optimal observation time before LT to risk stratify those who would benefit from LT.

SUMMARY

There is considerable interest in expanding LT criteria for patients beyond Milan criteria. In the context of organ shortage, expanding HCC criteria will impact the entire LT waitlist and should be carefully weighed against the effect on patients without HCC and patients with HCC within Milan or UNOS-DS. Limits to LT do exist, but these limits are not determined solely by tumor size and number. Response to LRT, dynamic tumor behavior, serum biomarkers, and imaging also play a role in risk stratification and selection of patients who may be appropriate for LT. With careful selection practices, certain patients with larger tumors can do well with LT and should not be excluded a priori based on tumor size or number alone. External factors outside of tumor burden and biology may also change the calculus and risk assessment. Centers need to consider local organ shortages, anticipated wait time, and potential availability of a living donor.

CLINICS CARE POINTS

- Tumor size and number alone are not the sole determinants of post-LT outcome.
- Survival thresholds for patients with HCC should be comparable with nontumor patients.
- In expanding criteria for HCC, transplant centers should consider the overall impact on the liver transplant waitlist, local organ shortage, anticipated wait time, and potential availability of living donation.
- Noninvasive serum markers and radiographic features can represent tumor biology and differentiation and independently predict HCC recurrence and post-LT survival.
- Combining biomarkers with tumor size and number can improve risk stratification for potential LT candidates with HCC exceeding Milan criteria and identify patients who will meet the acceptable survival threshold for DDLT or LDLT.

DISCLOSURE

The authors have nothing to disclose.

REFERENCES

1. Mazzaferro V, Regalia E, Doci R, et al. Liver transplantation for the treatment of small hepatocellular carcinomas in patients with cirrhosis. N Engl J Med 1996; 334(11):693–9.
2. OPTN policy notice: clarification of HCC downstaging protocol for standard exceptions. 2019. Available at: https://optn.transplant.hrsa.gov/media/3123/policynotice_20190801_liver.pdf. Accessed May 30, 2020.
3. Kwong A, Kim WR, Lake JR, et al. OPTN/SRTR 2018 annual data report: liver. Am J Transplant 2020;20(Suppl s1):193–299.
4. Singal AG, Lampertico P, Nahon P. Epidemiology and surveillance for hepatocellular carcinoma: new trends. J Hepatol 2020;72(2):250–61.
5. Clavien P-A, Lesurtel M, Bossuyt PMM, et al. Recommendations for liver transplantation for hepatocellular carcinoma: an international consensus conference report. Lancet Oncol 2012;13(1):e11–22.
6. Mehta N, Heimbach J, Harnois DM, et al. Validation of a risk estimation of tumor recurrence after transplant (RETREAT) score for hepatocellular carcinoma recurrence after liver transplant. JAMA Oncol 2017;3(4):493–500.
7. Mazzaferro V, Llovet JM, Miceli R, et al. Predicting survival after liver transplantation in patients with hepatocellular carcinoma beyond the Milan criteria: a retrospective, exploratory analysis. Lancet Oncol 2009;10(1):35–43.
8. Brondfield MN, Dodge JL, Hirose R, et al. Unfair advantages for hepatocellular carcinoma patients listed for liver transplant in short-wait regions following 2015 hepatocellular carcinoma policy change. Liver Transpl 2020;26(5):662–72.

9. Llovet JM, Burroughs A, Bruix J. Hepatocellular carcinoma. Lancet 2003; 362(9399):1907–17.

10. Kulik LM, Fisher RA, Rodrigo DR, et al. Outcomes of living and deceased donor liver transplant recipients with hepatocellular carcinoma: results of the A2ALL cohort. Am J Transplant 2012;12(11):2997–3007.

11. Bhangui P, Vibert E, Majno P, et al. Intention-to-treat analysis of liver transplantation for hepatocellular carcinoma: living versus deceased donor transplantation. Hepatology 2011;53(5):1570–9.

12. Liang W, Wu L, Ling X, et al. Living donor liver transplantation versus deceased donor liver transplantation for hepatocellular carcinoma: a meta-analysis. Liver Transpl 2012;18(10):1226–36.

13. Lai Q, Vitale A, Iesari S, et al. Intention-to-treat survival benefit of liver transplantation in patients with hepatocellular cancer: hepatology, Vol. XX, No. X, 2017. Hepatology 2017;66(6):1910–9.

14. Assalino M, Terraz S, Grat M, et al. Liver transplantation for hepatocellular carcinoma after successful treatment of macrovascular invasion: a multi-center retrospective cohort study. Transplant Int 2020;33(5):567–75.

15. Yao FY, Ferrell L, Bass NM, et al. Liver transplantation for hepatocellular carcinoma: expansion of the tumor size limits does not adversely impact survival. Hepatology 2001;33(6):1394–403.

16. Silva M, Moya A, Berenguer M, et al. Expanded criteria for liver transplantation in patients with cirrhosis and hepatocellular carcinoma. Liver Transpl 2008;14(10): 1449–60.

17. Sapisochin G, Goldaracena N, Laurence JM, et al. The extended Toronto criteria for liver transplantation in patients with hepatocellular carcinoma: a prospective validation study. Hepatology 2016;64(6):2077–88.

18. Otto G, Herber S, Heise M, et al. Response to transarterial chemoembolization as a biological selection criterion for liver transplantation in hepatocellular carcinoma. Liver Transpl 2006;12(8):1260–7.

19. Mehta N, Dodge JL, Grab JD, et al. National experience on down-staging of hepatocellular carcinoma before liver transplant: influence of tumor burden, AFP and wait time. Hepatology 2019. https://doi.org/10.1002/hep.30879. hep.30879.

20. Yao FY, Kerlan RK, Hirose R, et al. Excellent outcome following down-staging of hepatocellular carcinoma prior to liver transplantation: an intention-to-treat analysis. Hepatology 2008;48(3):819–27.

21. Sinha J, Mehta N, Dodge JL, et al. Are there upper limits in tumor burden for down-staging of hepatocellular carcinoma to liver transplant? Analysis of the all-comers protocol. Hepatology 2019;70(4):1185–96.

22. Mehta N, Dodge JL, Roberts JP, et al. Validation of the prognostic power of the RETREAT score for hepatocellular carcinoma recurrence using the UNOS database. Am J Transplant 2018;18(5):1206–13.

23. Mahmud N, Hoteit MA, Goldberg DS. Risk factors and center-level variation in hepatocellular carcinoma understaging for liver transplantation. Liver Transpl 2020. https://doi.org/10.1002/lt.25787.

24. Lai Q, Avolio AW, Graziadei I, et al. Alpha-fetoprotein and modified response evaluation criteria in solid tumors progression after locoregional therapy as predictors of hepatocellular cancer recurrence and death after transplantation: alpha-Fetoprotein Increase and m RECIST Progression. Liver Transpl 2013. https://doi.org/10.1002/lt.23706.

25. Kim DJ, Clark PJ, Heimbach J, et al. Recurrence of hepatocellular carcinoma: importance of mRECIST response to chemoembolization and tumor size. Am J Transplant 2014;14(6):1383–90.

26. Roberts JP, Venook A, Kerlan R, et al. Hepatocellular carcinoma: ablate and wait versus rapid transplantation. Liver Transpl 2010;16(8):925–9.

27. Mehta N, Heimbach J, Lee D, et al. Wait time of less than 6 and greater than 18 months predicts hepatocellular carcinoma recurrence after liver transplantation: proposing a wait time "sweet spot. Transplantation 2017;101(9):2071–8.

28. Ishaque T, Massie AB, Bowring MG, et al. Liver transplantation and waitlist mortality for HCC and non-HCC candidates following the 2015 HCC exception policy change. Am J Transplant 2019;19(2):564–72.

29. Berry K, Ioannou GN. Serum alpha-fetoprotein level independently predicts post-transplant survival in patients with hepatocellular carcinoma. Liver Transpl 2013; 19(6):634–45.

30. Hameed B, Mehta N, Sapisochin G, et al. Alpha-fetoprotein level >1000 ng/mL as an exclusion criterion for liver transplantation in patients with hepatocellular carcinoma meeting the Milan criteria. Liver Transpl 2014;20(8):945–51.

31. Duvoux C, Roudot-Thoraval F, Decaens T, et al. Liver transplantation for hepatocellular carcinoma: a model including α-fetoprotein improves the performance of Milan criteria. Gastroenterology 2012;143(4):986–94.e3 [quiz: e14–5].

32. Mehta N, Dodge JL, Roberts JP, et al. Alpha-fetoprotein decrease from >1,000 to <500 ng/mL in patients with hepatocellular carcinoma leads to improved post-transplant outcomes. Hepatology 2019;69(3):1193–205.

33. Halazun KJ, Tabrizian P, Najjar M, et al. Is it time to abandon the Milan criteria?: results of a bicoastal US collaboration to redefine hepatocellular carcinoma liver transplantation selection policies. Ann Surg 2018;268(4):690–9.

34. Giard J-M, Mehta N, Dodge JL, et al. Alpha-fetoprotein slope >7.5 ng/mL per month predicts microvascular invasion and tumor recurrence after liver transplantation for hepatocellular carcinoma. Transplantation 2018;102(5):816–22.

35. Halazun KJ, Najjar M, Abdelmessih RM, et al. Recurrence after liver transplantation for hepatocellular carcinoma: a new MORAL to the story. Ann Surg 2017; 265(3):557–64.

36. Chaiteerakij R, Zhang X, Addissie BD, et al. Combinations of biomarkers and Milan criteria for predicting hepatocellular carcinoma recurrence after liver transplantation. Liver Transpl 2015;21(5):599–606.

37. Yang SH, Suh K-S, Lee HW, et al. The role of (18)F-FDG-PET imaging for the selection of liver transplantation candidates among hepatocellular carcinoma patients. Liver Transpl 2006;12(11):1655–60.

38. Lee JW, Paeng JC, Kang KW, et al. Prediction of tumor recurrence by 18F-FDG PET in liver transplantation for hepatocellular carcinoma. J Nucl Med 2009; 50(5):682–7.

39. Hsu C-C, Chen C-L, Wang C-C, et al. Combination of FDG-PET and UCSF criteria for predicting HCC recurrence after living donor liver transplantation. Transplantation 2016;100(9):1925–32.

40. Fujiki M, Takada Y, Ogura Y, et al. Significance of des-gamma-carboxy prothrombin in selection criteria for living donor liver transplantation for hepatocellular carcinoma. Am J Transplant 2009;9(10):2362–71.

41. Kaido T, Ogawa K, Mori A, et al. Usefulness of the Kyoto criteria as expanded selection criteria for liver transplantation for hepatocellular carcinoma. Surgery 2013;154(5):1053–60.

42. Lee SD, Lee B, Kim SH, et al. Proposal of new expanded selection criteria using total tumor size and (18)F-fluorodeoxyglucose - positron emission tomography/computed tomography for living donor liver transplantation in patients with hepatocellular carcinoma: the National Cancer Center Korea criteria. World J Transplant 2016;6(2):411–22.
43. Mazzaferro V, Sposito C, Zhou J, et al. Metroticket 2.0 model for analysis of competing risks of death after liver transplantation for hepatocellular carcinoma. Gastroenterology 2018;154(1):128–39.
44. Lai Q, Vitale A, Halazun K, et al. Identification of an upper limit of tumor burden for downstaging in candidates with hepatocellular cancer waiting for liver transplantation: a West-East Collaborative effort. Cancers (Basel) 2020;12(2). https://doi.org/10.3390/cancers12020452.
45. Millonig G, Graziadei IW, Freund MC, et al. Response to preoperative chemoembolization correlates with outcome after liver transplantation in patients with hepatocellular carcinoma. Liver Transpl 2007;13(2):272–9.
46. Todo S, Furukawa H, Tada M. Japanese Liver Transplantation Study Group. Extending indication: role of living donor liver transplantation for hepatocellular carcinoma. Liver Transpl 2007;13(11 Suppl 2):S48–54.
47. Takada Y, Uemoto S. Liver transplantation for hepatocellular carcinoma: the Kyoto experience. J Hepatobiliary Pancreat Sci 2010;17(5):527–32.
48. Shirabe K, Aishima S, Taketomi A, et al. Prognostic importance of the gross classification of hepatocellular carcinoma in living donor-related liver transplantation. Br J Surg 2011;98(2):261–7.
49. Bertuzzo VR, Cescon M, Ravaioli M, et al. Analysis of factors affecting recurrence of hepatocellular carcinoma after liver transplantation with a special focus on inflammation markers. Transplantation 2011;91(11):1279–85.
50. Halazun KJ, Hardy MA, Rana AA, et al. Negative impact of neutrophil-lymphocyte ratio on outcome after liver transplantation for hepatocellular carcinoma. Ann Surg 2009;250(1):141–51.
51. Limaye AR, Clark V, Soldevila-Pico C, et al. Neutrophil-lymphocyte ratio predicts overall and recurrence-free survival after liver transplantation for hepatocellular carcinoma. Hepatol Res 2013;43(7):757–64.
52. Kornberg A, Witt U, Schernhammer M, et al. Combining 18F-FDG positron emission tomography with up-to-seven criteria for selecting suitable liver transplant patients with advanced hepatocellular carcinoma. Sci Rep 2017;7(1):14176.
53. Ye Y-F, Wang W, Wang T, et al. Role of [18F] fluorodeoxyglucose positron emission tomography in the selection of liver transplantation candidates in patients with hepatocellular carcinoma. Hepatobiliary Pancreat Dis Int 2017;16(3):257–63.

Frailty and Sarcopenia in Patients Pre– and Post–Liver Transplant

Yedidya Saiman, MD, PhD[a], Marina Serper, MD, MS[a,b],*

KEYWORDS

- Frailty • Sarcopenia • Liver transplantation • Malnutrition • Cirrhosis

KEY POINTS

- Frailty and/or sarcopenia are present in greater than half of patients undergoing liver transplantation (LT) evaluation. Although significant overlap exists between frailty and sarcopenia, they are unique clinical entities with different pathophysiology.
- The presence of either frailty or sarcopenia is associated with worse pre- and post-LT outcomes independent of the Model for End-Stage Liver Disease (MELD) and other complications of end-stage liver disease.
- Multiple tools to diagnose frailty and sarcopenia have been developed and are beginning to be incorporated into routine clinical practice.
- Nutritional supplementation and exercise may be important in slowing or reversing the effects of frailty and sarcopenia leading to improved muscle mass, but are not enough to reverse their clinical impact.

INTRODUCTION

Initially defined among older adults, frailty and sarcopenia are now appreciated in all forms of chronic diseases including end-stage liver disease (ESLD).[1] Greater than 50% of patients with ESLD screen positive for frailty and/or sarcopenia, which are associated with increased morbidity and mortality in the pre– and post–liver transplant (LT) settings.[1,2] Recently, there has been an upsurge of interest in understanding the pathogenesis of frailty and sarcopenia, refining the diagnostic criteria in patients with ESLD while further elucidating the relationship between the two. Furthermore, there is

Author contributions: All authors contributed to the writing of the article, critical revision, and approval of the final article.
a Division of Gastroenterology and Hepatology, University of Pennsylvania Perelman School of Medicine, 3400 Civic Center Boulevard, Philadelphia, PA 19104, USA; b Department of Medicine, Corporal Michael J Crescenz VA Medical Center, 3900 Woodland Ave, Philadelphia, PA, 19104, USA
* Corresponding author. Division of Gastroenterology and Hepatology, University of Pennsylvania Perelman School of Medicine, 3400 Civic Center Boulevard, Philadelphia, PA 19104.
E-mail address: marinas2@pennmedicine.upenn.edu

an increased emphasis on early diagnosis and implementation of clinical interventions to delay the devastating effects of frailty and sarcopenia thereby improving patients' chances to survive until and after LT. This review focuses on the effects of frailty and sarcopenia in the pre- and post-LT period in patients with ESLD. Despite multiple similarities between frailty and sarcopenia they are not the same. We aim to highlight shared and distinct themes between the two entities focusing on assessment and diagnosis, pathogenesis, clinical outcomes, and treatment.

DEFINITIONS OF FRAILTY AND SARCOPENIA

Frailty has classically been defined as an age-related syndrome of decreased physiologic reserve associated with disability resulting in poor health outcomes, reduced quality of life, and death.[3,4] Multiple factors contribute to frailty including decline in physiologic systems, poor cognition, and social isolation. Therefore, frailty is associated with advanced age, poor nutritional status, and comorbid conditions impacting cognitive function (**Fig. 1**).[3,5] Similar to frailty, sarcopenia was initially understood to be an age-associated loss of muscle mass and function, although its prevalence in nearly all forms of chronic disease is now well-established.[1,6] Sarcopenia arises from a change in muscle biology resulting in decreased muscle mass and function from altered metabolic and endocrine physiology (see **Fig. 1**). Sarcopenia is a major component of frailty, although they are distinct. Frailty is a clinical diagnosis comprising physical, mental, and psychosocial components, whereas sarcopenia is a physiologic change in the metabolic and endocrine function of muscle.

ASSESSMENT AND DIAGNOSIS
Frailty

Perhaps the most important tool in diagnosing frailty and sarcopenia is astute clinical suspicion and appropriate consideration of risk factors. Multiple assessment tools initially developed for evaluating frailty in older adults have been investigated in patients with liver disease (**Table 1**), which are easily administered, although rely on significant self-reporting.[9] The Liver Frailty Index (LFI) was adapted from existing frailty

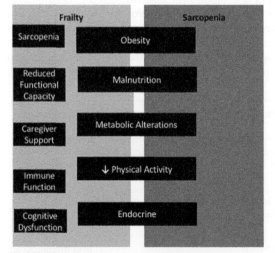

Fig. 1. Factors contributing to frailty and sarcopenia and associated clinical outcomes.

Table 1
Assessment tools for frailty and sarcopenia

Assessment Tool	Components
Frailty	
Fried Frailty Index	Weakness, exhaustion, weight loss, low activity, slow speed
Short Physical Performance Battery	Three performance-based tests: repeated chair stands, balance, and gait speed
Rockwood Frailty Index	Up to 70 items relating to comorbidities, changes in physical functioning, and neurologic signs
Clinical Frailty Scale	Modified from the Rockwood Clinical Frailty Scale; linear scale from score 1 (very fit) to 9 (terminally ill)
Braden Scale	Skin sensory perception, moisture, activity, mobility, nutrition, friction This scale was developed for risk assessment of pressure ulcers
Liver Frailty Index	Grip strength, chair stands, balance; specifically developed in ESLD
Six-minute-walk distance	Distance walked in 6-min
Gait speed	Gait speed, can use assistive mobility device if required
Activities of daily living	Feeding, toileting, dressing, bathing, transfers
Sarcopenia[7]	
Anthropometry	
Handgrip strength	Best performance of 3 trials of nondominant hand strength using a dynamometer
Six-minute-walk distance	Distance walked in 6-min
Midupper arm circumference	Circumference of flexed midupper arm
Triceps skinfold	Skin thickness measured with a skinfold caliper at midpoint between lateral projection of acromion process and inferior margin of olecranon process
Midarm muscle circumference	MAMC = MUAC (cm) −3.142 × TSF thickness (cm)
Indirect measurements	
Bioelectrical impedance analysis	Calculates lean (muscle) mass and fat mass by assessing body composition
Dual-energy x-ray absorptiometry	Measures relative attenuation of 2 x-ray energies through the body
Direct measurements	
Thigh muscle ultrasound[8]	Compression and featherweight thickness of thigh muscle at midpoint from the patella to the iliac crest; corrected for patient height
Computed tomography, abdominal	Total skeletal muscle mass at L3-level; corrected for patient height
MRI, abdominal	Total abdominal muscle mass, variable location based on study

Abbreviations: MAMC, midarm muscle circumference; MUAC, midupper arm circumference; TSF, triceps skinfold.
Adapted from Laube R, Wang H, Park L, et al. Frailty in advanced liver disease. Liver Int. 2018;38(12):2117-2128; with permission.

scores to specifically focus on patients with ESLD. The LFI measures physical function through performance-based tests and has been validated in multiple studies and enhances the LT waitlist mortality prediction over Model for End-Stage Liver Disease (MELD)-Na alone.[10,11] However, it is unknown whether frailty in this setting directly leads to increased mortality, or rather results in patients being passed over for organs, therefore increasing their waitlist mortality.

Sarcopenia

Multiple modalities have been adopted to assess muscle mass and sarcopenia in patients with liver disease, but few are used in routine clinical practice. Evaluation of muscle mass by anthropometric measurements, and direct and indirect measurements of muscle have all been studied in patients with ESLD (see **Table 1**).[12,13] Skeletal Muscle Index, defined as total abdominal muscle area at the L3 level from abdominal computed tomography scans and normalized to height, is the most widely used method to estimate total skeletal muscle mass. However, specific reference values/cutpoints to diagnosis sarcopenia remain elusive. Carey and colleagues[13] established sex-specific thresholds (50 cm^2/m^2 for men, 39 cm^2/m^2 for women) to diagnosis sarcopenia as a predictor of pre-LT waitlist removal or on-waitlist mortality; however, in a validation study by Kappus and colleagues[14] that used the same sex-specific cutoffs, there was no significant difference in pre-LT mortality and delisting. Such discrepancies underlie the challenge in interpreting the relationship between sarcopenia and pre-LT outcomes using current methodologies. These limitations reflect the methodology used to assess sarcopenia (use of a single computed tomography image from cross-sectional data) and patient selection.

Emerging techniques to assess sarcopenia are being established. These include the implementation of machine learning algorithms to automatically quantify L3 Skeletal Muscle Index[15,16] and use of MRI. MRI, however, is technically more challenging, although it can provide additional information regarding muscle function and performance. Future, prospective studies evaluating the utility of these techniques is required.

Although not directly a measure of frailty or sarcopenia, evidence of malnutrition alone should compel assessment of frailty and sarcopenia.[17] In LT patients evaluated for malnutrition by the Subjective Global Assessment, greater than 50% demonstrated moderate or severe malnutrition, thereby necessitating a baseline assessment and development of a nutritional management plan in all LT candidates.[18,19]

PATHOGENESIS OF FRAILTY AND SARCOPENIA IN CIRRHOSIS
Frailty

Despite advances in understanding the clinical implications of frailty and sarcopenia, the biologic underlying mechanisms and pathophysiology in liver disease are not well-described. Frailty results from the cumulative decline of multiple organ systems. In ESLD, liver failure, combined with neuromuscular, endocrine, immune, and skeletal muscle dysfunction, together promote frailty.[3] In patients deemed as "prefrail" (LFI between 3.2 and 4.4), an acute insult may disturb the underlying balance leading to development of overt frailty.[10] Increased loss of hippocampal neurons with resultant impairment of neuronal function is seen in elderly frail patients and in cirrhosis with hepatic encephalopathy (HE).[20–24] Low-grade chronic inflammation, observed in age-related frailty, is associated with elevated levels of interleukin-6, C-reactive protein, and tumor necrosis factor-α, all of which are dysregulated in patients with cirrhosis.

Skeletal muscle dysfunction and sarcopenia further increases one's risk of development of frailty.[3]

Sarcopenia

Sarcopenia in cirrhosis develops as a consequence of parallel mechanisms leading to severe muscle loss and dysfunction (**Box 1**). A proposed mechanism possibly unique to the development of sarcopenia in patients with ESLD is the development of hyperammonemia. Hyperammonemia develops as a consequence of hepatic dysfunction, decreased nitrogen clearance, and portosystemic shunting. Loss of hepatic ammonia detoxification leads to muscle disposal of ammonia through mitochondrial metabolism to glutamine and glutamate. This process is ATP-demanding and results in cataplerosis and subsequent branched-chain amino acid (BCAA) catabolism to replenish tricarboxylic acid cycle intermediates.[25,26]

Hyperammonemia further results in loss of muscle through inhibition of muscle protein synthesis through increased myostatin activation. Myostatin, a member of the transforming growth factor-β superfamily, is implicated in muscle protein synthesis and proteolysis through a nuclear factor-κB–dependent pathway.[25,27] Ammonia also disrupts mitochondrial ATP production through generation of reactive oxygenase species (ROS) promoting electron leak at mitochondrial complex III, impaired cellular respiration, and ROS-mediated cellular damage, a process similar to the effects of nitric oxide.[26] Finally, hyperammonemia-associated protein nitration results in elevated levels of muscle autophagy further leading to loss of muscle mass.[27]

Hepatic dysfunction leads to alteration in muscle secreted hormones and metabolites. These changes exacerbate liver disease while simultaneously inhibiting muscle turnover and regeneration.[28] Impaired glucose homeostasis in liver disease and insulin

---

Box 1
Pathogenesis of sarcopenia

Nutritional
  Decreased intake
  Malabsorption
  Vitamin deficiency

Physical inactivity
  Decreased aerobic exercise
  Decreased resistance exercise

Hyperammonemia
  Hepatic encephalopathy
  Increased myostatin
  Mitochondrial dysfunction
  Increased muscle autophagy and proteolysis

Inflammatory
  Low-grade systemic endotoxemia
  Low-grade systemic inflammation

Hormonal
  Decreased testosterone
  Decreased growth hormone

Metabolic
  Increased protein catabolism
  Increased insulin resistance
  Anabolic resistance

resistance associated with nonalcoholic fatty liver disease (NAFLD) or nonalcoholic steatohepatitis (NASH) further promote sarcopenia.[29] Similarly, activation of the ubiquitous signaling molecule, p38 mitogen-activated protein kinase (p38-MAPK), by ROS leads to loss of muscle stem cells required muscle regeneration.[28]

Multiple studies have demonstrated an association between sarcopenia and HE and sarcopenia is associated with minimal HE and future development of overt HE.[30] The relationship likely results from increased circulating ammonia levels. Although ammonia is only one component of HE, decreased muscle mass in sarcopenia triggers a vicious cycle. Increased glutamine release from muscle catabolism drives increased production of glutamic acid and ammonia from the small intestines and kidneys resulting in increased circulating ammonia and driving HE and sarcopenia.

Diet and Gastrointestinal Function

There are several reasons patients with ESLD may develop malnutrition. Dietary restrictions, most notably sodium restrictions, make food less palatable. This can then be compounded by ESLD-associated micronutrient deficiencies, which leads to altered taste sensation. Altered cognition associated with HE may lead to decreased oral intake. Limited gastric accommodation to oral intake associated with abdominal ascites and high rates of small intestinal bacterial overgrowth lead to decreased appetite, generalized discomfort, inadequate nutritional intake, and subsequent malnutrition.[31]

Nutrient Deficiency

Micronutrient deficiencies are common in ESLD, particularly vitamin D. In the context of sarcopenia, vitamin D has important effects in maintaining muscle mass and strength. Greater than 50% of patients with ESLD have vitamin D deficiency,[32] although the relative contribution to frailty and sarcopenia remains unclear. The benefits of vitamin D supplementation, however, have not been evaluated in ESLD. Additionally, nutrient deficiencies in fat-soluble vitamins (A, D, E, and K) and B vitamins (thiamine, folic acid, pyridoxine, and cobalamin) are prevalent in patient with cirrhosis. No studies have looked specifically at nutrient deficiency and frailty and sarcopenia, although the range of clinical symptoms associated with micronutrient deficiency is likely to impact patient frailty.[33]

Anabolic Resistance

Patients with liver disease develop anabolic resistance secondary to inflammatory stimuli and metabolic perturbations leading to decreased muscle protein synthesis and increased proteolysis even when nutritionally optimized.[34] As such nutritional interventions alone may not be sufficient to overcome ESLD-associated sarcopenia and specific interventions to overcome anabolic resistance are required.

PHYSICAL ACTIVITY AND PERFORMANCE IN FRAILTY AND SARCOPENIA

Decreased physical activity is a driver of frailty and sarcopenia, and predicts outcomes in ESLD independent of frailty and sarcopenia.[35] Poor physical activity and performance is an indirect indicator of cardiac function, obesity, and insulin resistance, which are all associated with frailty.[35] Indicators of physical performance including 6-minute-walk distance (6-MWD), 30-second chair stands, isometric knee extension, and maximal step length correlate with frailty even after adjustment for MELD.[36] The same is not true in sarcopenia, where indicators of physical performance are poorly correlated to muscle mass and changes in muscle mass and strength are not linear.[37,38] Furthermore, increased periods of immobility associated with frequent hospitalizations, HE, and poor energy promote muscle unloading and disuse atrophy further driving muscle loss.[39]

CLINICAL OUTCOMES ASSOCIATED WITH FRAILTY AND SARCOPENIA IN TRANSPLANT PATIENTS

Quality of Life

The impact of frailty on patient-reported outcomes and quality/satisfaction of life is evident in patients with ESLD. Frailty leads to decreased mobility, independence, and increased likelihood of HE, all of which contributes to decreased quality of life.[40] Tapper and colleagues[41] demonstrated in patients with compensated cirrhosis that frailty measured by performance of activities of daily life, chair-stands, and number of falls is associated with a decrease in health-related quality of life (HRQoL). The association even in patients with compensated cirrhosis underscores the importance of identifying and managing frailty at early stages of disease. Despite similar data on the effect of sarcopenia on quality of life in elderly patients, no study has specifically evaluated sarcopenia independent of frailty as a predictor of HRQoL in cirrhosis.

Pre–Liver Transplant

Frailty and sarcopenia in ESLD are associated with increased length of time on waitlist, death or removal from waitlist, and pre-LT morbidity independent of MELD score. Comparison between studies is challenging given the alternate methodologies used to assess frailty or sarcopenia, but nearly all studies demonstrate similar conclusions. Frailty is a predictor of waitlist mortality because each 1-unit increase in the FFI is associated with a 45% increase in MELD adjusted waitlist mortality.[42] Furthermore, frailty defined by the Clinical Frailty Scale is associated with increased rate of unplanned hospitalization (odds ratio, 3.6).[43] Similarly, data from 6-MWD testing demonstrates that each 0.1 m/s decrease in gait speed was associated with 22% increase in hospitalization days.[2,43] In addition to increased overall hospitalization, presence of frailty predicted postdischarge admission to rehabilitation center and 30-day readmission rates.[43,44] Conversely, each 100-m increase in the 6-MWD was associated with improved survival (hazard ratio [HR], 0.48).[45] Similar to frailty sarcopenia is independently and significantly associated with death on LT waitlist with a 2.0- to 2.4-fold higher risk of death.[46]

Despite the poor outcomes associated with frailty and sarcopenia neither are a consideration for waitlisting for an LT. As such, multiple groups have proposed adding a frailty or sarcopenia index to current MELD scoring systems. This would improve risk prediction over MELD-alone by indirectly accounting for clinical manifestations associated with frailty and sarcopenia. Accounting for frailty using the LFI, Lai and colleagues[10] demonstrated improved risk prediction at low and high MELD-Na scores. However, the MELD-Sarcopenia score only demonstrated improved mortality predictions in patients with low MELD scores (<15).[47] It must be noted whether adding frailty to the MELD score would change waitlist outcomes, because frail patients may be passed over for organs because of their frail status, thereby increasing waitlist mortality. If this is the case, increasing waitlist priority may not change their outcomes.

Post–Liver Transplant

Presence of frailty pre-LT defined by the LFI is associated with increased post-transplant hospital length of stay (LOS) and readmission within 3 months, but not death within the first year.[48] Similarly, patients with sarcopenia have increased post-LT LOS (40 vs 25 days) and higher 90-day incidence of bacterial infections (odds ratio, 4.6 between lowest and highest tertile of psoas muscle area).[49]

Patients with the lowest psoas muscle area had significantly decreased survival compared with those with the highest at 1 year (49.7% vs 87.0%). Even more surprising is that the effects of sarcopenia endure up to 3 years post-LT because again patients with the lowest psoas muscle area had decreased survival (26.4% vs 77.2%).[50] Nonetheless, these findings are not consistent across all studies because Montano-Loza and colleagues[51] demonstrated decreased median post-LT survival in patients with sarcopenia, although this was not significant, perhaps underlying the different modalities used in assessment of sarcopenia.[25] Data have shown that a 10% increase in muscle mass leads to sex-specific decrease in hospital LOS (10% in men, 3% in women), intensive care unit LOS (12% in men, 4% in women), and total days of intubation (13% in men, 7% in women). This suggests that even modest muscle mass preservation can have a significant clinical impact.[52] The risks of sarcopenia are further highlighted in patients undergoing living donor LT. Lower MELD scores associated with living donor LT are nonetheless overshadowed by low muscle mass resulting in increased post-LT mortality (HR, 2.06) and sepsis (HR, 5.31) in patients with sarcopenia.[53]

Only 16% of patients demonstrate resolution of sarcopenia post-LT, with similar data emerging from patients with frailty.[1,48] Multiple factors are likely associated with persistent frailty post-LT, including ongoing comorbidities, postsurgical complications, and failure in improvement of sarcopenia. Progressive muscle loss post-LT leads to development of de novo sarcopenia in approximately 25% of patients. This suggests that hepatic dysfunction is not the sole driver of sarcopenia. Long-standing ESLD may permanently alter skeletal muscle thereby driving ongoing sarcopenia that cannot simply be reversed by transplant.[1] Although body weight may improve this is usually in the form of increased fat mass and not lean muscle mass. Together, this contributes to a failure of skeletal muscle regeneration even in the absence of hepatic dysfunction. This may signify a unique entity or simply ongoing muscle loss in patients who underwent LT before obtaining a diagnosis of sarcopenia.[1]

Obesity

The convergence of obesity and sarcopenia, termed sarcopenic obesity, is particularly troublesome in patients with NASH cirrhosis. In addition to more advanced/aggressive liver disease sarcopenic obesity predicts worse outcomes than either sarcopenia or obesity alone in cadaveric and living donor transplant patients, suggesting an additive effect independent of increased cardiometabolic risks.[54] Haugen and colleagues[55] report that the prevalence of frailty in ESLD is independent of body mass index, but the risk of waitlist mortality in frail patients increased with body mass index.

CLINICAL MANAGEMENT OF FRAILTY AND SARCOPENIA

Treatment of patients with frailty and sarcopenia remains challenging because there are no targeted therapies and few clinical studies in patients with cirrhosis. The therapeutic options for patients with frailty or sarcopenia overlap because studies largely do not distinguish between them. Therapeutic interventions focus on increased caloric intake, metabolite/micronutrient supplementation, exercise, and management of underlying complications of liver disease affecting nutritional intake (**Table 2**). Additionally, interventions enhancing short-term memory attention and processing may have additional benefit specifically in patients with frailty.[56]

Table 2
Therapeutic strategies for frailty and sarcopenia in patients with ESLD

Intervention	Administration	Mechanism
High calorie and protein diet	Caloric intake of ≥35 kcal/kg/d and protein intake ≥1.5 g/kg/d	Improves nitrogen balance Decreases skeletal muscle proteolysis
Late-evening snack	≥50 g of complex carbohydrate snack/meal with protein before bed	Decreases lipid oxidation and improves nitrogen balance Decreases skeletal muscle proteolysis during overnight fasting
BCAA supplementation	BCAA 0.25 g/kg/d	Activates muscle protein synthesis through mTOR signaling pathway Decreases muscle autophagy Promotes ammonia metabolism
HMB supplementation	HMB 3 g/d in divided doses	Stimulates mTOR pathway Decreases muscle proteolysis Decreases muscle autophagy Increases protein synthesis
Physical activity	Aerobic and/or resistance exercise, moderate intensity	Increases mTOR activation via IGF-1 and phosphatidic acid leading to decreased muscle breakdown Increases expression of follistatin
Testosterone supplement	Testosterone IM or gel for patients with low serum testosterone	Inhibits myostatin through activation of androgen receptors in muscle Activates mTOR pathway
Zinc supplement	150–200 mg of elemental zinc/d	Improves zinc deficiency associated symptoms including altered taste, loss of appetite, and encephalopathy
Vitamin D supplement	Vitamin D 600–1000 IU/d for vitamin D levels <20 ng/mL, to reach >30 ng/mL	Prevents negative effects of vitamin D deficiency on musculoskeletal system
Long-term ammonia lowering strategies	Rifaximin, lactulose, LOLA, anaplerotic agents	Downregulates myostatin-mediated pathways Decreases muscle autophagy Improves muscle contractility

(continued on next page)

Table 2
(continued)

Intervention	Administration	Mechanism
SIBO treatment	Antibiotics – rifaximin, low FODMAP diet, prokinetics	Improves gastrointestinal discomfort May improve nutrient absorption
Reversal of portal hypertension	TIPS placement	Reduces HVPG Improves ascites May reduce metabolic rate
Antagonizing myostatin-mediated pathway	Myostatin antagonists, follistatin, mTOR agonists	Downregulates myostatin medication pathway Enhances mTOR signaling

Abbreviations: FODMAPS, fermentable oligosaccharides, disaccharides, monosaccharides, and polyols; HMB, β-hydroxy-β-methylbutyrate; HVPG, hepatic venous portal gradient; IGF, insulin-like growth factor; LOLA, L-ornithine-L-aspartate; mTOR, mammalian target of rapamycin; SIBO, small intestinal bacterial overgrowth; TIPS, transjugular intrahepatic portosystemic shunt.

Adapted from Bunchorntavakul C, Reddy KR. Review article: malnutrition/sarcopenia and frailty in patients with cirrhosis. Alimentary pharmacology & therapeutics. 2020;51(1):64-77; with permission.

Nutrition

Optimal caloric intake for patients with liver disease ranges from 35 to 45 kcal/g and 1.2 to 1.5 g/kg protein daily.[57] However, approaches need to be individualized. Although frailty and sarcopenia associated with alcoholic liver disease may simply be treated by alcohol cessation and nutritional supplementation, the approach to patients with other diseases (eg, hepatitis C virus, autoimmune) need to be different.[58] One of the most challenging cohorts of patients with ESLD to treat are those with sarcopenic obesity in which caloric restriction and protein consumption must be balanced to induce weight loss yet prevent further progression of sarcopenia.[59] Underlying these discussions is that despite these broad recommendations, there is minimal evidence to suggest that simple increased caloric and protein intake improves frailty or sarcopenia.

More targeted nutritional interventions including BCAA are associated with improved muscle mass in healthy and elderly individuals.[60] They supply increased carbon for ammonia metabolism into glutamine by muscle reducing total body ammonia load and improving muscle mass.[61] Studies comparing extended durations of defined caloric intake with or without BCAA supplementation demonstrate a reduction in composite of death by any cause (HR, 0.67), and improvement in serum albumin and HRQoL.[62] Although the improvements in HRQoL may signify a subsequent improvement in frailty, none of these studies directly measured muscle strength or mass.[63] In a similar study patients receiving BCAA demonstrated a small yet significant increase in midarm muscle circumference, whereas others showed an improvement in handgrip strength but not muscle mass after 28-days of supplementation, perhaps underscoring the need for longer-term administration.[64]

Dietary supplementation with β-hydroxy-β-methylbutyrate, a leucine metabolite, decreases muscle mass loss and improves muscle mass and strength in geriatric patients.[65] Recent studies have demonstrated an improvement in appendicular muscle mass handgrip strength at 12 weeks and 12 months after LT.[66] Additional interventional studies to assess 12 week of β-hydroxy-β-methylbutyrate supplementation on fat-free mass in patients with cirrhosis are currently underway.

Pharmacologic

No pharmacologic treatments for frailty or sarcopenia are currently recommended, although small trials have focused on improving muscle mass and strength. Testosterone increases muscle mass through muscle fiber hypertrophy and increased satellite cell number.[67] Testosterone is suppressed in up to 90% of patients with cirrhosis and exogenous supplementation improves muscle mass, but not survival.[68] Angiotensin-converting enzyme inhibitors have shown promise by improving endothelial function and angiogenesis while simultaneously reducing inflammation and promoting skeletal muscle glucose uptake.[69] No studies have been done in patients with cirrhosis, although clinical trials in age-related sarcopenia are ongoing.[70]

Ascites Management

Management of ESLD complications also shows utility in management of frailty and sarcopenia. Aggressive ascites management with diuretics or transjugular intrahepatic portosystemic shunt allows for improved gastric accommodation, increased oral intake, and may improve metabolic rate.[71] Transjugular intrahepatic portosystemic shunt placement for refractory ascites or variceal bleeding improves muscle mass at 6 months post-procedure.[72] Additionally, data from initial clinical trials of the automated low-flow ascites pump in patients with refractory ascites demonstrated an overall improvement in nutritional status, midarm muscle circumference, and hand-grip force over patients undergoing repeat large-volume paracentesis.[73]

Exercise

All forms of exercise in patients with ESLD are beneficial. Aerobic training improves cardiopulmonary performance, a measure of frailty, whereas resistance training has direct beneficial effects on sarcopenia.[35] Small studies have looked at the role of increasing daily steps together with nutritional interventions leading to an improvement in hepatic insulin sensitivity and an increase in HRQoL. Zenith and colleagues[74] showed that patients with Child-Turcotte-Pugh (CTP) A/B and low MELD scores who performed 8 weeks of aerobic exercise demonstrated improved oxygen uptake, which correlates to pre- and post-LT survival, thigh muscle thickness, and improved fatigue.[75] Similarly, Román and colleagues[76] found that moderate aerobic exercise with leucine supplementation led to improvements in 6-MWD (365 m to 445 m), thigh circumference, and HRQoL testing. Additionally, 12 weeks of supervised progressive resistance training in patients with CTP-A/B cirrhosis led to an increase in muscle strength (13% in treatment vs 4% in control group).[77] In patients with NASH, low-to-moderate intensity exercise led to weight loss and an improvement in hepatic function, but not in sarcopenia, underlying the importance of frequency and intensity of exercise regiments.[78]

Despite the promising results of these studies, they largely exclude patients with CTP-C cirrhosis and high MELD scores limiting the ability to apply these findings to many patients listed for transplantation. Although beyond the scope of this review, several excellent articles have recently summarized the clinical work-up and precautions of prescribing exercise regiments to patients with ESLD.[79]

CLINICAL CHALLENGES IN FRAILTY AND SARCOPENIA

Several challenges currently face the clinical management of patients with liver disease and frailty/sarcopenia. Much focus is given to patients undergoing LT, although the diagnosis is likely overlooked in patients with compensated cirrhosis not yet requiring LT evaluation. This is nonetheless likely the most opportune time to initiate observation and management of frailty and sarcopenia. Longitudinal changes in frailty are associated with poor transplant outcomes, a framework that may be able to be applied to patients with stable cirrhosis. This would potentially allow for early interventions thereby preventing future hepatic decompensations in particular in patients with NAFLD. NAFLD and sarcopenia each drive the progression of the other and improvement in sarcopenia in patients otherwise not eligible for liver transplantation may promote improvement in mortality and quality of life. With the development of newer tools to assess frailty, and the broad appreciation of its importance, identification and early interventions are being considered in many patients. Unfortunately, there remains a lack of consensus and clinical tools to specifically diagnose sarcopenia. Furthermore, diagnosis and patient education regarding frailty and sarcopenia is time consuming and may be beyond the scope of transplant physicians. Addressing these issues requires development of multidisciplinary teams to provide nutritional and exercise coaching and self-motivation techniques to elicit appropriate behavioral changes in patients with cirrhosis.

SUMMARY

Frailty and sarcopenia are highly prevalent in ESLD and strong predictors of patient morbidity and mortality in the pre- and post-LT periods. They are distinctly unique entities, although inherently intertwined and with shared underlying etiologies. Accurate and timely diagnosis remains critical to implement appropriate nutritional and exercise-based therapies to improve patient outcomes, but the absence of consensus in diagnosing sarcopenia in particular remains a challenge. Furthermore, a greater understanding of the underlying pathophysiology of these potentially modifiable risk factors is needed to develop targeted therapeutic strategies. Ongoing research is focused on developing methods to diagnose frailty and sarcopenia in routine clinical settings and understand the elements that are reversible to improve outcomes in patients with ESLD.

CLINICS CARE POINTS

- Frailty, malnutrition, and sarcopenia are common. Multiple brief and validated tools exist to measure them in clinical practice.
- Protein intake for patients with liver disease is important and should be individualized with the help of a registered dietitian.
- Physical activity including aerobic exercise and resistance training can improve muscle strength and should be encouraged.
- Aggressive treatment of hepatic encephalopathy may improve muscle breakdown.

DISCLOSURE

The authors have nothing to disclose.

FUNDING

M. Serper receives funding from the National Institutes of Health award (1K23 DK1158907-03).

REFERENCES

1. Bhanji RA, Takahashi N, Moynagh MR, et al. The evolution and impact of sarcopenia pre- and post-liver transplantation. Aliment Pharmacol Ther 2019;49(6): 807–13.
2. Dunn MA, Josbeno DA, Tevar AD, et al. Frailty as tested by gait speed is an independent risk factor for cirrhosis complications that require hospitalization. Am J Gastroenterol 2016;111(12):1768–75.
3. Laube R, Wang H, Park L, et al. Frailty in advanced liver disease. Liver Int 2018; 38(12):2117–28.
4. Fried LP, Tangen CM, Walston J, et al. Frailty in older adults: evidence for a phenotype. J Gerontol A Biol Sci Med Sci 2001;56(3):M146–56.
5. Fried LP, Ferrucci L, Darer J, et al. Untangling the concepts of disability, frailty, and comorbidity: implications for improved targeting and care. J Gerontol A Biol Sci Med Sci 2004;59(3):255–63.
6. Bhanji RA, Carey EJ, Yang L, et al. The long winding road to transplant: how sarcopenia and debility impact morbidity and mortality on the waitlist. Clin Gastroenterol Hepatol 2017;15(10):1492–7.
7. Beaudart C, McCloskey E, Bruyère O, et al. Sarcopenia in daily practice: assessment and management. BMC Geriatr 2016;16(1):170.
8. Isaka M, Sugimoto K, Yasunobe Y, et al. The usefulness of an alternative diagnostic method for sarcopenia using thickness and echo intensity of lower leg muscles in older males. J Am Med Dir Assoc 2019;20(9):1185.e1-8.

9. Lai JC, Volk ML, Strasburg D, et al. Performance-based measures associate with frailty in patients with end-stage liver disease. Transplantation 2016;100(12): 2656–60.

10. Lai JC, Covinsky KE, Dodge JL, et al. Development of a novel frailty index to predict mortality in patients with end-stage liver disease. Hepatology 2017;66(2): 564–74.

11. Lai JC, Covinsky KE, McCulloch CE, et al. The liver frailty index improves mortality prediction of the subjective clinician assessment in patients with cirrhosis. Am J Gastroenterol 2018;113(2):235–42.

12. Bunchorntavakul C, Reddy KR. Review article: malnutrition/sarcopenia and frailty in patients with cirrhosis. Aliment Pharmacol Ther 2020;51(1):64–77.

13. Carey EJ, Lai JC, Sonnenday C, et al. A North American expert opinion statement on sarcopenia in liver transplantation. Hepatology 2019;70(5):1816–29.

14. Kappus MR, Wegermann K, Bozdogan E, et al. Use of skeletal muscle index as a predictor of wait list mortality in patients with end-stage liver disease. Liver Transpl 2020;26(9):1090–9.

15. Burns JE, Yao J, Chalhoub D, et al. A machine learning algorithm to estimate sarcopenia on abdominal CT. Acad Radiol 2020;27(3):311–20.

16. Wang NC, Zhang P, Tapper EB, et al. Automated measurements of muscle mass using deep learning can predict clinical outcomes in patients with liver disease. Am J Gastroenterol 2020;115(8):1210–6.

17. Tandon P, Raman M, Mourtzakis M, et al. A practical approach to nutritional screening and assessment in cirrhosis. Hepatology 2017;65(3):1044–57.

18. Stephenson GR, Moretti EW, El-Moalem H, et al. Malnutrition in liver transplant patients: preoperative subjective global assessment is predictive of outcome after liver transplantation. Transplantation 2001;72(4):666–70.

19. Hasse J, Strong S, Gorman MA, et al. Subjective global assessment: alternative nutrition-assessment technique for liver-transplant candidates. Nutrition 1993; 9(4):339–43.

20. García-García R, Cruz-Gómez Á J, Urios A, et al. Learning and memory impairments in patients with minimal hepatic encephalopathy are associated with structural and functional connectivity alterations in hippocampus. Sci Rep 2018;8(1): 9664.

21. Clegg A, Young J, Iliffe S, et al. Frailty in elderly people. Lancet 2013;381(9868): 752–62.

22. Leng S, Chaves P, Koenig K, et al. Serum interleukin-6 and hemoglobin as physiological correlates in the geriatric syndrome of frailty: a pilot study. J Am Geriatr Soc 2002;50(7):1268–71.

23. Hubbard RE, O'Mahony MS, Savva GM, et al. Inflammation and frailty measures in older people. J Cell Mol Med 2009;13(9b):3103–9.

24. Dirchwolf M, Ruf AE. Role of systemic inflammation in cirrhosis: from pathogenesis to prognosis. World J Hepatol 2015;7(16):1974–81.

25. Ebadi M, Bhanji RA, Mazurak VC, et al. Sarcopenia in cirrhosis: from pathogenesis to interventions. J Gastroenterol 2019;54(10):845–59.

26. Davuluri G, Allawy A, Thapaliya S, et al. Hyperammonaemia-induced skeletal muscle mitochondrial dysfunction results in cataplerosis and oxidative stress. J Physiol 2016;594(24):7341–60.

27. Qiu J, Thapaliya S, Runkana A, et al. Hyperammonemia in cirrhosis induces transcriptional regulation of myostatin by an NF-kappaB-mediated mechanism. Proc Natl Acad Sci U S A 2013;110(45):18162–7.

28. Dasarathy S. Myostatin and beyond in cirrhosis: all roads lead to sarcopenia. J Cachexia Sarcopenia Muscle 2017;8(6):864–9.

29. Cleasby ME, Jamieson PM, Atherton PJ. Insulin resistance and sarcopenia: mechanistic links between common co-morbidities. J Endocrinol 2016;229(2): R67–81.

30. Nardelli S, Gioia S, Faccioli J, et al. Sarcopenia and cognitive impairment in liver cirrhosis: a viewpoint on the clinical impact of minimal hepatic encephalopathy. World J Gastroenterol 2019;25(35):5257–65.

31. Theocharidou E, Dhar A, Patch D. Gastrointestinal motility disorders and their clinical implications in cirrhosis. Gastroenterol Res Pract 2017;2017:8270310.

32. Malham M, Jørgensen SP, Ott P, et al. Vitamin D deficiency in cirrhosis relates to liver dysfunction rather than aetiology. World J Gastroenterol 2011;17(7):922–5.

33. Kozeniecki M, Ludke R, Kerner J, et al. Micronutrients in liver disease: roles, risk factors for deficiency, and recommendations for supplementation. Nutr Clin Pract 2020;35(1):50–62.

34. Morton RW, Traylor DA, Weijs PJM, et al. Defining anabolic resistance: implications for delivery of clinical care nutrition. Curr Opin Crit Care 2018;24(2):124–30.

35. Bhanji RA, Montano-Loza AJ, Watt KD. Sarcopenia in cirrhosis: looking beyond the skeletal muscle loss to see the systemic disease. Hepatology 2019;70(6): 2193–203.

36. Williams FR, Berzigotti A, Lord JM, et al. Review article: impact of exercise on physical frailty in patients with chronic liver disease. Aliment Pharmacol Ther 2019;50(9):988–1000.

37. Goodpaster BH, Park SW, Harris TB, et al. The loss of skeletal muscle strength, mass, and quality in older adults: the health, aging and body composition study. J Gerontol A Biol Sci Med Sci 2006;61(10):1059–64.

38. Yadav A, Chang YH, Carpenter S, et al. Relationship between sarcopenia, six-minute walk distance and health-related quality of life in liver transplant candidates. Clin Transplant 2015;29(2):134–41.

39. Wall BT, Dirks ML, van Loon LJ. Skeletal muscle atrophy during short-term disuse: implications for age-related sarcopenia. Ageing Res Rev 2013;12(4):898–906.

40. Derck JE, Thelen AE, Cron DC, et al. Quality of life in liver transplant candidates: frailty is a better indicator than severity of liver disease. Transplantation 2015; 99(2):340–4.

41. Tapper EB, Baki J, Parikh ND, et al. Frailty, psychoactive medications, and cognitive dysfunction are associated with poor patient-reported outcomes in cirrhosis. Hepatology 2019;69(4):1676–85.

42. Lai JC, Feng S, Terrault NA, et al. Frailty predicts waitlist mortality in liver transplant candidates. Am J Transplant 2014;14(8):1870–9.

43. Tandon P, Tangri N, Thomas L, et al. A rapid bedside screen to predict unplanned hospitalization and death in outpatients with cirrhosis: a prospective evaluation of the clinical frailty scale. Am J Gastroenterol 2016;111(12):1759–67.

44. Tapper EB, Finkelstein D, Mittleman MA, et al. Standard assessments of frailty are validated predictors of mortality in hospitalized patients with cirrhosis. Hepatology 2015;62(2):584–90.

45. Carey EJ, Steidley DE, Aqel BA, et al. Six-minute walk distance predicts mortality in liver transplant candidates. Liver Transpl 2010;16(12):1373–8.

46. Montano-Loza AJ, Meza-Junco J, Prado CM, et al. Muscle wasting is associated with mortality in patients with cirrhosis. Clin Gastroenterol Hepatol 2012;10(2): 166–73, 173.e1.

47. Montano-Loza AJ, Duarte-Rojo A, Meza-Junco J, et al. Inclusion of sarcopenia within MELD (MELD-sarcopenia) and the prediction of mortality in patients with cirrhosis. Clin Transl Gastroenterol 2015;6:e102.
48. Lai JC, Segev DL, McCulloch CE, et al. Physical frailty after liver transplantation. Am J Transplant 2018;18(8):1986–94.
49. Krell RW, Kaul DR, Martin AR, et al. Association between sarcopenia and the risk of serious infection among adults undergoing liver transplantation. Liver Transpl 2013;19(12):1396–402.
50. Englesbe MJ, Patel SP, He K, et al. Sarcopenia and mortality after liver transplantation. J Am Coll Surg 2010;211(2):271–8.
51. Montano-Loza AJ, Meza-Junco J, Baracos VE, et al. Severe muscle depletion predicts postoperative length of stay but is not associated with survival after liver transplantation. Liver Transpl 2014;20(6):640–8.
52. DiMartini A, Cruz RJ Jr, Dew MA, et al. Muscle mass predicts outcomes following liver transplantation. Liver Transpl 2013;19(11):1172–80.
53. Masuda T, Shirabe K, Ikegami T, et al. Sarcopenia is a prognostic factor in living donor liver transplantation. Liver Transpl 2014;20(4):401–7.
54. Kamo N, Kaido T, Hamaguchi Y, et al. Impact of sarcopenic obesity on outcomes in patients undergoing living donor liver transplantation. Clin Nutr 2019;38(5):2202–9.
55. Haugen CE, McAdams-DeMarco M, Verna EC, et al. Association between liver transplant wait-list mortality and frailty based on body mass index. JAMA Surg 2019;154(12):1103–9.
56. Ng TP, Feng L, Nyunt MS, et al. Nutritional, physical, cognitive, and combination interventions and frailty reversal among older adults: a randomized controlled trial. Am J Med 2015;128(11):1225–36.e1.
57. Mazurak VC, Tandon P, Montano-Loza AJ. Nutrition and the transplant candidate. Liver Transplant 2017;23(11):1451–64.
58. Marroni CA, Fleck AM Jr, Fernandes SA, et al. Liver transplantation and alcoholic liver disease: history, controversies, and considerations. World J Gastroenterol 2018;24(26):2785–805.
59. Bhanji RA, Narayanan P, Allen AM, et al. Sarcopenia in hiding: the risk and consequence of underestimating muscle dysfunction in nonalcoholic steatohepatitis. Hepatology 2017;66(6):2055–65.
60. Rasmussen BB, Wolfe RR, Volpi E. Oral and intravenously administered amino acids produce similar effects on muscle protein synthesis in the elderly. J Nutr Health Aging 2002;6(6):358–62.
61. Dam G, Ott P, Aagaard NK, et al. Branched-chain amino acids and muscle ammonia detoxification in cirrhosis. Metab Brain Dis 2013;28(2):217–20.
62. Muto Y, Sato S, Watanabe A, et al. Effects of oral branched-chain amino acid granules on event-free survival in patients with liver cirrhosis. Clin Gastroenterol Hepatol 2005;3(7):705–13.
63. Les I, Doval E, García-Martínez R, et al. Effects of branched-chain amino acids supplementation in patients with cirrhosis and a previous episode of hepatic encephalopathy: a randomized study. Am J Gastroenterol 2011;106(6):1081–8.
64. Uojima H, Sakurai S, Hidaka H, et al. Effect of branched-chain amino acid supplements on muscle strength and muscle mass in patients with liver cirrhosis. Eur J Gastroenterol Hepatol 2017;29(12):1402–7.
65. Flakoll P, Sharp R, Baier S, et al. Effect of beta-hydroxy-beta-methylbutyrate, arginine, and lysine supplementation on strength, functionality, body composition, and protein metabolism in elderly women. Nutrition 2004;20(5):445–51.

66. Lattanzi B, Giusto M, Albanese C, et al. The effect of 12 weeks of β-hydroxy-β-methyl-butyrate supplementation after liver transplantation: a pilot randomized controlled study. Nutrients 2019;11(9):2259.
67. Sinha-Hikim I, Roth SM, Lee MI, et al. Testosterone-induced muscle hypertrophy is associated with an increase in satellite cell number in healthy, young men. Am J Physiol Endocrinol Metab 2003;285(1):E197–205.
68. Sinclair M, Grossmann M, Hoermann R, et al. Testosterone therapy increases muscle mass in men with cirrhosis and low testosterone: a randomised controlled trial. J Hepatol 2016;65(5):906–13.
69. Morley JE. Pharmacologic options for the treatment of sarcopenia. Calcif Tissue Int 2016;98(4):319–33.
70. Band MM, Sumukadas D, Struthers AD, et al. Leucine and ACE inhibitors as therapies for sarcopenia (LACE trial): study protocol for a randomised controlled trial. Trials 2018;19(1):6.
71. Dasarathy J, Alkhouri N, Dasarathy S. Changes in body composition after transjugular intrahepatic portosystemic stent in cirrhosis: a critical review of literature. Liver Int 2011;31(9):1250–8.
72. Plauth M, Schütz T, Buckendahl DP, et al. Weight gain after transjugular intrahepatic portosystemic shunt is associated with improvement in body composition in malnourished patients with cirrhosis and hypermetabolism. J Hepatol 2004;40(2):228–33.
73. Stirnimann G, Banz V, Storni F, et al. Automated low-flow ascites pump for the treatment of cirrhotic patients with refractory ascites. Therap Adv Gastroenterol 2017;10(2):283–92.
74. Zenith L, Meena N, Ramadi A, et al. Eight weeks of exercise training increases aerobic capacity and muscle mass and reduces fatigue in patients with cirrhosis. Clin Gastroenterol Hepatol 2014;12(11):1920–6.e2.
75. Bernal W, Martin-Mateos R, Lipcsey M, et al. Aerobic capacity during cardiopulmonary exercise testing and survival with and without liver transplantation for patients with chronic liver disease. Liver Transpl 2014;20(1):54–62.
76. Román E, Torrades MT, Nadal MJ, et al. Randomized pilot study: effects of an exercise programme and leucine supplementation in patients with cirrhosis. Dig Dis Sci 2014;59(8):1966–75.
77. Aamann L, Dam G, Borre M, et al. Resistance training increases muscle strength and muscle size in patients with liver cirrhosis. Clin Gastroenterol Hepatol 2020; 18(5):1179–87.e6.
78. Hallsworth K, Adams LA. Lifestyle modification in NAFLD/NASH: facts and figures. JHEP Rep 2019;1(6):468–79.
79. Tandon P, Ismond KP, Riess K, et al. Exercise in cirrhosis: translating evidence and experience to practice. J Hepatol 2018;69(5):1164–77.

Advances in Rejection Management
Prevention and Treatment

Claire R. Harrington, MD[a], Guang-Yu Yang, MD, PhD[b],
Josh Levitsky, MD[c,d,*]

KEYWORDS

- T-cell mediated rejection • Antibody-mediated rejection • Biomarkers of rejection
- Immunosuppression minimization • Tolerance

KEY POINTS

- There are 3 main categories of rejection defined by the Banff Working group: T-cell–mediated rejection, antibody-mediated rejection, and chronic rejection.
- Preventing rejection is one of the most important parts of managing liver transplant recipients and involves vigilant monitoring for initial signs of rejection as well as improving medication compliance.
- First-line treatment is high-dose steroids. When patients are refractory to high-dose steroids, an antibody-mediated rejection needs to be considered as a diagnosis.
- There are currently no noninvasive, cost-effective, and highly accurate assays to monitor and guide management of rejection in liver transplant recipients.
- New research has emerged in the biomarkers of rejection, including serum proteins, peripheral blood lymphocytes, complement proteins, microRNA, and peripheral blood mononuclear cells.

INTRODUCTION

The history of liver transplantation had a challenging beginning in 1963 with survival rates ranging from hours to days.[1] These grim survival rates were secondary to an inadequate understanding of the acute host rejection of foreign tissue and early technical surgical complications. The use of long-term immunosuppressive strategies had

[a] Department of Medicine, Northwestern University Feinberg School of Medicine, 676 North St. Clair Street, Suite 2330, Chicago, IL 60611, USA; [b] Department of Pathology, Northwestern University Feinberg School of Medicine, 251 E Huron St. Chicago, IL 60611, USA; [c] Division of Gastroenterology and Hepatology, Northwestern University Feinberg School of Medicine, 676 North St. Clair Street, Suite 1400, Chicago, IL 60611, USA; [d] Comprehensive Transplant Center, Northwestern University Feinberg School of Medicine, 676 North St. Clair Street, Suite 1900, Chicago, IL 60611, USA
* Corresponding author.
E-mail address: josh.levitsky@nm.org

Clin Liver Dis 25 (2021) 53–72
https://doi.org/10.1016/j.cld.2020.08.003   liver.theclinics.com

limited impact owing to this restricted survival time, but consisted of techniques varying from thymectomy, splenectomy, actinomycin C, and azaserine along with a mainstay of treatment consisting of azathioprine and prednisone.[1] These strategies were largely adopted from renal allografts that preceded liver transplantation by about a decade.[2] Within the next 4 years, surgical techniques improved, as did survival, with a 19-month-old girl surviving 13 months with her transplant in 1967.[3] For the next decade, azathioprine and prednisone were the mainstays of therapy, as well as heterologous antilymphocyte globulin, which had been shown to be effective in renal transplantation.[4] There was also experimentation with irradiation of the transplanted livers to treat rejection.[3]

As the struggle of improving surgical techniques and early rejection survival was being addressed, the importance of balancing prolonged immunosuppression after transplantation became the next battleground. Azathioprine doses were limited by bone marrow suppression, thus providing overall inadequate immunosuppression.[5] Cyclosporine replaced azathioprine as the mainstay of treatment in the 1980s, when it proved to be a more potent, targeted immunosuppressant with fewer bone marrow effects.[6] The drawback of cyclosporine, though, was nephrotoxicity and an array of other adverse side effects.[6] The field took another leap with the development of tacrolimus in the 1990s.[5] It was found to not only be effective as a salvage therapy for patients who could either not tolerate or failed cyclosporine, but also as a primary immunosuppressant in conjunction with steroids.[5] It has since been found to be superior to cyclosporine in improving patient mortality and decreasing steroid-resistant rejection.[7] Largely owing to advances in calcineurin inhibitor (CNI) therapy, 1-year survival rates rapidly increased from the 67% in the 1980s to 90% in 2017.[8] Today, death or need for retransplantation owing to any sort of rejection is uncommon during the first 10 years after transplantation.[9]

The tacrolimus registration trials of 1994[10] revealed a significant concern for mainly nephrotoxicity and neurotoxicity. This led to drugs being developed to be used as adjuncts such as mycophenolate mofetil (MMF), which was used to decrease nephrotoxicity by allowing for minimization of tacrolimus and cyclosporine doses and systemic trough levels.[11] There are a variety of newer medications being trialed to reduce CNI exposure, which are discussed elsewhere in this article. Despite this development, tacrolimus remains the key immunosuppressive agent for liver recipients to this day (Fig. 1).

It was previously thought that there were 4 main types of rejection: hyperacute rejection, acute rejection, chronic rejection (CR), and humoral rejection. There has been a shift in redefining liver transplant rejection, mainly by the Banff Working group defining the main categories as T-cell–mediated rejection (TCMR), which also includes

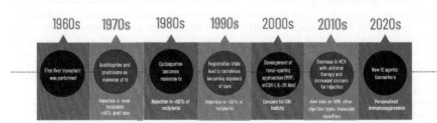

Fig. 1. History of immunosuppression in liver transplantation. AMR, antibody-medicated rejection; HCV, hepatitis c virus; IL-2R Abs, interleukin-2 receptor antibodies; IS, immunosuppression; mTOR-I, mammalian target of rapamycin inhibitors; tx, treatment.

plasma cell-rich rejection as a subtype, antibody-mediated rejection (AMR), and chronic rejection (CR).[12,13] Therefore, efforts have been made to establish diagnostic criteria to distinguish between each type involving histopathology, clinical findings, as well as various serum studies.

We first outline each type of rejection and their distinguishing features. We then focus on prevention of rejection, including methods for monitoring for rejection, and then discuss treatment options according to the various types of rejection.

T-CELL–MEDIATED REJECTION

TCMR, as its name suggests, is characterized by predominantly T-cell infiltrates. TCMR is further separated into loosely defined time classifications of early (varying from within 90 days of transplant to <6 months) and late (usually >6 months).[12–14] Severity is based on the distribution and severity of inflammation,[15] extent of tissue damage,[16] and signs of vascular injury.[12,17] These episodes of rejection can be further characterized by histologic grade of the degree of portal, bile ducts (ductulitis), and venous endothelial inflammation (endotheliitis).[12] This is used to create a composite score called the rejection activity index (RAI)[13] which guides management, as discussed elsewhere in this article.

Early TCMR histologically presents with ductulitis, portal or central venous endotheliitis, and/or mixed portal inflammation (lymphocytes, eosinophils, etc) with little to no inflammatory activity in the hepatocytes abutting the connective tissue of the portal triad, called the interface plate.[13] In contrast, late TCMR can present with interface or lobular hepatitis, plasma cell infiltrates, and perivenulitis, defined as inflammation in the area historically known as zone 3 or centrilobular area of the liver surrounding the central vein, and typically less ductulitis.[18]

Early TCMR is the most common type of rejection and it occurs in 10% to 40% of liver transplant recipients and is most common within the first month of being transplanted.[19,20] It was initially believed that early TCMR was not a significant risk factor for mortality[21,22] or graft loss.[22] This thought was in stark contrast with other solid organ transplants and was thought to be because the antidonor immune response was less potent in the liver compared with other organs, as well as the capacity of the liver to regenerate from injury.[21,23] New data from the more recent era has emerged, though, that indicates that early TCMR is associated with an increased risk of graft failure and death in liver transplant recipients.[15] Therefore, the clinical importance of preventing and treating early TCMR is even more vital.

About 10% of recipients can develop plasma cell-rich rejection usually late (>6 months) after transplantation.[12,24] This result is considered an atypical presentation of TCMR and is pathologically very similar to primary autoimmune hepatitis.[25] Criteria for diagnosis require (1) portal and/or perivenular infiltration of plasma cells (defined as >30%) with interface and/or perivenular necroinflammatory activity that involves a majority of portal tracts and (2) original disease causing liver failure to be other than autoimmune hepatitis. The third criterion, lymphocytic cholangitis, is not required but ideally present. This type of rejection has also been seen in interferon-treated and less so in recipients with direct-acting antiviral–treated hepatitis C.[26]

ANTIBODY-MEDIATED REJECTION

The most recently defined category of rejection is AMR, which is less common in liver versus other organ transplant recipients.[12] This is thought to be because the liver is a tolerogenic organ compared with other organs,[19,23] with several potential immunobiological mechanisms outside the scope of this review. The diagnosis of AMR is mainly considered in patients thought to have TCMR that is not responding to standard therapy or unexplained graft failure.[13] When AMR does occur, it can be hyperacute (typically ABO incompatible), acute, or chronic. Both diagnostic criteria for acute and chronic heavily rely on the presence of donor-specific antibodies (DSA), complement component 4d (C4d) staining, and histopathologic findings.[12]

Acute AMR usually occurs within the first few weeks after transplantation.[12] According to the most recent criteria released by the Banff Working Group in 2016, the recipient must meet all 4 criteria: (1) histopathology defined as endothelial cell hypertrophy or enlargement, capillary dilation, leukocyte sludging, and edema,[12] (2) positive serum DSA, (3) diffuse microvascular C4d deposition (most specifically portal vein and sinusoidal endothelial cell staining),[27] and (4) reasonable exclusion of other insults such as obstructive cholangiopathy.[12] These criteria are important because superimposed TCMR is common and so these criteria help to define mixed AMR and TCMR rejection episodes.[27] A subset of acute AMR is ABO-incompatible orthotopic liver transplant rejection, previously known as hyperacute rejection, which is extremely rare. In these episodes of rejection, histology reveals similar endothelial cell hypertrophy, but also has periportal hepatocyte coagulative necrosis along with red blood cell congestion and hemorrhage.[28]

The criteria for a diagnosis of chronic AMR are less clear and it is essentially a diagnosis of exclusion. Its histopathology consists of at least mild mononuclear portal and/or perivenular inflammation with interface involvement, as well as some degree of fibrosis. The other 3 criteria required for diagnosis are recent circulating HLA DSA in the past 3 months, at least focal C4d-positive (>10% portal tract microvasculature), and exclusion of other possible etiologies for insult.[12] The clinical picture is also helpful and is usually a recipient that is not adequately immunosuppressed with persistent serum DSA positivity.[29] Even with these criteria, it is difficult to diagnose chronic AMR owing to a lack of specificity because many of these findings can be seen in transplant recipients with no clinical or biochemical evidence of rejection.[12] Further confounding the diagnosis is, similar to acute AMR, a potential simultaneous episode of TCMR.[30]

CHRONIC REJECTION

Although CR can also be separated into early and late CR, this corresponds with varying histopathologic findings and not timing after transplantation.[17] However, these lines are even further blurred because biopsies can be mixed by having both early and late features.[31,32] The pathophysiology is thought to be a combination of direct immunologic injury and indirect ischemic damage secondary to an obliterative arteriopathy.[31] The distinguishing factor between TCMR and CR are the more fibrotic, irreversible, and less inflammatory characteristics of CR with targeting of primarily the bile ducts (previously known as the vanishing bile duct syndrome), hepatic artery, and the terminal hepatic venules and surrounding liver tissue.[17] Early CR is characterized by less than 50% duct loss and perivenular mononuclear inflammation with associated hepatocyte dropout and fibrosis.[33] Late CR is characterized by greater than 50% duct loss and progression of perivenular fibrosis involving the centrilobular area.[33] Other findings include hepatocyte ballooning and intrasinusoidal foam cell clusters.[17] Unfortunately, similar to chronic AMR, late CR has many nonspecific findings that are not uniformly present in all cases.[31,32] This factor is of clinical importance because the findings that are consistent with late CR have also been associated with a high likelihood of graft failure.[32] These findings are bile duct loss in greater than 50% of the portal tracts, severe perivenular fibrosis, and small arterial loss[32] (**Fig. 2**).

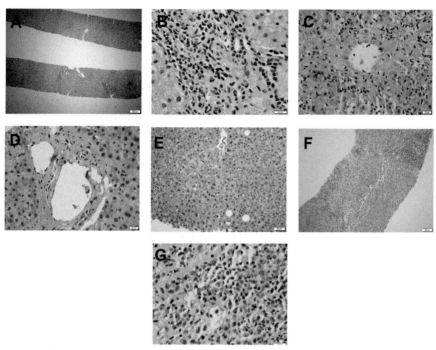

Fig. 2. Pathology. Focal mild acute cellular rejection. (*A*) Low-power view of needle biopsy of liver showing a few portal areas with mild portal inflammation. (*B*) High-power view showing mild portal inflammation is mainly composed of lymphocytes with occasional eosinophils and minimal ductulitis. Severe acute cellular rejection. (*C*) Showing perivenulitis and necrosis with lymphocyte infiltration. Chronic cellular rejection. (*D*) Loss of bile duct in the portal area. (*E*) Cytoplasmic and canalicular cholestasis. Plasma cell hepatitis. (*F*) Extensive portal and lobular inflammation with bridging necrosis. (*G*) High-power view showing sheet pattern of plasma cell infiltration in the portal area.

PREVENTION

Prevention of rejection is arguably the most important part of managing a post liver transplant patient. Two vital components for avoiding rejection are vigilant monitoring for initial signs of rejection to provide early interventions and improving medication compliance. Anecdotally, it has been noted that early rejection is not usually based on patient compliance, but secondary to insufficient immunosuppression, whereas later episodes of rejection are mainly due to patient adherence and more sparse monitoring. However, certain subsets of recipients (younger, autoimmune liver disease, prior rejections) have higher risks despite adequate monitoring and adherence[14,16] (**Fig. 3**).

The first step in rejection prevention is appropriately screening transplant candidates. Dobbels and colleagues[34] reported that pretransplant factors such as lower social support, lower conscientiousness, and lack of a stable relationship were predictors for post-transplant complications such as rejection and graft loss. Therefore, a thorough pretransplant screen is necessary to choose appropriate transplant candidates as the first step in allocating the limited resource of transplantable livers. However, this selection process should be wary of allocating a limited life-saving resource based predominantly on socioeconomic factors, subsequently causing an inequity of access weighted against the poor and minorities.[35]

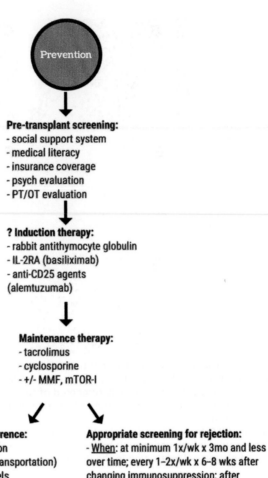

Fig. 3. Prevention. IL-2RA, interleukin-2 receptor antagonists; MMF, mycophenolate mofetil; mTOR-1, mammalian target of rapamycin inhibitors; OT, occupational therapy; PT, physical therapy.

When a patient is deemed an appropriate candidate for transplant, there is always a concern that insufficient immunosuppression will trigger early rejection within a few days of transplantation. Studies have evaluated induction immunosuppression therapy at the time of transplant, although this is only used in 20% to 25% of liver transplant recipients, again, owing to the tolerogenic nature of the liver.[36] The theoretic benefit behind induction immunosuppression is to provide additional prophylaxis against rejection in the acute period within the first few weeks after transplantation, when the risk of rejection is known to be highest.[36] In addition, because many patients have kidney dysfunction before and after transplantation, induction therapy may provide immunosuppressive coverage allowing the delay in use of nephrotoxic CNI therapy. The mechanism of action for effective induction therapy is either lymphocyte depleting or lymphocyte inhibiting.[36] There are several types of induction therapies, including rabbit antithymocyte globulin (ATG; which replaced the earlier anti-CD3 monoclonal antibody), IL-2 receptor antagonists such as basiliximab, and anti-CD52 agents such as alemtuzumab.[36,37] There has been some evidence that shows that induction therapy is associated with improved long-term graft survival and decreased rates of acute rejection.[37] Unfortunately, other than lymphocyte and neutrophil counts on a regular complete blood count, there are no assays that can measure the effectiveness of these agents, making their safety and efficacy challenging to monitor.[38] Lymphocyte-depleting therapies are especially associated with a higher risk for opportunistic infections and malignant complications such as post-transplant lymphoproliferative disease, making broad prophylaxis against both bacteria and viruses an essential part of patients' regimens.[39]

After the acute period following transplantation, patient adherence to laboratory monitoring and immunosuppressive regimens is one of the most consistently reported determinants of outcomes after transplant, including rejection and graft loss.[40,41] This factor is clinically significant because nonadherence is quite prevalent, ranging from 15% to 40% in the long term after liver transplantation.[40,41] Studies have shown that a lack of adherence correlates with a lack of social support, a lack of daily structure, limited literacy, depression, decreased physical health, and decreased cognitive function.[40,42] It is important to evaluate the reason for nonadherence by first considering the social determinants of health, such as an inability to afford the medication or limitations surrounding transportation and access. There could be confusion about how to take the medication or a misunderstanding about the significance of the medication. In older patients, there may be an inability to remember to take the medication. Depression and apathy can also inhibit patient adherence. Once the reason(s) for nonadherence is identified, a multidisciplinary approach is necessary to address all the risk factors and maximize adherence. A team should include social workers to help access benefits, physical therapists, occupational therapists, psychologists and therapists, among many others. Recent studies have focused on electronic monitoring feedback as a method for improving adherence, but future research is needed to elucidate the effect that these feedback systems have on clinical outcomes.[43]

Another known risk factor for increased nonadherence is an increased number of medications.[42] Because tacrolimus has become the mainstay of therapy in most liver transplant recipients,[5,7] it is of utmost importance to make taking this medication as convenient as possible. Extended-release once-daily tacrolimus formulations have been shown to be equally efficacious as twice-a-day dosing in liver transplant recipients.[44] Although consolidation of tacrolimus is helpful, liver transplant recipients are usually taking several other drugs, including anti-infection prophylaxis. They also tend to have complex medication regimens owing to metabolic and cardiovascular comorbidities, including hypertension, hyperlipidemia, and diabetes.[45] This situation is enhanced by nonalcoholic fatty liver disease becoming the most common diagnosis of patients listed for liver transplantation.[46] Owing to these complex medication regimens, it has been shown that medication and health literacy are also a significant factors in medication adherence.[40] To increase medication and health literacy, tools can be used, such as improved medication labels, simplified patient instructions, and close follow-up of at-risk patients.[47]

An additional challenge in the post-transplant period is balancing underimmunosuppression and overimmunosuppression. Immunosuppression, especially CNIs, are associated with well-known adverse effects, including increased cardiovascular disease, metabolic syndrome, kidney injury, opportunistic and community-acquired infections, and malignancy.[13,38] Therefore, the goal of immunosuppression should be aimed at minimizing the dose and number of drugs to prevent associated toxicities while still preventing rejection. Unfortunately, the ability to wean immunosuppression is limited by a lack of an effective way to monitor for rejection during this weaning period.

The most specific way to monitor for rejection is biopsy, but serial biopsies are invasive and financially impractical.[48] Because of this, surveillance liver biopsies have fallen out of favor.[49] Therefore, the most common method currently used are liver function tests and measuring immunosuppressive drugs levels.[48] Unfortunately, there is no standardized therapeutic range for CNIs (tacrolimus and cyclosporine), the most common primary immunosuppressants.[50] This lack is because the serum concentration of immunosuppressants is not consistently a reflection of the patient's cellular immunity.[38,51] The primary method of monitoring, however, is via trough levels of both cyclosporine and tacrolimus.[52] There has been some interest in the use of area under the concentration time–curve as an alternative for monitoring.[52] Although the area under the concentration time–curve has been seen to be a better method to optimize dosing of cyclosporine, the need for multiple blood draws has inhibited it from becoming a ubiquitous method of monitoring.[53] Area under the concentration time–curve monitoring has also been explored with tacrolimus, but has not been used in clinical practice.[52] MMF and sirolimus also have trough levels that are now available, but have the same flaws as CNIs.[52] Therefore, there have been many efforts to create a more accurate, but noninvasive way, to monitor for rejection, which will be discussed elsewhere in this article.

There is also no general consensus on the frequency of screening laboratory tests for monitoring. Because early TCMR is the most frequent type of rejection, it has been suggested to evaluate liver enzymes along with trough drug levels every 1 to 2 weeks until 3 to 6 months after transplantation.[16] Unfortunately, liver injury tests are nonspecific in rejection and can either show an increase in the transaminases or a cholestatic pattern; other etiologies such as vascular and biliary complications may be the reason for these elevations.[51] As noted elsewhere in this article, to prevent immunosuppressant toxicity, there is a theoretic incentive to wean immunosuppressant therapy, although there are no existing data demonstrating improved clinical outcomes with such a strategy. It is important, however, that liver injury tests are stable preceding any decrease in immunosuppression.[13] This factor is especially significant because it has been shown that patients with changes made in the preceding weeks were at higher risk for episodes for rejection.[14] Therefore, it is recommended that patients be monitored closely after any change in their immunosuppression regimen.[14]

Later after transplant (>1 year), rejection becomes less common, but it might be indicated to screen for rejection when patients are exposed to certain triggers, such as vaccinations. We know that antigen-dependent immune responses can lead to allograft rejection.[54] Therefore, there is a theoretic risk of vaccination-induced graft rejection.[55] There have been conflicting data, mostly in the kidney transplant population, that vaccination against influenza has been associated with an increase in anti-HLA antibodies that would theoretically increase the risk of rejection.[56,57] This risk of rejection with influenza vaccination has not been seen in larger studies.[58] It would be reasonable, though, to monitor for rejection by trending serum liver injury tests more frequently after exposure to an immune system-triggering insult.

There is increasing thought that antigen-independent injury can lead to inflammation that can also have downstream effects of rejection.[54] In transplanted organs, antigen-independent injury is mostly from the ischemia–reperfusion injury that the liver experiences perioperatively, which leads to the release of cytokines among many other inflammatory mediators.[54] An additional complication is biliary stricture, because the bile ducts are very sensitive to ischemia; it is solely supplied by the hepatic artery. It has been shown that biliary complications correlate with an increased risk of acute rejection thought to be due to the triggering of an inflammatory response.[19]

There has also been research regarding the risk factors associated with rejection that could be screened for to categorize patients as high risk for rejection for initiating closer monitoring. Several risk factors for early TCMR exist, including younger recipient age, HLA-DR mismatch, cytomegalovirus mismatch, older donor age, and patients with autoimmune liver diseases such as primary biliary cirrhosis and sclerotic cholangitis; however, not all of these factors are consistent throughout the literature and are controversial.[14,19,59] It would be reasonable to consider more frequent or invasive monitoring of these higher risk patients both in the short and long term after transplantation. There also may be an indication for closer monitoring based on the genetic profile of the patient, which will be discussed elsewhere in this article.

Although protocol liver biopsies have fallen out of favor, there may be some usefulness for them in higher risk populations and pediatric recipients.[60,61] What has been shown is that, even in the setting of normal liver injury tests, allograft biopsies have revealed histologic and clinically significant abnormalities in both pediatric and adult liver transplant populations.[49,61,62] Sanada and colleagues[61] showed in their pediatric population that at 5 years after transplantation, biopsies were able to significantly detect graft fibrosis that was reversible with uptitration of immunosuppression. This phenomenon was also seen in the adult population with nonalcoholic fatty liver disease, as well as patients with a history of primary biliary cholangitis.[62] Therefore, although there are no clear data that show that protocol liver allograft biopsies improve patient or graft outcomes, there may be some potential usefulness for them in these higher risk patient population; longer term outcome data are needed.

TREATMENT
T-Cell–Mediated Rejection

For liver transplant recipients who do develop TCMR, the standard of care depends on the severity of the RAI score[13] (**Fig. 4**). An RAI score of less than 4 is defined as mild, an RAI score of 4 to 6 is moderate, and an RAI score of greater than 7 to 9 is severe.[13]

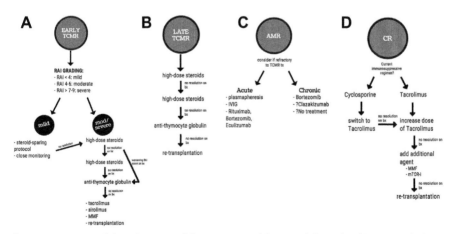

Fig. 4. Treatments. (*A*) Early TCMR. (*B*) Late TCMR. (*C*) AMR. (*D*) CR. bx, biopsy; IVIG, intravenous immunoglobulin; mTOR-I, mammalian target of rapamycin inhibitors.

There is some argument for withholding treatment in mild TCMR, or simply a mild increase in baseline immunosuppression, owing to its potential to self-resolve and the associated side effects of more potent immunosuppressive treatment.[63] The first-line treatment of moderate and severe RAI-scored TCMR are corticosteroids. There is a paucity of data about the optimal dose of steroids, however, and so there continues to be minor interinstitutional variability in dosage of steroids. In 2002, Volpin and colleagues[64] conducted the first and only study in the literature comparing different regimens of methylprednisolone in the treatment of early TCMR in liver transplant recipients. In this study, they compared 1-g pulses of methylprednisolone for 3 days followed by a baseline dose of 20 mg on the fourth day versus 1000 mg the first day, 200 mg on the second day, and then tapered by 40 mg every day for 5 days until the baseline dose of 20 mg was reached on the seventh day. Ultimately, they found that the group that only received 1 dose of 1000 mg followed by a 6-day taper to 20 mg/d of methylprednisolone fared better (defined by a higher rate of resolution of early TCMR), and that this regimen was associated with a lower rate of infectious complications, both bacterial and viral.[64]

Approximately 60% to 90% of early TCMR episodes respond to a single round of high-dose corticosteroids.[64] Owing to the efficacy of steroids, a second round of high-dose steroids, if the patient continues to have evidence of rejection on repeat biopsy, may be required in 10% to 15% of cases of early TCMR.[64] The effectiveness of steroid treatments in these cases of rejection have been shown to be more responsive in patients who are on maintenance tacrolimus at higher levels, and thus it is recommended to increase baseline immunosuppression in patients with TCMR during and after the steroid treatment.[10] Only 5% to 15% of patients are deemed steroid resistant, with persistent early TCMR on repeat biopsy despite courses of high-dose steroids or simply worse rejection on repeat biopsy after the first steroid course.[20,64] In these cases, there are options for second-line treatment.

Several studies have shown resolution of steroid-resistant rejection with treatment with ATG.[19,20,65] The most common side effects experienced include fever and chills with ATG, as well as arthralgias, abdominal pain, leukopenia, and anemia.[20] The main long-term risks after ATG administration are opportunistic infections and malignancy, such as post-transplant lymphoproliferative disorder.[65] Other options for steroid-resistant cases include increasing baseline therapy of tacrolimus, sirolimus, and MMF.[59,66–68] It was initially thought that anti–IL-2 agents such as basiliximab would be beneficial in steroid-resistant acute rejection,[69] but it has been shown that IL-2 receptor blockers are not efficacious as second-line therapy for acute rejection.[13]

Late TCMR tends to be more refractory to treatment compared with early TCMR, and this refractoriness could either be related to being a more severe entity or that it is diagnosed later in the course, with patients being less monitored over time and perhaps less adeherent.[16] It is associated with younger age, female sex, previous graft failure, autoimmune disease, primary biliary cholangitis, primary sclerosing cholangitis, and noncompliance indicated by low serum levels of immunosuppressants, emphasizing the need for encouragement of compliance with post-transplant patients.[14,16] The algorithm for treatment is the same as early TCMR with steroids as first line, but instead of a 90% response rate in early TCMR,[64] 1 study only showed 22% of late TCMR responding to pulsed high-dose steroids.[14] Conversely, a review of liver transplant recipients in Western Canada showed that only 5% of late TCMR episodes were steroid resistant and required rabbit ATG.[70] The wide differences in responses is likely due to the variability in histologic and biochemical severity, and the timing of presentation after transplantation. For steroid-resistant cases, ATG has been used.[71] Historically, rabbit ATG has been used for steroid-resistant cases, but owing to its considerable side effect profile,[72] it is no longer an option. Late TCMR that only has a partial response to steroids or is steroid resistant is clinically significant because these patients are at a higher risk of developing CR and graft loss.[14,16,70] Data are limited owing to the low frequency, but it is clear that an emphasis on compliance and prevention of late TCMR is of utmost importance.

Plasma cell-rich rejection is uncommon but now increasingly reported in the literature. Treatment is similar to the treatment of autoimmune hepatitis, although one could use the treatment of early or late TCMR in more severe cases.[24] The recommendation is for prednisone 20 mg to 40 mg daily with consideration of additional immunosuppressive therapy, such as azathioprine, 1 to 2 mg/kg daily.[73] The dose of prednisone should be tapered over a time period of 4 to 8 weeks, ultimately ending with a maintenance therapy of 5 to 10 mg/d.[73] This maintenance dose of prednisone in addition to the standard primary immunosuppression has been shown to decrease risk of progressive liver disease, retransplantation, and mortality.[74] There is a paucity of data owing to the rarity of this type of rejection, but there are new data suggesting the use of MMF as a substitute for azathioprine for treatment.[75] There is also a small case series suggesting that mammalian target of rapamycin inhibitors, such as sirolimus and everolimus, may have some usefulness in difficult-to-treat cases.[76] There is clearly a need for larger multicenter studies to further elucidate the best treatment options.

Antibody-Mediated Rejection

There is a paucity of data in the management of acute and even fewer data on chronic AMR. The diagnosis usually occurs when a patient is refractory to treatment with standard of treatment for TCMR and usually is due to the fact that mild acute AMR usually presents in combination with TCMR.[13,77] Most of the management of AMR is theoretic and experimental owing to the small number of cases and mainly based on experience in the kidney transplant population.[77] The mainstay of treatment is plasmapheresis and intravenous immunoglobulin to theoretically remove the antibodies mediating the rejection process.[69] The other modalities that have been experimented with all work against B cells and plasma cells, which are the main cell type in the pathophysiology of AMR. Examples include rituximab (an anti-CD20 antibody), bortezomib (used in the treatment of multiple myeloma; a protease inhibitor that acts against B cells and plasma cells), and eculizumab (a monoclonal antibody that is a complement inhibitor that activates the humoral immune system and, thus, B cells).[69] In late AMR, bortezomib may be preferable to rituximab because rituximab is known to not specifically affect plasma cells.[78] In terms of chronic AMR, there is a recent study investigating clazakizumab, a monoclonal antibody that inhibits the activation of the inflammatory mediator, IL-6.[79] A pilot trial by Eskandary and colleagues[79] theorizes that clazakizumab will inhibit DSA-mediated inflammation and thus act as a treatment of chronic AMR, but the trial will need to be completed and applicable to liver transplant recipients. It is unknown if aggressive therapies should be used in chronic AMR because the risks of therapy may outweigh the benefits. Therefore, the outcomes of chronic AMR need to be better defined before increasingly aggressive treatments are pursued.

Chronic Rejection

The mainstay of treatment for CR is optimization of immunosuppression. The only effective approach that has been shown is switching from cyclosporine to tacrolimus as the primary immunosuppressant, noting that cyclosporine is rarely used now as first-line therapy.[69] Other options include increasing the dose of tacrolimus for patients who are already on tacrolimus therapy or adding an additional immunosuppressive agent, although there are not much data showing that these methods are effective.[69,80] Examples of additional immunosuppressive agents are mammalian target of rapamycin inhibitors (sirolimus or everolimus) and MMF that have been shown to be able to reverse CR, especially if early, in up to 60% of patients, but the studies and experience are quite small in nature.[81] Unfortunately, a significant percentage of patients do not respond to an increased level of immunosuppression and ultimately require retransplantation.[80] Steroids or lymphodepletional therapies have been shown to have no usefulness in CR.[69] It is also important to consider the diagnosis of chronic AMR in cases of CR although, as noted elsewhere in this article, the appropriate treatment and management of these cases are unclear.

BIOMARKERS OF REJECTION

There are currently no noninvasive, economical, and highly accurate assays to monitor and guide management of rejection in liver transplant recipients.[69] There have been efforts to create tests to monitor for rejection based on both antigen-specific and nonspecific assays.[51]

Some examples of antigen-specific assays include donor specific assays, which is part of the diagnosis of AMR, as noted in the Introduction. There is literature to support that limiting dilution assays can be used to more closely quantify the recipient's antigen-specific immune response to a donor stimulus, so theoretically could be used to titrate immunosuppression.[82] The limiting factor of this test is that the assays often requires a significant amount of cells and blood.[38,51] Mixed lymphocyte reaction assays help to estimate the in vitro response to direct recognition of allogeneic molecules, but has not been validated in the clinical population and are complicated and time consuming to perform.[82] Enzyme-linked immunosorbent assay has also been proposed, but are limited owing to their labor-intensive nature and questionable reproducibility.[83] There are also antigen nonspecific assays such as cytokine genetic polymorphisms, monitoring regulatory T cells, and gene expression. Unfortunately, none of these methods have been able to be verified for use in the clinical setting.[48] There has been a surge in the research in this area, although primarily in nonhepatic organs such as kidney and heart transplantation, but also in liver transplantation more recently.

Studies in liver transplant recipients initially focused on DNA biomarkers that portended an increased or decreased risk for various types of rejection.[84–91] This process could be useful to categorize patients at higher risk for rejection, and so therefore be monitored more closely for rejection. Studies have found that recipient DNA with increased levels of HLA-DR3, tumor necrosis factor-2, CC chemokine 3L1, and glutathione S-transferase T1 are at higher risk for either early TCMR or CR.[84,89,91] These DNA markers have not been used in clinical practice yet and, unfortunately, DNA is a fixed variable and has lower usefulness in serial clinical management and immune monitoring.

Therefore, there has been a shift to evaluate for biomarkers that can be obtained serially to predict acute rejection and guide management. These biomarkers include serum proteins, peripheral blood lymphocytes, complement proteins, microRNA, and peripheral blood mononuclear cells.[92–96] Shaked and colleagues[95] showed that microRNA levels could be used to not only diagnose early TCMR, but also diagnose rejection up to 40 days before any clinical expression of rejection. Similarly, Levitsky and colleagues[97] revealed that globin-reduced RNA could be detected up to 90 days before an episode of early TCMR compared with non-AR patient. This outcome is promising because these assays could replace the more invasive liver biopsy as well as allow for immunosuppression titration during minimization before any clinical evidence of rejection.

Proteoforms, which is a measure of intact proteins, have also been explored as a biomarker for rejection because it is thought to be closer to the resultant phenotype and may be more accurate in rejection monitoring.[98] Toby and colleagues[96] showed that specific proteoforms were more common in patients with evidence of early TCMR compared with patients with no evidence of rejection and vice versa. Proteoforms that were elevated in patients with active evidence of early TCMR included thymosin-beta 4 and thymosin-beta 10, which are thought to activate hepatic stellate cells responsible for liver fibrosis[99] **(Table 1)**.

Interestingly, the liver's unique tolerogenic characteristics allows a window into the molecular factors that contribute to developing tolerance and in some cases the ability to discontinue immunosuppression.[19,23] The main "tolerance signatures" discovered thus far could also be used for future personalization of immunosuppression: blood immunophenotypic assays (CD4+CD25^{high} FOXP3+ cells and Vδ1/Vδ2 cell ratios), cytokine gene profiles (natural killer, γδ T cell, Th17 cells, and CD8$^+$ receptor genes), and genomic microarrays.[38,96] DNA markers and specific proteoforms that correlate with a decreased risk of early TCMR may lead to minimization of inflammation, cytokine signaling, and improvement of cytoskeletal regulation.[96] For instance, the proteoform CXCL4, which blocks Th17 differentiation, is more common in patients without any evidence of acute rejection compared with those with early TCMR.[96] Similarly, the proteoforms profilin 1, cofilin 1, filamin A, and cytoplasmic actin 1, which all act as actin-binding proteins to help with cytoskeletal regulation, are all abundant in patients with healthy graft function.[96] In the same vein, DNA markers such as tumor growth factor-beta 1 gene polymorphisms (anti-inflammatory)[85] and HLA-C (inhibits natural killer cells)[86,88] are seen to be protective from episodes of rejection. These markers could help to identify patients who are candidates for more aggressive immunosuppression minimization or even full withdrawal.

SUMMARY AND FUTURE DIRECTIONS

There are several aspects of current rejection management in need of further elucidation.

1. The usefulness of induction therapy and other novel immunosuppressive agents in prevention of acute rejection in the setting of known adverse effects.[39]
2. More data on the management of acute and chronic AMR, plasma cell-rich rejection, and CR. It would be beneficial to conduct multicenter studies owing to the rarity of each of these types.
3. The clinical usefulness of noninvasive biomarkers in immunosuppression management and rejection to personalize immunosuppression therapies.

Ultimately, further clarification of the immunopathology of rejection and personalization of immunosuppression would be very helpful to the management of liver transplant recipients. The development of more effective ways to monitor for risk factors of rejection or detect rejection before there is any clinical evidence will likely improve graft and patient survival. This process can be modeled after key developments that have been seen in the kidney transplant population, including the use of gene expression.[100] With improved graft life and survival of liver transplant recipients, the new frontier of rejection management is focused on immunosuppression minimization, withdrawal, and personalization.

Table 1
Biomarkers of liver graft injury and rejection

Author	Phenotype	Source	Biomarker	Increased Risk (+)/Protective (−)
Evans et al,[84] 2001	CR	Recipient DNA	HLA-DR3, TNF-2	+
Gomez-Mateo et al,[85] 2006	AR	Recipient DNA	TGFβ-1	−
Moya-Quiles et al,[86] 2007	AR	Recipient DNA	HLA-Cw*07	−
Sindhi et al,[87] 2008	AR	Recipient DNA	rs9296068 SNP	+
Hanvesakul et al,[88] 2008	Injury	Donor DNA	Donor HLA-C	−
Li et al,[89] 2012	AR	Recipient DNA and mRNA	CCL3L1 gene	+
Karimi et al,[90] 2011	AR	Recipient DNA	IL-6, IFN-γ	+
Kamei et al,[91] 2013	AR	Donor and recipient DNA	GSTT1 genotype	+
Massoud et al,[92] 2011	AR	Recipient serum proteins	C4, C1q	+
Fan et al,[93] 2012	AR	Recipient PBL	Th17 cells (CD4+, IL17+)	+
Farid et al,[94] 2012	Injury	Recipient serum and biopsy	miRNA (122, 148a, 194)	+
Shaked et al,[95] 2017	AR vs non-AR	Recipient miRNA	miRNA (hsa-miR-483-3p, hsa-miR-885-5p)	±
Toby et al,[96] 2017	AR vs non-AR	Recipient PBMC	Proteoforms	±
Levitsky et al,[97] 2020	AR vs non-AR	Recipient mRNA	36 gene panel	±

+, increased risk; −, protective.

Abbreviations: AR, acute rejection; C1q, complement component 1q; C4, complement component 4; CCL, CC chemokine; CD4, cluster of differentiation 4; DNA, deoxyribonucleic acid; GST, glutathione S-transferase; HLA, human leukocyte antigen; IFN-γ, interferon-gamma; IL, interleukin; miRNA, microRNA; mRNA, messenger ribonucleic acid; PBL, peripheral blood lymphocytes; PBMC, peripheral blood mononuclear cells; SNP, single nucleotide polymorphism; TGF, tumor growth factor; Th, T helper type; TNF, tumor necrosis factor.

Data from Refs.[84-97]

CLINICS CARE POINTS

- Early TCMR is the most common type of rejection with new data showing that it may be associated with an increased risk of graft failure and death in liver transplant recipients.
- Allow the severity of the RAI score guide initial management of early TCMR.
- Consider AMR as a diagnosis in patients not responding to standard TCMR therapy or have unexplained graft failure.
- The only effective approach to the treatment of CR in the literature is switching from cyclosporine to tacrolimus as the primary immunosuppressant.
- Encouraging patient adherence and addressing social determinants of health can help prevent rejection and graft loss.

DISCLOSURE

Dr J. Levitsky is a consultant, stockholder, and recipient of research funds from Viracor, Eurofins, and Transplant Genomics Inc.; Dr J. Levitsky is a consultant, speaker, and recipient of research funds from Novartis. Dr C.R. Harrington and Dr G-Y. Yang have nothing to disclose.

REFERENCES

1. Starzl T, Marchioro TL, Vonkaulla KN, et al. Homotransplantation of the liver in humans. Surg Gynecol Obstet 1963;117:659–76.
2. Starzl T, Marchioro TL, Brittain RS, et al. Problems in renal homotransplantation. JAMA 1964;187:734–40.
3. Starzl T, Groth CG, Brettschneider L, et al. Orthotopic homotransplantation of the human liver. Ann Surg 1968;168:392–415.
4. Starzl T, Marchioro TL, Porter KA, et al. The use of heterologous antilymphoid agents in canine renal and liver homotransplantation and in human renal homotransplantation. Surg Gynecol Obstet 1967;124(2):301–8.
5. Starzl T, Todo S, Fung J, et al. 506 for liver, kidney, and pancreas transplantation. Lancet 1989;2(8670):1000–4.
6. Calne R, Rolles K, White DJ, et al. Cyclosporin A initially as the only immunosuppressant in 34 recipients of cadaveric organs: 32 kidneys, 2 pancreases, and 2 livers. Lancet 1979;2(8151):1033–6.
7. Muduma G, Saunder R, Odeyemi I, et al. Systematic review and meta-analysis of tacrolimus versus ciclosporin as primary immunosuppression after liver transplant. PLoS One 2016;11(11):e0160421.
8. National UNOS STAR file: liver data [DVD] united network for organ sharing; 1985-2017.
9. Daniel K, Eickhoff J, Lucey MR. Why do patients die after a liver transplantation? Clin Transplant 2017;31(3). https://doi.org/10.1111/ctr.12906.
10. U.S. Multicenter FK506 Liver Study Group. A comparison of tacrolimus (FK506) and cyclosporine for immunosuppression in liver transplantation. N Engl J Med 1994;331(17):1110–5.
11. Reich D, Clavien PA, Hodge EE. MMF renal dysfunction after liver transplantation working group. Mycophenolate mofetil for renal dysfunction in liver transplant recipients on cyclosporine or tacrolimus: randomized, prospective, multicenter pilot study results. Transplantation 2005;80(1):18–25.

12. Demetris A, Bellamy C, Hübscher SG, et al. 2016 comprehensive update of the Banff Working Group on Liver Allograft Pathology: introduction of antibody-mediated rejection. Am J Transplant 2016;16(10):2816–35.
13. Charlton M, Levitsky J, Agel B, et al. International liver transplantation society consensus statement on immunosuppression in liver transplant recipients. Transplantation 2018;102(5):727–43.
14. Thurairajah P, Carbone M, Bridgestock H, et al. Late acute liver allograft rejection; a study of its natural history and graft survival in the current era. Transplantation 2013;95(7):955–9.
15. Levitsky J, Goldberg D, Smith AR, et al. Acute rejection increases risk of graft failure and death in recent liver transplant recipients. Clin Gastroenterol Hepatol 2017;15(4):584–93.e2.
16. Mor E, Gonwa TA, Husberg BS, et al. Late-onset acute rejection in orthotopic liver transplantation–associated risk factors and outcome. Transplantation 1992;54(5):821–4.
17. Blakolmer K, Jain A, Ruppert K, et al. Chronic liver allograft rejection in a population treated primarily with tacrolimus as baseline immunosuppression: long-term follow-up and evaluation of features for histopathological staging. Transplantation 2000;69(11):2330–6.
18. Banff Working Group, Demetris AJ, Adeyi O, Bellamy COC, et al. Liver biopsy interpretation for causes of late liver allograft dysfunction. Hepatology 2006; 44(2):489–501.
19. Dogan N, Husing-Kabar A, Schmidt HH, et al. Acute allograft rejection in liver transplant recipients: incidence, risk factors, treatment success, and impact on graft failure. J Int Med Res 2018;46(9):3979–90.
20. Aydogan C, Sevmis S, Aktas S, et al. Steroid-resistant acute rejections after liver transplant. Exp Clin Transplant 2010;8(2):172–7.
21. Charlton M, Seaberg E. Impact of immunosuppression and acute rejection on recurrence of hepatitis C: results of the national institute of diabetes and digestive and kidney diseases liver transplantation database. Liver Transpl Surg 1999;5(4 Suppl 1):S107–14.
22. Jain A, Reyes J, Kashyap R. Long-term survival after liver transplantation in 4,000 consecutive patients at a single center. Ann Surg 2000;232:490–500.
23. Starzl T. Immunosuppressive therapy and tolerance of organ allografts. N Engl J Med 2008;358(4):407–11.
24. Stirnimann G, Ebadi M, Czaja AJ, et al. Recurrent and de novo autoimmune hepatitis. Liver Transpl 2019;25(1):152–66.
25. Demetris A, Sebagh M. Plasma cell hepatitis in liver allografts: variant of rejection or autoimmune hepatitis? Liver Transpl 2008;14(6):750–5.
26. Levitsky J, Fiel MI, Norvell JP, et al. Risk for immune-mediated graft dysfunction in liver transplant recipients with recurrent HCV infection treated with pegylated interferon. Gastroenterology 2012;142(5):1132–9.e1.
27. O'Leary J, Michelle Shiller S, Bellamy C, et al. Acute liver allograft antibody-mediated rejection: an inter-institutional study of significant histopathological features. Liver Transpl 2014;20(10):1244–55.
28. Haga H, Egawa H, Shirase T, et al. Periportal edema and necrosis as diagnostic histological features of early humoral rejection in ABO-incompatible liver transplantation. Liver Transpl 2004;10(1):16–27.
29. Del Bello A, Congy-Jolivet N, Muscari F, et al. Prevalence, incidence and risk factors for donor-specific anti-HLA antibodies in maintenance liver transplant patients. Am J Transplant 2014;14(4):867–75.

30. Yamada H, Kondou H, Kimura T, et al. Humoral immunity is involved in the development of pericentral fibrosis after pediatric live donor liver transplantation. Pediatr Transplant 2012;16(8):858–65.
31. Oguma S, Belle S, Starzl TE, et al. A histometric analysis of chronically rejected human liver allografts: insights into the mechanisms of bile duct loss: direct immunologic and ischemic factors. Hepatology 1989;9(2):204–9.
32. Blakolmer K, Jain A, Ruppert K, et al. Chronic liver allograft rejection in a 1000+ Tacrolimus-treated cohort with a median follow-up of more than 5 years. Transplantation 2000;69(11):2330–6.
33. Neil D, Hubscher SG. Histologic and biochemical changes during the evolution of chronic rejection of liver allografts. Hepatology 2002;35(3):639–51.
34. Dobbels F, Vanhaecke J, Dupont L, et al. Pretransplant predictors of posttransplant adherence and clinical outcome: an evidence base for pretransplant psychosocial screening. Transplantation 2009;87(10):1497–504.
35. Kaswala D, Zhang J, Liu A, et al. A Comprehensive analysis of liver transplantation outcomes among ethnic minorities in the United States. J Clin Gastroenterol 2020;54(3):263–70.
36. Rostaing L, Saliba F, Calmus Y, et al. Review article: use of induction therapy in liver transplantation. Transplant Rev 2012;26(4):246–60.
37. Penninga L, Wettergren A, Wilson CH, et al. Antibody induction versus placebo, no induction, or another type of antibody induction for liver transplant recipients. Cochrane Database Syst Rev 2014;(6):CD010253.
38. Levitsky J. Next level of immunosuppression: drug/immune monitoring. Liver Transpl 2011;17:S60–5.
39. Page E, Kwun J, Oh B, et al. Lymphodepletional strategies in transplantation. Cold Spring Harb Perspect Med 2013;3(7):a015511.
40. Serper M, Patzer RE, Reese PP, et al. Medication misuse, nonadherence, and clinical outcomes among liver transplant recipients. Liver Transpl 2015; 21(1):22–8.
41. Burra P, Germani G, Gnoato F, et al. Adherence in liver transplant recipients. Liver Transpl 2011;17(7):760–70.
42. Prendergast M, Gaston RS. Optimizing medication adherence: an ongoing opportunity to improve outcomes after kidney transplantation. Clin J Am Soc Nephrol 2010;5(7):1305–11.
43. van Heuckelum M, van den Ende CHM, Houterman AEJ, et al. The effect of electronic monitoring feedback on medication adherence and clinical outcomes: a systematic review. PLoS One. 2017;12(10):e0185453.
44. Kim S, Lee SD, Kim YK, et al. Conversion of twice-daily to once-daily tacrolimus is safe in stable adult living donor liver transplant recipients. Hepatobiliary Pancreat Dis Int 2015;14(4):374–9.
45. Watt K, Pedersen RA, Kremers WK, et al. Evolution of causes and risk factors for mortality post-liver transplant: results of the NIDDK long-term follow-up study. Am J Transplant 2010;10(6):1420–7.
46. Zamora-Valdes D, Watt KD, Kellogg TA, et al. Long-term outcomes of patients undergoing simultaneous liver transplantation and sleeve gastrectomy. Hepatology 2018;68(2):485–95.
47. Clement S, Ibrahim S, Crichton N, et al. Complex interventions to improve the health of people with limited literacy: a systematic review. Patient Educ Couns 2009;75(3):340–51.

48. Israeli M, Klein T, Brandhorst G, et al. Confronting the challenge: individualized immune monitoring after organ transplantation using the cellular immune function assay. Clin Chim Acta 2012;413(17–18):1374–8.
49. Mells G, Neuberger J. Protocol liver allograft biopsies. Transplantation 2008; 85(12):1686–92.
50. Class II special controls guidance document: cyclosporine and tacrolimus assays; draft guidance for industry and FDA. Devices DoCL; 2002.
51. Sood S, Testro AG. Immune monitoring post liver transplant. World J Transplant 2014;4(1):30–9.
52. Mohammadpour N, Elyasi S, Vahdati N, et al. A review on therapeutic drug monitoring of immunosuppressant drugs. Iran J Basic Med Sci 2011;14(6): 485–98.
53. Jorga A, Holt D, Johnston A. Therapeutic drug monitoring of cyclosporine. Transplant Proc 2004;36(2):S396–403.
54. Mori D, Kreisel D, Fullerton JN, et al. Inflammatory triggers of acute rejection of organ allografts. Immunol Rev 2014;258(1):132–44.
55. Valour F, Conrad A, Ader F, et al. Vaccination in adult liver transplantation candidates and recipients. Clin Res Hepatol Gastroenterol 2020;44(2):126–34.
56. Baluch A, Humar A, Eurich D, et al. Randomized controlled trial of high-dose intradermal versus standard-dose intramuscular influenza vaccine in organ transplant recipients. Am J Transplant 2013;13(4):1026–33.
57. Katerinis I, Hadaya K, Duquesnoy R, et al. De novo anti-HLA antibody after pandemic H1N1 and seasonal influenza immunization in kidney transplant recipients. Am J Transplant 2011;11(8):1727–33.
58. Fernandez-Ruiz M, Lumbreras C, Arrazola MP, et al. Impact of squalene-based adjuvanted influenza vaccination on graft outcome in kidney transplant recipients. Transpl Infect Dis 2015;17(2):314–21.
59. Wu L, Tam N, Deng R, et al. Steroid-resistant acute rejection after cadaveric liver transplantation: experience from one single center. Clin Res Hepatol Gastroenterol 2014;38(5):592–7.
60. Sheikh A, Chau KY, Evans HM. Histological findings in protocol biopsies following pediatric liver transplant: low incidence of abnormalities at 5 years. Pediatr Transplant 2018;22(5):e13212.
61. Sanada Y, Matsumoto K, Urahashi T, et al. Protocol liver biopsy is the only examination that can detect mid-term graft fibrosis after pediatric liver transplantation. World J Gastroenterol 2014;20(21):6638–50.
62. Abraham S, Poterucha JJ, Rosen CB, et al. Histologic abnormalities are common in protocol liver allograft biopsies from patients with normal liver function tests. Am J Surg Pathol 2008;32(7):965–73.
63. Dousset B, Hubscher SG, Padbury RT, et al. Acute liver allograft rejection - is treatment always necessary? Transplantation 1993;55(3):529–34.
64. Volpin R, Angeli P, Galioto A, et al. Comparison between two high- dose methylprednisolone schedules in the treatment of acute hepatic cellular rejection in liver transplant recipients: a controlled clinical trial. Liver Transpl 2002;8(6): 527–34.
65. Lee J, Lee J, Lee JJ, et al. Efficacy of rabbit anti-thymocyte globulin for steroid-resistant acute rejection after liver transplantation. Medicine (Baltimore) 2016; 95(23):e3711.
66. Pfitzmann R, Klupp J, Langrehr JM, et al. Mycophenolate mofetil for immunosuppression after liver transplantation: a follow-up study of 191 patients. Transplantation 2003;76(1):130–6.

67. Mártinez J, Pulido LB, Bellido CB, et al. Rescue immunosuppression with mammalian target of rapamycin inhibitor drugs in liver transplantation. Transplant Proc 2010;42(2):641–3.
68. Coelho F, Coelho RF, Massarollo PC, et al. Use of tacrolimus in rescue therapy of acute and chronic rejection in liver transplantation. Rev Hosp Clin Fac Med Sao Paulo 2003;58(3):141–6.
69. Shaik I, Carmody IC, Chen PW. Treatment of acute and chronic rejection. In: Busuttil RW, Klintmalm GBG, editors. Transplantation of the liver. 3rd edition. Philadelphia: Saunders 2015. p. 1317–28.
70. Ramji A, Yoshida EM, Bain VG, et al. Late acute rejection after liver transplantation: the Western Canada experience. Liver Transpl 2002;8(10):945–51.
71. Nakanishi C, Kawagishi N, Sekiguchi S, et al. Steroid-resistant late acute rejection after a living donor liver transplantation: case report and review of the literature. Tohoku J Exp Med 2007;211(2):195–200.
72. Moini M, Schilsky ML, Tichy EM. Review on immunosuppression in liver transplantation. World J Hepatol 2015;7(10):1355–68.
73. Liberal R, Longhi MS, Grant CR, et al. Autoimmune hepatitis after liver transplantation. Clin Gastroenterol Hepatol 2012;10(4):346–53.
74. Salcedo M, Vaquero J, Bañares R, et al. Response to steroids in de novo autoimmune hepatitis after liver transplantation. Hepatology 2002;35(2):349–56.
75. Zachou K, Gatselis N, Papadamou G, et al. Mycophenolate for the treatment of autoimmune hepatitis: prospective assessment of its efficacy and safety for induction and maintenance of remission in a large cohort of treatment-naive patients. J Hepatol 2011;55(3):636–46.
76. Kerkar N, Dugan C, Rumbo C, et al. Rapamycin successfully treats posttransplant autoimmune hepatitis. Am J Transplant 2005;5(5):1085–9.
77. Hogen R, DiNorcia J, Dhanireddy K. Antibody-mediated rejection: what is the clinical relevance? Curr Opin Organ Transplant 2017;22(2):97–104.
78. Kim P, Demetris AJ, O'Leary JG. Prevention and treatment of liver allograft & antibody-mediated rejection and the role of the 'two-hit hypothesis'. Curr Opin Organ Transplant 2016;21(2):209–18.
79. Eskandary F, Durr M, Budde K, et al. Clazakizumab in late antibody-mediated rejection: study protocol of a randomized controlled pilot trial. Trial 2019; 20(1):37.
80. Jain A, Demetris AJ, Kashyap R, et al. Does tacrolimus offer virtual freedom from chronic rejection after primary liver transplantation? Risk and prognostic factors in 1,048 liver transplantations with a mean follow-up of 6 years. Liver Transpl 2001;7(7):623–30.
81. Neff G, Montalbano M, Slapak-Green G, et al. A retrospective review of sirolimus (Rapamune) therapy in orthotopic liver transplant recipients diagnosed with chronic rejection. Liver Transpl 2003;9(5):477–83.
82. Truong D, Bourdeaux C, Wiers G, et al. The immunological monitoring of kidney and liver transplants in adult and pediatric recipients. Transpl Immunol 2009; 22(1–2):18–27.
83. Reding R, Gras J, Truong DQ, et al. The immunological monitoring of alloreactive responses in liver transplant recipients: a review. Liver Transpl 2006; 2006(3):373–83.
84. Evans P, Smith S, Hirschfield G, et al. Recipient HLA-DR3, tumour necrosis factor-alpha promoter allele-2 (tumour necrosis factor-2) and cytomegalovirus infection are interrelated risk factors for chronic rejection of liver grafts. J Hepatol 2001;34(5):711–5.

85. Gomez-Mateo J, Marin L, Lopez-Alvarez MR, et al. TGF-beta1 gene polymorphism in liver graft recipients. Transpl Immunol 2006;17(1):55–7.
86. Moya-Quiles M, Alvarez R, Miras M, et al. Impact of recipient HLA-C in liver transplant: a protective effect of HLA-C2*07 on acute rejection. Hum Immunol 2007;68(1):51–8.
87. Sindhi R, Higgs BW, Weeks DE, et al. Genetic variants in major histocompatibility complex-linked genes associated with pediatric liver transplant rejection. Gastroenterology 2008;135(3):830–9.
88. Hanvesakul R, Spencer N, Cook M, et al. Donor HLA-C genotype has a profound impact on the clinical outcome following liver transplantation. Am J Transplant 2008;8(9):1931–41.
89. Li H, Xie HY, Zhou L, et al. Copy number variation in CCL3L1 gene is associated with susceptibility to acute rejection in patients after liver transplantation. Clin Transplant 2012;26(2):314–21.
90. Karimi M, Daneshmandi S, Pourfathollah AA, et al. Association of IL-6 promoter and IFN-gamma gene polymorphisms with acute rejection of liver transplantation. Mol Biol Rep 2011;38(7):4437–43.
91. Kamei H, Masuda S, Nakamura T, et al. Impact of glutathione S-transferase T1 gene polymorphisms on acute cellular rejection in living donor liver transplantation. Transpl Immunol 2013;28(1):14–7.
92. Massoud O, Heimbach J, Viker K, et al. Noninvasive diagnosis of acute cellular rejection in liver transplant recipients: a proteomic signature validated by enzyme-linked immunosorbent assay. Liver Transpl 2011;17(6):723–32.
93. Fan H, Li LX, Han DD, et al. Increase of peripheral Th17 lymphocytes during acute cellular rejection in liver transplant recipients. Hepatobiliary Pancreat Dis Int 2012;11(6):606–11.
94. Farid W, Pan Q, van der Meer AJ, et al. Hepatocyte-derived microRNAs as serum biomarkers of hepatic injury and rejection after liver transplantation. Liver Transpl 2012;18(3):290–7.
95. Shaked A, Chang BL, Barnes MR, et al. An ectopically expressed serum miRNA signature is prognostic, diagnostic, and biologically related to liver allograft rejection. Hepatology 2017;65(1):269–80.
96. Toby T, Abecassis M, Kim K, et al. Proteoforms in peripheral blood mononuclear cells as novel rejection biomarkers in liver transplant recipients. Am J Transplant 2017;17(9):2458–67.
97. Levitsky J, Asrani S, Schiano T, et al. Discovery and validation of a novel blood-based molecular biomarker of rejection following liver transplantation. Am J Transplant 2020;20(8):2173–83.
98. Savaryn J, Catherman AD, Thomas PM, et al. The emergence of top-down proteomics in clinical research. Genome Med 2013;5(6):53.
99. Kim J, Jung Y. Thymosin beta 4 is a potential regulator of hepatic stellate cells. Vitam Horm 2016;102:121–49.
100. Friedewald J, Kurian SM, Heilman RL, et al. Clinical trials in organ transplantation. Development and clinical validity of a novel blood-based molecular biomarker for subclinical acute rejection following kidney transplant. Am J Transplant 2019;19(1):98–109.

Expanding Role of Donation After Circulatory Death Donors in Liver Transplantation

Kristopher P. Croome, MD, MS*, C. Burcin Taner, MD

KEYWORDS

- DCD • HCC • Non–heart beating • Ischemic cholangiopathy • Allocation

KEY POINTS

- The number of donation after circulatory death (DCD) liver transplants (LTs) performed annually in the United States has continued to grow since 2012.
- Outcomes with DCD LT have continued to show improvement with better donor and recipient selection.
- There has been a paradigm shift from viewing recipients as "not sick enough for a DCD" to viewing recipients as "too sick for a DCD."
- Changes to liver allocation likely will increase the number of DCDs being pursued for patients with an hepatocellular carcinoma exception.
- Lack of a robust safety net for ischemic cholangiopathy after DCD LT remains one of the major barriers to more broad utilization in the United States.

EXPANSION, CONTRACTION, AND RE-EXPANSION

The first liver transplants (LTs) performed by Dr Thomas Starzl all were from donors who were declared deceased based on irreversible cessation of cardiorespiratory function. These donors thus represented the first donation after circulatory death (DCD) donors.[1] With the development of the Harvard criteria for brain death in 1968 and the acceptance of declaration of death according to neurologic criteria as a legal entity, most countries, including the United States, almost exclusively utilized donation after brain death (DBD) donors until the 1990s.[2] Groups in Pittsburgh and Wisconsin began to describe a renewed utilization of DCD LTs in the mid-1990s.[3,4] Excitement surrounding DCD LTs resulted in expanded utilization from 1994 to 2007 (**Fig. 1**). Given the markedly improved results with DBD LTs most transplant centers were achieving by the year 2000, many centers applied the same principles and concepts they were

The article did not receive any funding.
Department of Transplant, Mayo Clinic Florida, 4500 San Pablo Road, Jacksonville, FL 32224, USA
* Corresponding author.
E-mail address: croome.kristopher@mayo.edu

Clin Liver Dis 25 (2021) 73–88
https://doi.org/10.1016/j.cld.2020.08.005
1089-3261/21/© 2020 Elsevier Inc. All rights reserved.

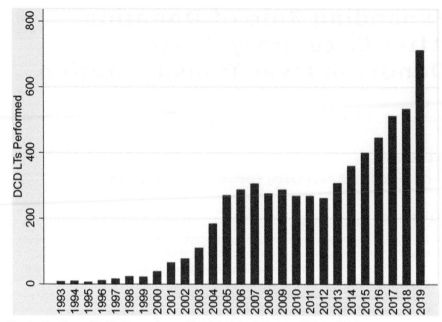

Fig. 1. Number of DCD LTs performed in the United States, 1993 to 2019.

utilizing with DBD LTs to DCD LTs. By the mid-2000s, reports were beginning to emerge describing inferior results and high rates of graft loss with DCD LTs. These inferior results were ascribed to high rates of biliary complications (specifically ischemic cholangiopathy [IC]) as well as increased rates of primary nonfunction and hepatic artery thrombosis.[5–8] During that same time period, the regulatory landscape for solid organ transplantation dramatically changed in 2007, when new Conditions of Participation were issued by the Centers for Medicare & Medicaid Services (CMS).[9,10] Under the new rules, minimum risk-adjusted post-transplant graft and patient survival rates were required for Medicare certification and reimbursement. Due to the described inferior results with DCD LTs and the concomitant increased regulatory scrutiny of graft and patient survival rates, a contraction in the utilization of DCD LTs was observed from 2007 until 2012 (see **Fig. 1**).

With time, large single-center series began to demonstrate that equivalent or near-equivalent results between DCD LTs and DBD LTs could be achieved through both modifications of procurement techniques and careful donor selection as well as donor-recipient matching.[11–14] These large single-center experiences suggested that in order to achieve acceptable results with DCD LTs, DCD liver grafts should not be thought of as interchangeable with DBD liver grafts. As more data emerged demonstrating that acceptable results with DCD LT can be achieved with appropriate donor and recipient selection,[15–18] the number of DCD LTs performed annually has continued to grow from 2012 to 2019 (see **Fig. 1**). A study published in 2016 reviewing the US national experience with DCD LT demonstrated that in addition to increasing volumes, a sequential improvement in US national graft and patient survival after DCD LTs has been observed over time.[19] That study demonstrated an evolution in the collective understanding of how to utilize DCD liver grafts. Concomitant with the improvement in outcomes, there was a decrease in the proportion of DCD liver grafts utilized for recipients with specific characteristics: in the intensive care unit (ICU) at the time of transplant, on a ventilator at the time of transplant, listed for redo-LT, and listed with primary sclerosing cholangitis as the primary diagnosis. There also was an observed decrease in donor warm ischemia time (DWIT) and cold ischemia time (CIT).

Despite the national improvement with DCD LTs and increase in the number of DCD LTs performed, substantial variability in the utilization of DCD livers currently still exists across the country.[20] This variability in DCD liver utilization has been shown to have no correlation with median Model for End-stage Liver Disease (MELD) score at transplant (MMaT).[20] It has been known for many years that a significant amount DCD liver graft utilization in the United States has been driven by a few high-utilization centers.[21] Encouragingly, in 2019, a substantial increase in DCD LT volumes was seen across the country, with increases as high as 700% in United Network for Organ Sharing (UNOS) regions that had notoriously had low numbers of DCD LTs. Theses data may suggest that utilization of DCD liver grafts is becoming more ubiquitous.

PARADIGM SHIFT FROM "NOT SICK ENOUGH FOR A DONATION AFTER CIRCULATORY DEATH" TO "TOO SICK FOR A DONATION AFTER CIRCULATORY DEATH"

As the inferior results with DCD LTs began to emerge in the mid-2000s, there was a prevailing sentiment at many transplant centers that DCD liver grafts should be utilized for only the sickest LT candidates, because these candidates were desperate enough to warrant the increased risks of IC and graft loss. Patients with lower MELD scores (albeit obviously being sick enough to warrant an LT) or patients with a standard malignancy exception often were viewed as "not sick enough for a DCD." This concept was supported by several publications that utilized modeling to demonstrate which recipients would benefit from a DCD LT.[22–24] This rationale subsequently was shown to be flawed for multiple reasons. First, although the greatest survival benefit for taking any liver graft always is seen in the patient who is facing imminent death, in many countries where programs also are responsible for maintaining a benchmark of post-LT outcomes, all organ offers involve an assessment of benefit, utility, resource consumption, and futility. Second, these modeling studies inputted data for the rates of IC and graft failure that were several orders of magnitude higher than those that have been achieved in large single-center reports with DCD LTs.[15–18] Yet experienced DCD LT centers have demonstrated that IC rates and graft survival similar to DBD LT can be achieved with careful donor-recipient selection. Therefore, it is incorrect to presume that the outcomes with DCD LTs do not vary depending on which recipient is selected. Third, these models assume that "waiting for a better organ offer" is a legitimate strategy for a patient with a lower MELD score. The reality of the current environment with limited availability of liver grafts is that those candidates with lower MELD scores may be waiting for a better offer that never comes or alternatively waiting until they become sick enough that their MELD score increases dramatically. This approach undoubtedly increases resource consumption, decreases success of DCD LTs, and more importantly increases risk of morbidity and mortality before and after LTs.

With experience it has become clear that recipient selection is equally if not more important than donor selection in order to achieve optimal outcomes with DCD LT. Previously published registry studies (using Scientific Registry of Transplant Recipients [SRTR] from the US and UK national registries) have demonstrated that the following recipient characteristics are associated with increased hazard of graft loss after DCD LT: recipient in the ICU, recipient on ventilator, elevated MELD score, advanced recipient age, and recipient undergoing retransplantation.[25–27]

The importance of donor-recipient matching in DCD LT has been formalized in several donor-recipient matching scores that have been developed.[27–29] The most recent of these scores, based on a large cohort of DCD LTs, is the UK DCD Risk Index (**Fig. 2**).[27] This score is based on 2 donor (donor age and donor body mass index), 2 ischemic time (functional DWIT and CIT), and 3 recipient (recipient age, recipient MELD, and retransplantation status) variables. With these variables, a score between 0 and 27 is generated. DCD LTs in the low-risk group (score ≤5) had a 1-year graft survival rate of greater than 95%, compared with greater than 85% in the moderate risk group (score 6–10) and less than 40% in the futile group (score >10). The investigators advocate avoidance of DCD LTs for the futile group.

A previous publication from the authors' group demonstrated that transplant programs with higher median donor risk index (DRI) and higher DCD liver graft utilization displayed MELD score distributions that were distributed normally and platykurtic[30] (**Fig. 3**). These centers were able to successfully utilize a high number of DCD liver grafts through donor-recipient matching. This was compared with programs with low median DRI and lower DCD utilization that displayed MELD score distributions that were highly negatively skewed and leptokurtic because of primarily utilizing standard criteria donor (SCD) DBD liver grafts (**Fig. 4**). By utilizing higher DRI organs that were declined by other centers, normally distributed and platykurtic transplant centers were able to transplant lower MELD score patients despite being located in high MMaT locations.

When evaluating the appropriateness of an LT recipient for a DCD LT, some general principles to follow are

1. Minimize recipient surgical complexity in order to ensure that the liver implantation is as smooth as possible. Recipients undergoing a redo-LT, recipients with history of extensive upper abdominal surgery, or those who may require a complex vascular reconstruction should be avoided.
2. Minimize a tenuous environment for an already marginal graft. Subjecting the DCD liver graft to prolonged hypotension and necessity of significant vasopressor use may compound the ischemia that the liver already has suffered by nature of being a DCD.
3. Selecting a recipient who can tolerate early allograft dysfunction (EAD). Recipients who have high MELD scores and are in the ICU, recipients with a significant cardiac history, or recipients with compromised renal function may not be ideal candidates

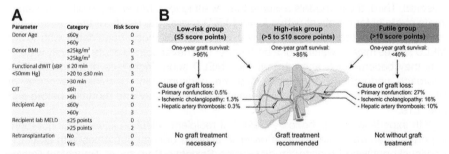

Parameter	Category	Risk Score
Donor Age	≤60y	0
	>60y	2
Donor BMI	≤25kg/m²	0
	>25kg/m²	3
Functional dWIT (sBP <50mm Hg)	≤ 20 min	0
	>20 to ≤30 min	3
	>30 min	6
CIT	≤6h	0
	>6h	2
Recipient Age	≤60y	0
	>60y	3
Recipient lab MELD	≤25 points	0
	>25 points	2
Retransplantation	No	0
	Yes	9

Low-risk group (≤5 score points)
One-year graft survival: >95%
Cause of graft loss:
- Primary nonfunction: 0.5%
- Ischemic cholangiopathy: 1.3%
- Hepatic artery thrombosis: 0.3%
No graft treatment necessary

High-risk group (>5 to ≤10 score points)
One-year graft survival: >85%
Graft treatment recommended

Futile group (>10 score points)
One-year graft survival: <40%
Cause of graft loss:
- Primary nonfunction: 27%
- Ischemic cholangiopathy: 16%
- Hepatic artery thrombosis: 10%
Not without graft treatment

Fig. 2. The UK DCD Risk index. (*A*) Parameters with respective scores. (*B*) DCD outcomes based on score. sBP, systolic blood pressure. (*Adapted from* Schlegel A, Kalisvaart M, Scalera I, Laing RW, Mergental H, Mirza DF, Perera T, Isaac J, Dutkowski P, Muiesan P. The UK DCD Risk Score: A new proposal to define futility in donation-after-circulatory-death liver transplantation. J Hepatol. 2018 Mar;68(3):456-464; with permission.)

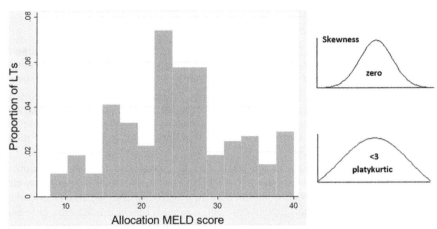

Fig. 3. Example of the MELD distribution of a transplant program in a high MELD location with a median DRI of 1.7 (normal distribution and platykurtic). (*From* Croome KP, Lee DD, Burns JM, Keaveny AP, Taner CB. Intraregional model for end-stage liver disease score variation in liver transplantation: Disparity in our own backyard. Liver Transpl. 2018 Apr;24(4):488-496; with permission.)

because they may not be able to tolerate EAD, which is seen at a higher frequency in recipients of DCD compared with DBD LT.[31–34]

The improved outcomes of DCD LTs can be explained at least partially by the transplant communities' increased understanding of the importance of donor-recipient matching. This understanding highlights the paradigm shift from selecting patients using the principle of "not sick enough for a DCD" to "too sick for a DCD."

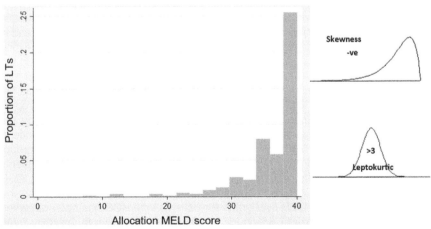

Fig. 4. Example of the MELD distribution of a transplant program in the same high MELD location with a median DRI of 1.3 (highly negatively skewed and leptokurtic). -ve, negative. (*From* Croome KP, Lee DD, Burns JM, Keaveny AP, Taner CB. Intraregional model for end-stage liver disease score variation in liver transplantation: Disparity in our own backyard. Liver Transpl. 2018 Apr;24(4):488-496; with permission.)

NEW LIVER ALLOCATION POLICY AND EXPANSION OF THE ROLE OF DONATION AFTER CIRCULATORY DEATH FOR HEPATOCELLULAR CARCINOMA

Historically, LT candidates with hepatocellular carcinoma (HCC) have experienced a substantial advantage in deceased donor liver allocation with lower waitlist mortality/dropout within 1 year of listing compared with those candidates without an HCC diagnosis.[35] HCC patients meeting criteria for exception received a MELD score of 28 after a 6-month waiting period and then had a ladder model of increasing exception scores every 3 months thereafter. This model provided some rationale for declining a DCD liver graft and waiting for a better liver offer as MELD score increased over time. Recent developments in liver organ allocation have changed the LT landscape substantially, particularly for patients with HCC MELD exceptions. The liver distribution system based on acuity circles went into effect on February 4, 2020.[36] This acuity circle allocation system replaces donation service area (DSA) and regional boundaries previously used in liver organ distribution with a system based on distance between donor hospital and transplant hospital. In addition to the recent implementation of the acuity circles system, HCC patients no longer have a ladder model of increasing exception scores over time and instead are given an exception score of median MMaT minus 3 (MMaT-3) for a 250 nautical-mile radius surrounding the listing center. Undoubtedly, this has resulted in decreased access to high-quality DBD organs for patients with HCC (according to UNOS data from January 1, 2020, to April 30, 2020, fewer than 100 HCC patients received an LT, compared with 150 per month in previous years). One potential option for this population may be increased utilization of DCD livers. This potential shift is congruent with the principle of using extended criteria organs in recipients with lower biological MELD scores, such as many HCC patients, because of the perception that these recipients are better able to tolerate an extended criteria organ.[37] The authors' group demonstrated in a previous publication that after the implementation of the Share 35 policy more HCC patients have received livers from DCD donors,[38] potentially the result of the highest-quality organs being preferentially utilized by higher MELD score recipients with broader sharing.

Initially the utilization of DCD liver grafts for LT candidates with HCC was met with some trepidation.[39] It was postulated that the rate of HCC recurrence could be elevated in patients receiving a DCD graft based on biologic possibility that ischemia reperfusion injury is associated with stimulation of growth in micromestastases and in increasing the adhesion of tumor cells in several nontransplant studies.[40,41] Despite these initial concerns, a large single-center study demonstrated no difference in the rate of recurrence of HCC between DCD LTs and DBD LTs (12.3% and 12.1%, respectively).[42] In addition, if ischemia reperfusion injury in the DCD grafts was felt to be an important factor in recurrence, it would be expected to see a higher proportion of initial site of recurrence to be the liver in the DCD LT recipients. In that study, the opposite was true, because the liver graft represented the first site of recurrence in 65% of recipients in the DBD group and only 37% of recipients in the DCD group. Other recent studies also have demonstrated excellent results with HCC recipients receiving DCD liver grafts, with no increase in recurrence compared with DBD LTs.[43–45]

Increased utilization of DCD liver grafts for patients with HCC has been observed within the United States from 7.6% in 2002 to 35.9% in 2015 (**Fig. 5**). A similar trend of increased utilization of DCD liver grafts for patients with HCC has been observed within the United Kingdom from 0% in 1997 to 34% in 2016.[46] It is likely that this trend will increase in the United States with the new allocation system. With all patients who are listed for an HCC exception receiving MMaT-3, not only will access to SCD DBD

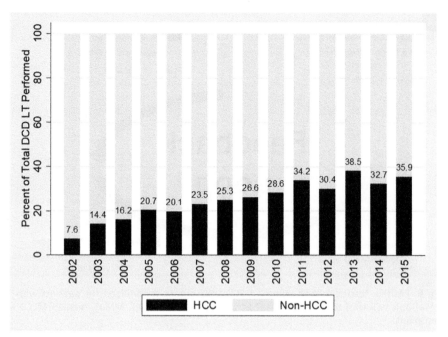

Fig. 5. Percent of DCD LT in the United States utilized for patients with HCC from 2002 to 2015.

organs be reduced but also there will be a positive feedback loop, where, if SCD DBD organs are utilized for patients with a MMaT-3, it will lead to a lower MMaT at the next recalibration (**Fig. 6**). Because exception score patients make up historically between 25% and 46% of patients transplanted, the MMaT theoretically could be lowered by 3 MELD points at each recalibration until it becomes virtually impossible to get a non–extended criteria donor (ECD) organ for an exception MELD score patient.[30] In many areas of the country, MMaT historically has tended to approach the exception MELD score. Therefore, for each HCC exception LT performed, it will become harder to get future HCC exception cases transplanted. Because DCD donors and DBD donors greater than or equal to age 70 years do not count toward calculation of MMaT at each calibration, they can be utilized for HCC exception patients without lowering MMaT for future recalibrations. In addition, in the newly adopted acuity circle system, livers from DCD donors are allocated earlier in the match sequence to transplant centers closer to the donor hospital compared with liver donor allocation for DBD donors less than 70 years of age. For livers from DCD donors, after initial offers to Status 1A and 1B candidates, the initial distribution sequence is as follows:

- Compatible candidates with a MELD score or pediatric end-stage liver disease (PELD) score of 15 or higher, listed at transplant hospitals within a 150 nautical-mile radius of the donor hospital
- Compatible candidates with a MELD score or PELD score of 15 or higher, listed at transplant hospitals within a 250 nautical-mile radius of the donor hospital
- Compatible candidates with a MELD score or PELD score of 15 or higher, listed at transplant hospitals within a 500 nautical-mile radius of the donor hospital

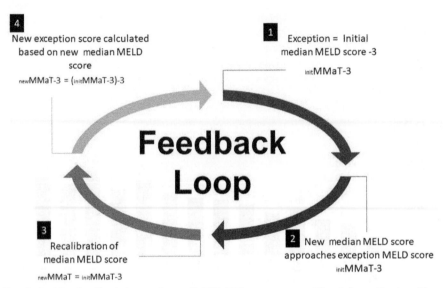

4
New exception score calculated
based on new median MELD
score

$_{new}$MMaT-3 = ($_{init}$MMaT-3)-3

1 Exception = Initial
median MELD score -3

$_{init}$MMaT-3

Feedback Loop

3
Recalibration of
median MELD score

$_{new}$MMaT = $_{init}$MMaT-3

2 New median MELD score
approaches exception MELD score
$_{init}$MMaT-3

Fig. 6. Positive feedback loop where, if SCD DBD organs are utilized for patients with a MMaT-3, it will lead to a lower MMaT at the next recalibration. MMaT, median MELD at transplant.

EXPANDED CRITERIA DONOR—DONATION AFTER CIRCULATORY DEATH LIVER TRANSPLANT

As high-volume DCD LT centers have gained experience with DCD LTs, these centers have continued to expand donor criteria, including pursuing ECD DCD liver grafts with acceptable results. Pursuit of these organs should be undertaken cautiously at transplant centers with less experience with DCD LTs or with less experience in the utilization of marginal grafts; however, in highly selected cases in experienced centers, they can be utilized with acceptable outcomes.

Advanced DCD donor age has been shown in multiple registry studies to have a negative impact on graft survival.[25–27] Therefore, there is little disagreement that younger DCDs are "better"; however older DCDs are not necessarily "bad." A single-center study from the United Kingdom investigated the outcomes of DCD donors age greater than 60 years (N = 93) compared with those age less than or equal to 60 years (N = 222) and demonstrated no differences in graft or patient survival between the groups.[47] In that study, the rates of vascular, biliary, and overall complications were similar between the groups. More recently, the authors' group compared the outcomes of DCD LTs from donors age greater than or equal to 50 years (N = 155) and those with donor age less than 50 years (N = 316) in a multicenter US study.[48] No difference in graft survival was seen between the groups. Although the rate of IC was not statistically significant different between the groups, there was a slight trend of increased IC in the DCD donor age greater than or equal to 50 group (11.6%) compared with the DCD donor age less than 50 group (7.6%). Additionally, in that study, Cox regression analysis using national data obtained from SRTR was used to evaluate predictors of graft failure in DCD donor age greater than or equal to 50 years. Significant predictors of graft failure included a calculated MELD score greater than or equal to 30, recipient mechanical ventilation at the time of transplant, recipient medical condition (in ICU) and CIT. Another US study investigated the outcomes of ECD DCD livers, defined as those with 1 of the following factors: donor age greater than 50 years, donor body mass index greater than 35 kg/m^2, functional DWIT greater than 30 minutes, and donor liver macrosteatosis greater than 30%.[49] That study found that, in the era from 2003 to 2011, 1-year graft failure rate was as high as 25%; however, in the modern era, with introduction of changes to their DCD protocol, graft failure rate was reduced to 6%. The investigators concluded that with the optimization of perioperative conditions, ECD DCD livers can be transplanted successfully in select cases. A recent single-center study from Spain compared the outcomes of DCD LTs from donors successfully 70 years (N = 32) and those with a donor age less than 70 (N = 45).[50] No difference in graft survival was seen between the groups nor was there a significant difference in the rate of IC or retransplantation. Graft survival at 1-year, however, in the entire DCD cohort in that study was 72.7%, which may fall below acceptable standards for graft survival in some countries.

Given the potentially additive risk from using donor livers that are both steatotic and from a DCD donor, there is a paucity of data on the outcome of DCD LTs utilizing livers with macrosteatosis.[51] In a recent multicenter analysis, the outcomes of utilizing DCD liver grafts with macrosteatosis were investigated.[52] In that analysis, DCD donors with macrosteatosis less than 30% had no increase in perioperative complications and similar patient and graft survival compared with DCD donors with no steatosis. In contrast, DCD liver grafts with moderate macrosteatosis (30%–60%) had higher rates of postreperfusion syndrome, primary nonfunction, postreperfusion cardiac arrest, EAD, and acute kidney injury compared with DCD donors with no steatosis. The data on the utilization of DCD liver grafts with steatosis remains limited; therefore, extreme caution should be taken when utilizing these grafts, particularly when the degree of steatosis approaches 30% or greater.

Although technically not falling under the heading of ECD DCD, there has been some debate about the appropriateness of utilizing DCD grafts for candidates who need simultaneous liver kidney (SLK) transplant. Initial studies investigating the outcomes of SLK transplant using grafts from DCD donors described inferior outcomes compared with those using grafts from DBD donors (DBD-SLK).[53–55] A study looking at US national data from 2000 to 2010 demonstrated inferior patient, liver graft, and kidney graft survival for recipients of DCD-SLK compared with DBD-SLK transplant.[53] More recently, a study using updated US national data demonstrated that there has been a significant improvement in the results with DCD-SLKs in the modern era.[56] In the most recent era (2011–2018) in that study, DCD-SLK was compared with a propensity matched cohort of DBD-SLK and no differences in patient, liver graft, or kidney graft survival were observed. In addition, both bilirubin (0.5 mg/dL vs 0.5 mg/dL, respectively) and creatinine (1.2 mg/dL vs 1.2 mg/dL, respectively) at last follow-up were not different between the DCD-SLK and DBD-SLK groups. Donors used for DCD-SLK generally were younger with relatively shorter DWIT. In addition, a concomitant decrease in the proportion of patients in the ICU prior to DCD-SLK transplant was observed. It seems, therefore, that in select patients (not in the ICU prior to transplant) requiring an SLK, it may be appropriate to receive organs from younger DCD donors.

ISCHEMIC CHOLANGIOPATHY AND BARRIERS TO EXPANDING DONATION AFTER CIRCULATORY DEATH UTILIZATION AND CRITERIA IN THE UNITED STATES

The improved US national outcomes with DCD LTs are highly encouraging. Nonetheless, despite these improvements, IC remains the Achilles heel of DCD LTs. When discussing IC, it is important to stress a few points. First, IC is not unique to DCD LTs, as it has been described at rates of 2% to 4% with DBD LTs.[14–17] In addition, a certain rate of IC can be expected, even with the most experienced DCD LT protocols. Second, IC can present with a spectrum of clinical and radiologic severity after LT, ranging from mild ischemic changes to complete biliary necrosis.[57] Although severe cases of IC frequently require retransplantation, many cases can be managed effectively with percutaneous or endoscopic interventions and still yield acceptable long-term outcomes.[58–60] Several distinct radiologic patterns of IC have been described, which are associated with different clinical courses[61,62]:

- Diffuse necrosis: these patients have severe abnormalities of nearly the entire biliary system that are identified soon after transplant. These patients almost uniformly require retransplantation.
- Bilateral multifocal/multifocal progressive: these patients began with mild to moderate stenosis of the second-order and peripheral ducts and progressively worsen over time.
- Confluence dominant: these patients develop strictures confined to the biliary confluence, with relative preservation of the second-order and peripheral ducts. In this pattern, biliary abnormalities progress in severity over time but geographically never expanded beyond the hilar confluence. Many of these patients can be successfully managed long term with ERCP and stenting and frequently do not go on to need retransplantation.
- Minor form: these patients may display mild radiologic abnormalities consistent with early IC without development of clinical symptoms and never go on to develop more extensive strictures.

Initial series with DCD LTs demonstrated IC rates as high as 30%.[5–8] More recent single-center series from North America providing era-stratified data have described IC rates after DCD LTs ranging from 2.6% to 5.3%.[15–18] These data suggest that with strict donor and recipient selection, rates of IC similar to that observed with DBD LTs can be achieved. With more widespread DCD utilization in centers with less experience or with relaxation of selection criteria, it is inevitable that higher rates of IC should be expected. Unlike patients who develop primary nonfunction, who often have higher calculated MELD scores, or patients with early hepatic artery thrombosis, who receive MELD exception points, patients with IC often languish on the waiting list once relisted due to lower MELD scores. This difficulty in getting patients retransplanted as well as the fears of falling below CMS metrics for graft survival represent some of the major barriers to more widespread pursuit of DCD liver donors in the United States. Currently, a standard exception for IC after DCD LT does not exist. Guidelines for nonstandard IC exception as part of the National Review Board have been published by the Organ Procurement and Transplantation Network Liver and Intestine Committee.[63] These guidelines are as follows.

Prior DCD transplant that demonstrated 2 or more of the following criteria within 12 months of transplant should be considered for MELD exception:

- Persistent cholestasis as defined by abnormal bilirubin (greater than 2 mg/dL)
- Two or more episodes of cholangitis with an associated bacteremia requiring hospital admission
- Evidence of nonanastomotic biliary strictures not responsive to further treatment

A previous study demonstrated that patients relisted after DCD LT who received MELD exception points had better outcomes compared with those who were not granted exception points.[64] In the current climate, even patients who receive an IC exception from the National Review Board likely will get only MMaT-3, similar to most other standard exception patients. This will likely make it challenging to get these patients re-transplanted, since utilizing a marginal graft for patients who have IC and are a redo-LT, is likely not a wise decision.

If the transplant community as a whole wants to encourage more widespread acceptance of DCD liver grafts, changes to the exception score for patients with IC should be made so that these patients receive a score of MMaT not MMaT-3. A previous study from the authors' group demonstrated that mortality for patients relisted for biliary complications after DCD LT was higher than mortality/delisted rate for patients, with exception points for both HCC and hepatopulmonary syndrome at 3-month to 12-month time points (**Fig. 7**).[57] In addition, it should not be overlooked that waitlist patients who accept a DCD liver graft are allowing a higher number of DBD liver grafts to be available for other recipients on the waiting list.

One potential downside to providing a standardized exception scheme for relisting patients developing IC after DCD LT is that it may lead to over-aggressive pursuit of DCD LTs, resulting in higher rates of graft failure. Although this could be one result of providing an exception score safety net, programs still will be publicly accountable for their graft survival rates. The annual number of patients relisted for biliary complications after DCD LT nationally has remained relatively low (N = 15–30/y; 4%–5%).[57] Relisting trends undoubtedly would need to be monitored after implementation of any new standardized MELD exception score paradigm. The authors believe that the goal of developing a MELD exception score safety net should be to encourage the pursuit of DCD LT appropriately and not to reward programs who experience increased graft failure rates secondary to overly aggressive acceptance patterns. A structured approach to the timely access for retransplantation based on objective clinical and radiological criteria is warranted for those patients and programs who risk the development of IC. A standard exception score through the National Liver Review Board will

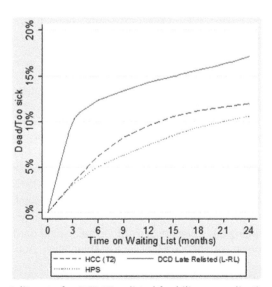

Fig. 7. Waitlist mortality rate for DCD LTs relisted for biliary complications (L-RL) compared with patients listed for HCC or hepatopulmonary syndrome. HPS, hepatopulmonary syndrome. (*From* Croome KP, Lee DD, Nguyen JH, Keaveny AP, Taner CB. Waitlist Outcomes for Patients Relisted Following Failed Donation After Cardiac Death Liver Transplant: Implications for Awarding Model for End-Stage Liver Disease Exception Scores. Am J Transplant. 2017 Sep;17(9):2420-2427; with permission.)

demonstrate a commitment to greater utilization and innovation in DCD LTs by the transplant community.[65]

SUMMARY

Better understanding of how to utilize DCD liver grafts has resulted in improved national outcomes and an increase in the number of DCD LTs being performed. The role of DCD liver grafts for patients with HCC likely will continue to expand given the recent allocation changes. As future technologies, such as machine perfusion, become increasingly available, the transplant community remains hopeful that the degree of risk associated with DCD LTs will be able to be modified in the positive direction, allowing for broadening of acceptable DCD donors. IC remains the Achilles heel of DCD LT and, although rates of IC have fallen dramatically with improved protocols, a certain rate of IC likely is unavoidable. Finally, if promoting expansion of DCD LTs is to be continued, development of a more robust safety net for patients who develop IC after DCD LT is warranted.

CLINICS CARE POINTS

- Recipient selection is as important as donor selection when utilizing DCD donors.
- With the new liver allocation policy, patients with HCC may represent ideal candidates for DCD donor livers.
- Not all patients that develop IC have similar clinical courses. Many patients with Confluence Dominant or Minor Forms of IC can be successfully managed long term with ERCP and stenting and frequently do not go on to need retransplantation.

DISCLOSURE

None of the authors have any conflict of interest to disclose.

REFERENCES

1. Starzl TE, Putnam CW. Experience in hepatic transplantation. Philadelphia: WB Saunders Company; 1969.
2. A definition of irreversible coma. Report of the ad hoc committee of the Harvard medical school to examine the definition of brain death. JAMA 1968;205(6): 337–40.
3. Casavilla A, Ramirez C, Shapiro R, et al. Experience with liver and kidney allografts from non-heart-beating donors. Transplantation 1995;59:197–203.
4. D'Alessandro AM, Hoffmann RM, Knechtle SJ, et al. Successful extrarenal transplantation from non-heart-beating donors. Transplantation 1995;59:977–82.
5. Foley DP, Fernandez LA, Leverson G, et al. Donation after cardiac death: the University of Wisconsin experience with liver transplantation. Ann Surg 2005;242(5): 724–31.
6. Skaro AI, Jay CL, Baker TB, et al. The impact of ischemic cholangiopathy in liver transplantation using donors after cardiac death: the untold story. Surgery 2009; 146(4):543–52 [discussion: 52–3].
7. de Vera ME, Lopez-Solis R, Dvorchik I, et al. Liver transplantation using donation after cardiac death donors: long-term follow-up from a single center. Am J Transplant 2009;9(4):773–81.

8. Jay C, Ladner D, Wang E, et al. A comprehensive risk assessment of mortality following donation after cardiac death liver transplant - an analysis of the national registry. J Hepatol 2011;55(4):808–13.

9. Hamilton TE. Improving organ transplantation in the United States–a regulatory perspective. Am J Transplant 2008;8(12):2503–5.

10. Medicare program; hospital conditions of participation: requirements for approval and re-approval of transplant centers to perform organ transplants; final rule. Fed Regist 2007;72(61):15198–280. To be codified at 42 CFR sec 405, 482, 488, 498. Available at: https://www.gpo.gov/fdsys/pkg/FR-2007-03-30/pdf/07-1435.pdf. Accessed December 22, 2015.

11. Grewal HP, Willingham DL, Nguyen J, et al. Liver transplantation using controlled donation after cardiac death donors: an analysis of a large single-center experience. Liver Transpl 2009;15(9):1028–35.

12. Dubbeld J, Hoekstra H, Farid W, et al. Similar liver transplantation survival with selected cardiac death donors and brain death donors. Br J Surg 2010;97(5):744–53.

13. Taner CB, Bulatao IG, Willingham DL, et al. Events in procurement as risk factors for ischemic cholangiopathy in liver transplantation using donation after cardiac death donors. Liver Transpl 2012;18(1):100–11.

14. Taner CB, Bulatao IG, Perry DK, et al. Asystole to cross-clamp period predicts development of biliary complications in liver transplantation using donation after cardiac death donors. Transpl Int 2012;25(8):838–46.

15. Croome KP, Lee DD, Perry DK, et al. Comparison of longterm outcomes and quality of life in recipients of donation after cardiac death liver grafts with a propensity-matched cohort. Liver Transpl 2017;23(3):342–51.

16. Laing RW, Scalera I, Isaac J, et al. Liver transplantation using grafts from donors after circulatory death: a propensity score-matched study from a single center. Am J Transplant 2016;16(6):1795–804.

17. Bohorquez H, Seal JB, Cohen AJ, et al. Safety and outcomes in 100 consecutive donation after circulatory death liver transplants using a protocol that includes thrombolytic therapy. Am J Transplant 2017;17(8):2155–64.

18. Kollmann D, Sapisochin G, Goldaracena N, et al. Expanding the donor pool: donation after circulatory death and living liver donation do not compromise the results of liver transplantation. Liver Transpl 2018;24(6):779–89.

19. Croome KP, Lee DD, Keaveny AP, et al. Improving national results in liver transplantation using grafts from donation after cardiac death donors. Transplantation 2016;100(12):2640–7.

20. Croome KP, Lee DD, Keaveny AP, et al. Noneligible donors as a strategy to decrease the organ shortage. Am J Transplant 2017;17(6):1649–55. This article describes the wide varyance in DCD liver graft utilization and suggests potential reasons for why this variance in seen.

21. Hobeika MJ, Menser T, Nguyen DT, et al. United States donation after circulatory death liver transplantation is driven by a few high-utilization transplant centers. Am J Transplant 2020;20(1):320–1.

22. Jay CL, Skaro AI, Ladner DP, et al. Comparative effectiveness of donation after cardiac death versus donation after brain death liver transplantation: Recognizing who can benefit. Liver Transpl 2012;18(6):630–40.

23. Taylor R, Allen E, Richards JA, et al. Liver Advisory Group to NHS Blood and Transplant. Survival advantage for patients accepting the offer of a circulatory death liver transplant. J Hepatol 2019;70(5):855–65.

24. Vinson AJ, Gala-Lopez B, Tennankore K, et al. The use of donation after circulatory death organs for simultaneous liver-kidney transplant: to DCD or Not to DCD? Transplantation 2019;103(6):1159–67.
25. Mateo R, Cho Y, Singh G, et al. Risk factors for graft survival after liver transplantation from donation after cardiac death donors: an analysis of OPTN/UNOS data. Am J Transplant 2006;6:791–6.
26. Mathur AK, Heimbach J, Steffick DE, et al. Donation after cardiac death liver transplantation: predictors of outcome. Am J Transplant 2010;10(11):2512–9.
27. Schlegel A, Kalisvaart M, Scalera I, et al. The UK DCD Risk Score: a new proposal to define futility in donation-after-circulatory-death liver transplantation. J Hepatol 2018;68(3):456–64.
28. Hong JC, Yersiz H, Kositamongkol P, et al. Liver transplantation using organ donation after cardiac death: a clinical predictive index for graft failure-free survival. Arch Surg 2011;146:1017–23.
29. Khorsandi S, Giorgakis E, Vilca-Melendez H, et al. Developing a donation after cardiac death risk index for adult and pediatric liver transplantation. World J Transplant 2017;7:203–12.
30. Croome KP, Lee DD, Burns JM, et al. Intraregional model for end-stage liver disease score variation in liver transplantation: Disparity in our own backyard. Liver Transpl 2018;24(4):488–96.
31. Olthoff KM, Kulik L, Samstein B, et al. Validation of a current definition of early allograft dysfunction in liver transplant recipients and analysis of risk factors. Liver Transpl 2010;16:943–9.
32. Croome KP, Lee DD, Croome S, et al. The impact of postreperfusion syndrome during liver transplantation using livers with significant macrosteatosis. Am J Transplant 2019;19(9):2550–9.
33. Chadha RM, Croome KP, Aniskevich S, et al. Intraoperative events in liver transplantation using donation after cardiac death donors. Liver Transpl 2019;25(12): 1833–40.
34. Lee DD, Singh A, Burns JM, et al. Early allograft dysfunction in liver transplantation with donation after cardiac death donors results in inferior survival. Liver Transpl 2014;20(12):1447–53.
35. Ishaque T, Massie AB, Bowring MG, et al. Liver transplantation and waitlist mortality for HCC and non-HCC candidates following the 2015 HCC exception policy change. Am J Transplant 2019;19(2):564–72.
36. New national liver and intestinal organ transplant system in effect. 2020. Available at: https://unos.org/policy/liver-distribution/. Accessed February 28, 2020.
37. Schaubel DE, Sima CS, Goodrich NP, et al. The survival benefit of deceased donor liver transplantation as a function of candidate disease severity and donor quality. Am J Transplant 2008;8:419–25.
38. Croome KP, Lee DD, Harnois D, et al. Effects of the share 35 rule on waitlist and liver transplantation outcomes for patients with hepatocellular carcinoma. PLoS One 2017;12(1):e0170673.
39. Croome KP, Wall W, Chandok N, et al. Inferior survival in liver transplant recipients with hepatocellular carcinoma receiving donation after cardiac death liver allografts. Liver Transpl 2013;19(11):1214–23.
40. van der Bilt JD, Kranenburg O, Nijkamp MW, et al. Ischemia/reperfusion accelerates the outgrowth of hepatic micrometastases in a highly standardized murine model. Hepatology 2005;42:165–75.
41. Doi K, Horiuchi T, Uchinami M, et al. Hepatic ischemia-reperfusion promotes liver metastasis of colon cancer. J Surg Res 2002;105:243–7.

42. Croome KP, Lee DD, Burns JM, et al. The use of donation after cardiac death allografts does not increase recurrence of hepatocellular carcinoma. Am J Transplant 2015;15(10):2704–11.

43. El-Gazzaz G, Hashimoto K, Quintini C, et al. Is Liver transplantation outcome worse for HCC patients using organ donation after cardiac death? [abstract]. Am J Transplant 2013;13(suppl 5).

44. Martinez-Insfran LA, Ramirez P, Cascales P, et al. Parrilla PEarly outcomes of liver transplantation using donors after circulatory death in patients with hepatocellular carcinoma: a comparative study. Transplant Proc 2019;51(2):359–64.

45. Goldkamp W, Vanatta J, Nair S, et al. Outcomes of patients with hepatocellular carcinoma receiving a donation after cardiac death liver graft [abstract]. Am J Transplant 2015;15(suppl 3).

46. Wallace D, Cowling TE, Walker K, et al. Short- and long-term mortality after liver transplantation in patients with and without hepatocellular carcinoma in the UK. Br J Surg 2020. https://doi.org/10.1002/bjs.11451.

47. Schlegel A, Scalera I, Thamara M, et al. Impact of donor age in donation after cardiac death liver Transplantation: is the cut-off "60" still of relevance? Liver Transpl 2018;24(3):352–62.

48. Croome KP, Mathur AK, Lee DD, et al. Outcomes of donation after circulatory death liver grafts from donors 50 years or older: a multicenter analysis. Transplantation 2018;102(7):1108–14.

49. Mihaylov P, Mangus R, Ekser B, et al. Expanding the donor pool with the use of extended criteria donation after circulatory death livers. Liver Transpl 2019;25(8):1198–208.

50. Cascales-Campos PA, Ferreras D, Alconchel F, et al. Controlled donation after circulatory death up to 80 years for liver transplantation: pushing the limit again. Am J Transplant 2020;20(1):204–12.

51. Croome KP, Lee DD, Taner CB. The "skinny" on assessment and utilization of steatotic liver grafts: a systematic review. Liver Transpl 2019;25(3):488–99.

52. Croome KP, Mathur AK, Mao S, et al. Peri-operative and longterm outcomes of utilizing donation after circulatory death liver grafts with macrosteatosis: a multicenter analysis. Am J Transplant 2020. https://doi.org/10.1111/ajt.15877.

53. Wadei HM, Bulatao IG, Gonwa TA, et al. Inferior long-term outcomes of liver-kidney transplantation using donation after cardiac death donors: single-center and organ procurement and transplantation network analyses. Liver Transpl 2014;20(6):728–35.

54. Alhamad T, Spatz C, Uemura T, et al. The outcomes of simultaneous liver and kidney transplantation using donation after cardiac death organs. Transplantation 2014;98(11):1190–8.

55. LaMattina JC, Mezrich JD, Fernandez LA, et al. Simultaneous liver and kidney transplantation using donation after cardiac death donors: a brief report. Liver Transpl 2011;17(5):591–5.

56. Croome KP, Mao S, Yang L, et al. Improved national results with simultaneous liver-kidney transplantation using donation after circulatory death donors. Liver Transpl 2020;26(3):397–407.

57. Croome KP, Lee DD, Nguyen JH, et al. Waitlist outcomes for patients relisted following failed donation after cardiac death liver transplant: implications for awarding model for end-stage liver disease exception scores. Am J Transplant 2017;17(9):2420–7.

58. Croome KP, McAlister V, Adams P, et al. Endoscopic management of biliary complications following liver transplantation after donation from cardiac death donors. Can J Gastroenterol 2012;26(9):607–10.
59. Zoepf T, Maldonado de Dechêne EJ, Dechêne A, et al. Optimized endoscopic treatment of ischemic-type biliary lesions after liver transplantation. Gastrointest Endosc 2012;76(3):556–63.
60. Hintze RE, Abou-Rebyeh H, Adler A, et al. Endoscopic therapy of ischemia-type biliary lesions in patients following orthotopic liver transplantation. Z Gastroenterol 1999;37:13–20.
61. Giesbrandt KJ, Bulatao IG, Keaveny AP, et al. Radiologic characterization of ischemic cholangiopathy in donation-after-cardiac-death liver transplants and correlation with clinical outcomes. AJR Am J Roentgenol 2015;205(5):976–84.
62. Lee HW, Suh KS, Shin WY, et al. Classification and prognosis of intrahepatic biliary stricture after liver transplantation. Liver Transpl 2007;13(12):1736–42.
63. eview. Available at: https://optn.transplant.hrsa.gov/media/2847/liver_guidance_adult_meld_201706.pdf Accessed April 4, 2020
64. Maduka RC, Abt PL, Goldberg DS. Use of model for end-stage liver disease exceptions for donation after cardiac death graft recipients relisted for liver transplantation. Liver Transpl 2015;21(4):554–60.
65. Abt PL, Goldberg DS. Retransplantation after a failed donation after circulatory determination of death liver transplant: MELD exception priority and second chances. Am J Transplant 2017;17(9):2240–2.

Optimizing the Selection of Patients for Simultaneous Liver-Kidney Transplant

Khurram Bari, MD, MS[a], Pratima Sharma, MD, MS[b],*

KEYWORDS

- Outcomes • Waiting list • MELD

KEY POINTS

- The proportion of patient undergoing simultaneous liver-kidney transplantation has increase significantly in Model for End Stage Liver Disease era compared with the era before the Model for End Stage Liver Disease.
- Current simultaneous liver-kidney transplantation policy takes into account standardized medical eligibility criteria for simultaneous liver-kidney transplantation listing.
- Current simultaneous liver-kidney transplantation policy provides a safety net option to prioritize kidney transplant after liver transplant recipients who are unlikely to recover their renal function within 60 to 365 days after liver transplant alone.
- Estimating renal function in end-stage liver disease is challenging.
- Measures should be taken to carefully select the simultaneous liver-kidney transplantation candidates to improve their outcomes.

INTRODUCTION

Simultaneous liver-kidney transplantation (SLKT) is an important option for liver transplant candidates with stage 4 chronic kidney disease (CKD) or end-stage renal disease, sustained acute kidney injury (AKI) deemed unlikely to recover after liver transplantation (LT), and those with metabolic diseases such as primary hyperoxaluria.[1] Since the adoption of Model for End-Stage Liver Disease (MELD) score-based allocation in 2002, the incidence of SLKT has increased from 2% to 3% in the pre-MELD era to 8% to 9% in the MELD era.[2,3] This system has engendered controversy within the transplant community because SLKT draw deceased donor kidneys from

[a] Division of Gastroenterology and Hepatology, University of Cincinnati, 231 Albert Sabin Way, ML 0595, MSB 7259, Cincinnati, OH 45267, USA; [b] Division of Gastroenterology and Hepatology, Michigan Medicine, University of Michigan, 3912 Taubman Center, 1500 East Medical Center Drive, Ann Arbor, MI 48109, USA
* Corresponding author. 3912 Taubman Center, 1500 East Medical Center Drive, Ann Arbor, MI 48109
E-mail address: pratimas@med.umich.edu

Clin Liver Dis 25 (2021) 89–102
https://doi.org/10.1016/j.cld.2020.08.006
1089-3261/21/Published by Elsevier Inc.
liver.theclinics.com

the kidney transplant candidate pool.[4,5] Owing to the safety net option in the current SLKT allocation implemented in August 2017, there was a 9% decrease in the SLKT rates between August 2017 and December 2018.

EVOLUTION OF SIMULTANEOUS LIVER-KIDNEY TRANSPLANTATION POLICY SINCE THE IMPLEMENTATION OF THE MODEL FOR END-STAGE LIVER DISEASE SCORE

The decision for SLKT listing is somewhat easier for LT candidates with stage 4 CKD or end-stage renal disease and inherited metabolic disease compared with those with sustained AKI deemed unlikely to recover after LT alone. There have been documented differences in center use of SLKT. Published data have demonstrated wide variability in SLKT rates across the United States, with the highest SLKT rates in Organ Procurement and Transplantation Network (OPTN)/United Network for Organ Sharing regions 1 and 7.[6]

Before August 2017, the OPTN policy did not specify any medical criteria for assessing kidney function when a kidney was allocated to a liver–kidney candidate. The policy simply stated that if the donor and the candidate are local, then the kidney will be allocated with the liver. This process became further complicated if the deceased donor kidney was offered to the SLKT candidate within the same region as the organ procurement organization. This pertains to the variations and nonstandardization of distribution practices and allowed paybacks at the organ procurement organization level within the region. Moreover, difficulty in assessing renal function in patients with cirrhosis, drawbacks associated with creatinine-based equations to assess the estimated glomerular filtration rate (GFR) and lack of prospective and granular data limited the development of evidence-based listing and transplant practices between February 2002 and July 2017. **Box 1** shows the evolution of SLKT allocation before August 2017.[2,7–9]

There were significant concerns owing to the absence of any specific policy addressing the allocation of the deceased donor kidneys in the context of simultaneous renal–nonrenal organ transplantation. The OPTN organized a Working Group in 2014 composed of members of multiple OPTN committees, including Kidney Transplantation, Liver and Intestinal Transplantation, Organ Procurement Organizations, Ethics, Minority Affairs, and Operations and Safety, to develop policy language to address the allocation of organs to individuals with end stage liver disease and renal dysfunction. The policy language developed through data review, discussion, deliberation, and compromise, and was ultimately ratified by the OPTN Board of Directors in June 2016, and was implemented August 10, 2017.[10,11]

CURRENT SIMULTANEOUS LIVER-KIDNEY TRANSPLANTATION ALLOCATION POLICY

The current SLKT policy has 2 important components: medical eligibility criteria and the option of a safety net.[1] The medical eligibility criteria are stratified by the presence of CKD, AKI, or select metabolic diseases (**Table 1**). The option of a safety net is for those LT recipients who do not recover renal function, or subsequently develop advanced, persistent renal dysfunction within 60 to 365 days of LT alone. Safety net candidates are assigned significant allocation priority in the kidney allocation system to receive an expedited kidney after liver transplant, appearing ahead of other local adult candidates (**Table 2**).

The data presented by Wiseman and Wilk[12] at the American Transplant Congress held in 2019 in Boston, Massachusetts, showed an absolute decrease of 6 SLKT per month in the first year after policy implementation compared with 1 year before August 2017. However, the kidney after liver transplant registration increased from

---

Box 1
Evolution of SLKT policy from 2002 to 2017

Davis and colleagues[9] (2007)
- CKD with GFR $\leq$30 mL/min
- AKI/HRS on dialysis for $\geq$6 wk; prolonged AKI (?): kidney biopsy with fixed damage

Eason and colleagues[8] (2008) Consensus Report
- CKD GFR $\leq$30 mL/min; CKD on kidney biopsy (>30% glomerulosclerosis/fibrosis)
- Other criteria: diabetes, hypertension, age >65 y, preexisting kidney disease: proteinuria, renal size, duration of elevated Cr
- AKI/HRS with Cr $\geq$2 mg/dL or dialysis $\geq$8 wk

OPTN Policy (3.5.10) (2009)
- CKD requiring dialysis (CMS 2728 form); CKD (GFR $\leq$30 mL/min MDRD6 or measured GFR, proteinuria >3 g/d)
- Sustained AKI with dialysis $\geq$6 wk; sustained AKI without dialysis (GFR $\leq$25 mL/min $\geq$6 wk)
- Sustained AKI: combination of time in analysis or GFR $\leq$25 mL/min for 6 wk
- Inherited metabolic disorders

Nadim and colleagues[2] (2012) Consensus Report
- Candidates with CKD for 3 mo: eGFR $\leq$40 mL/min (MDRD-6) or GFR $\leq$30 mL/min (iothalamate); proteinuria $\geq$2g a d; kidney biopsy: >30% global glomerulosclerosis or >30% interstitial fibrosis
- AKI deemed irreversible for $\geq$4 wk: stage 3 AKI: 3× increase in sCr from baseline; sCr $\geq$4.0 mg/dL with acute increase of $\geq$0.5 mg/dL/dialysis; eGFR $\leq$35 mL/min (MDRD-6 equation) or GFR $\leq$25 mL/min (iothalamate)/dialysis
- Inherited metabolic disorders

Data from Refs.[2,8,9]

3.6 per month 1 year before the policy was enacted to 11.7 per month after policy enactment. This increase was mainly seen owing to increased eligibility in the safety net kidney after liver candidates. The 6-month review after policy enactment showed an increase in kidney after LT from 1.4 per month to 7.3 per month.[12]

Table 1
Current SLKT policy

Transplant Nephrologist to Confirm Candidate Has *One* of the Following	Transplant Center Must Document *One* of the Following in the Medical Record
CKD with measured/estimated GFR $\leq$60 mL/min >90 d	Dialysis for ESRD Most recent estimated GFR/CrCl <30 mL/min at registration on kidney waiting list
Sustained AKI	Dialysis for 6 consecutive wk Estimated GFR/CrCl $\leq$25 mL/min for at least 6 consecutive wk Any combination of the above for 6 consecutive wk
Inherited metabolic disease	Hyperoxaluria Atypical HUS - mutations in factor H and possibly factor I Familial non-neuropathic systemic amyloid Methylmalonic aciduria

Abbreviations: CrCl, Creatinine Clearance; ESRD, end-stage renal disease; GFR, glomerular filtration rate; HUS, hemolytic uremic syndrome.

Table 2
Allocation scheme for kidney transplant after liver transplant safety net

Sequence A KDPI ≤20%	Sequence B KDPI 21%–34%	Sequence C KDPI 35%–85%	Sequence D KDPI >85%
Highly sensitized	Highly sensitized	Highly sensitized	Highly sensitized
0 ABDRmm	0 ABDRmm	0 ABDRmm	0 ABDRmm
Prior living donor	Prior living donor	Prior living donor	*Local SLKT safety net*
Local pediatrics	Local pediatrics	*Local SLKT safety net*	Local + regional
Local top 20% EPTS	*Local SLKT safety net*	Local	National
0 ABDRmm (all)	Local adults	Regional	
Local (all)	Regional pediatrics	National	
Regional pediatrics	Regional adults		
Regional (top 20%)	National pediatrics		
Regional (all)	National adults		
National pediatrics			
National (top 20%)			
National (all)			

Abbreviations: ABDRmm, A, B, DR mismatches; KDPI, Kidney Donor Profile Index.

CHALLENGES IN OPTIMIZING PATIENTS FOR SIMULTANEOUS LIVER-KIDNEY TRANSPLANTATION
Assessment of Renal Function Among Patients with Cirrhosis

The evaluation of renal function in patients with cirrhosis, whether owing to AKI or from CKD, is challenging. Measured GFR based on the clearance of exogenous markers including inulin, iothalamate, or iohexol is considered the gold standard. However, these measurements have several limitations in clinical practice because they are expensive, time consuming, and not feasible for dynamic assessment of renal function. Serum creatinine (sCr) and creatinine clearance measured by 24-hour urine collection are not reliable indicators because these factors are influenced by sex, race, age, body weight, and muscle mass, as well as worsening liver synthetic function.[13,14] Cystatin C is a low-molecular-weight protein produced by nucleated cells. It is exclusively cleared by glomerular filtration. In contrast with sCr, it is not dependent on age, sex, or muscle mass.[15]

Many sCr and cystatin C-based equations, including Cockcroft-Gault,[16] Modified Diet in Renal Disease (MDRD),[17] and Chronic Kidney Disease Epidemiology Collaboration,[15] overestimate renal function those with estimated GFR less than 40 mL/min/1.73 m^2 among patients with cirrhosis (**Table 3**).[18,19] The MDRD-6 equation estimates the renal function accurately in patients with cirrhosis and with least degree of overestimation. The MDRD-6 equation was superior to the MDRD-4 and Chronic Kidney Disease Epidemiology Collaboration equations, especially for those with estimated a GFR of less than 30 mL/min[18] However, in those with measured GFR greater than 30 to 40 mL/min, the MDRD-6 equation tends to underestimate the GFR. Regardless of these limitations, current OPTN policy recommends the use of either the estimated GFR using the MDRD-6 equation or measured GFR by iothalamate or iohexol methods for SLKT considerations.[1]

Many biomarkers have been studied to distinguish between the phenotypes of AKI and CKD. Urinary neutrophil gelatinase-associated lipocalin (NGAL) is a small protein produced by several cells and organs such as renal tubular cells, leukocytes, and hepatocytes. Its expression increases after ischemic and nephrotoxic insults.[20,21] Among those with hepatorenal syndrome (HRS), urinary NGAL was significantly higher in those with concomitant infections.[22] However, there is a significant overlap in

Table 3
Equations used to estimate GFR

Equation Title	Variables	Equation
Cockcroft-Gault[16]	Age, sCr, gender, weight	CrCl (male) = ideal body weight ([140−age)]/72 × sCr mg/dL]) CrCl (female) = 0.85 × ideal body weight ([140−age)]/72 × sCr mg/dL])
MDRD-4[17]	Age, sCr, gender, ethnicity	GFR = 186 × sCr (mg/dL)$^{-1.154}$ × age$^{-0.203}$ × 1.212 (if black) × 0.742 (if female)
MDRD-6[17]	Age, sCr, gender, ethnicity, BUN, albumin	GFR = 170 × sCr (mg/dL)$^{-0.999}$ × age$^{-0.176}$ × 1.180 (if black) × 0.762 (if female) × BUN$^{-0.170}$ × albumin$^{0.138}$
CKD-EPI[15]	Age, sCr, gender, ethnicity	GFR = 141 × min(sCr/κ, 1)^{α} × max(sCr/κ, 1)$^{-1.209}$ × 0.993^{Age} × 1.018 [if female] × 1.159 [if black]
CKD-EPI cystatin C[15]	Age, gender, cystatin C	eGFR = 133 × min(Scys/κ, 1)$^{-0.499}$ × max (Scys/0 κ, 1)$^{-1.328}$ × 0.996^{Age} × 0.932 [if female]
CKD-EPI creatinine cystatin C[15]	Age, gender, cystatin C, sCr, ethnicity	eGFR = 135 × min(sCr/κ, 1)^{α} × max(sCr/κ, 1)$^{-0.601}$ × min(Scys/κ, 1)$^{-0.375}$ × max(Scys/κ, 1)$^{-0.711}$ × 0.995^{Age} × 0.969 [if female] × 1.08 [if black]

Min: minimum of sCr/κ or 1, κ is 0.7 for females and 0.9 for males, α −0.329 for females and −0.411 for males. max, maximum of sCr/κ or 1, Scys, serum cystatin C.

Abbreviations: BUN, blood urea nitrogen; CKD-EPI, Chronic Kidney Disease Epidemiology Collaboration; CrCl, creatinine clearance; eGFR, estimate GFR.

Data from Refs.[15–17]

urinary NGAL values in patients with AKI owing to acute tubular necrosis (ATN) and HRS.[20,21,23] Because NGAL is also produced by leukocytes, it should be interpreted with caution in patients with infections, particularly urinary tract infection.[24] Several other biomarkers, such as IL-18, kidney injury molecule-1, and liver-type fatty acid-binding protein have been found to be less attractive in differentiating AKI phenotype in patients with liver cirrhosis.[20,25]

Difficulty in Identifying Those with Sustained Acute Kidney Injury for Simultaneous Liver-Kidney Transplantation Candidacy

Differentiation between the phenotypes of AKI in cirrhosis has therapeutic and prognostic implications including eligibility for SLKT. Patient with HRS usually improve their renal function after LT alone.[26–28] In 1 study, the cumulative incidence of renal nonrecovery among those who were on dialysis for less than 90 days before transplant was 8.9% at 6 months after LT.[26] Age, diabetes, a history of re-LT, and pre-LT dialysis duration were independently associated with renal nonrecovery.[26–28] These patients, if they have renal nonrecovery, can be listed for kidney transplant within 1 year of LT under the safety net option of the current SLKT policy. ATN, in contrast, is associated with intrinsic kidney changes, mainly owing to ischemic damage to the tubules after a hypotensive event such as variceal bleeding or sepsis. These patients usually require pretransplant renal replacement therapy and less likely to recover renal function after LT alone and should be considered for SLKT listing. **Table 4** shows the determination

Table 4
Determination of AKI phenotype

Clinical Feature	Diagnosis
History and physical	
Refractory ascites, chronic hypotension, hyponatremia, recent (within 1 wk) large volume paracentesis, active infection	Favors HRS-AKI diagnosis
Use of potential nephrotoxic agents (NSAIDs, aminoglycosides, iodinated contrast, vancomycin, foscarnet, etc), sepsis, renal ischemia, prolonged prerenal azotemia	Favors ATN-AKI diagnosis
Routine testing	
FeNa <1%, Urine sodium <10 mEq/L	Favors HRS diagnosis
FeNa >2%–3%, Urine red blood cell >50 cells per high power field (when no urinary catheter is in place), proteinuria >500 mg/d, casts	Favors ATN diagnosis
Novel biomarkers	
NGAL >220 μg/g creatinine	Favors ATN-AKI diagnosis
Renal ultrasound examination	
No urinary obstruction or renal parenchymal disease	Favors HRS-AKI diagnosis
Renal histology	
Normal renal tubules and glomeruli	Favors ATN-AKI
Response to treatment	
Good response to vasoconstrictors plus intravenous albumin	Favors HRS-AKI diagnosis

Abbreviations: ATN, acute tubular necrosis; FeNa, Fractional Excretion of Sodium; NSAIDs, nonsteroidal anti-inflammatory drugs.

of AKI phenotypes based on history, physical examination, and routinely available diagnostic testing.

AKI is seen in 20% of hospitalized patients with decompensated cirrhosis and should be managed aggressively (**Fig. 1**). Prerenal causes such as HRS and ATN are the major causes of AKI in patients with decompensated cirrhosis, whereas postrenal causes, IgA nephropathy, nephrotoxicity, and glomerulonephritis are less common.[29] Multiple criteria have been proposed for the diagnosis and staging of AKI constitute variation in creatinine (see **Table 4**).[30–33] Although previously defined as separate entity, the International Ascites Club[33] revised the definition of HRS in 2015 to incorporate it into a broad definition of AKI based on Kidney Disease Improving Global Outcomes criteria and further refined the definition in 2019 (**Table 5**).[32,33] These criteria define AKI in cirrhosis to have occurred within the past 7 days. It is important that most recent sCr value from the past 3 months and from before the hospitalization should be considered because 30% of the AKIs have occurred before hospitalization.[33–35] **Fig. 2** shows the proposed management of AKI in patients with cirrhosis.

Chronic Kidney Disease and Decompensated Cirrhosis

There is high prevalence of diabetes, hypertension, and cardiac disease in LT candidates with nonalcoholic fatty liver disease, thus increasing the risk and incidence of CKD. A recent review of OPTN data comparing recipients of SLKT with diagnosis of ATN or HRS versus recipients with diagnosis of diabetes or hypertension suggested

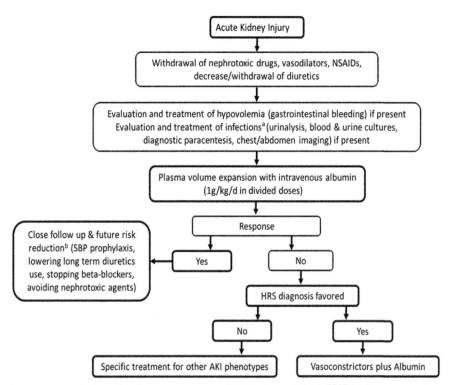

Fig. 1. Proposed algorithm for management of AKI in liver cirrhosis.[33,35] [a] Infectious work up dictated by clinical presentation, [b] future measures dictated by underlying etiology of AKI, NSAIDs, nonsteroidal anti-inflammatory drugs; HRS, hepatorenal syndrome; SBP, spontaneous bacterial prophylaxis. (*Adapted from* Angeli P, Gines P, Wong F, Bernardi M, Boyer TD, Gerbes A, Moreau R, et al. Diagnosis and management of acute kidney injury in patients with cirrhosis: revised consensus recommendations of the International Club of Ascites. Gut 2015;64:531-537; and Angeli P, Garcia-Tsao G, Nadim MK, Parikh CR. News in pathophysiology, definition and classification of hepatorenal syndrome: A step beyond the International Club of Ascites (ICA) consensus document. J Hepatol 2019;71:811-822; with permission).

that despite a lower acuity of illness, patients with hypertension and diabetes have inferior survival after SLKT than those with ATN or HRS.[36] LT candidates with CKD should undergo a detailed evaluation to determine the etiology and stage of CKD (**Table 6**) and receive optimal management based on the etiology.

PATIENT AND GRAFT SURVIVAL AFTER SIMULTANEOUS LIVER-KIDNEY TRANSPLANTATION

Gonwa and colleagues[37] showed better survival of SLKT recipients compared with those who received LT alone but had evidence of pre-LT renal dysfunction (sCr >1.99) or on renal replacement therapy Locke and colleagues[38] showed superior patient and graft survival for SLKT recipients who were on dialysis for greater than 12 weeks. An inverse probability of treatment weighted propensity score matched study comparing 1981 SLKT recipients with 5470 LT alone recipients with renal dysfunction (sCr >2.0 mg/dL) transplanted between 2002 and 2009 demonstrated a small but significant 3.7-month gain in 5-year mean post-

Table 5
Definitions and diagnostic criteria of AKI in liver cirrhosis

Definition of AKI	Increase in sCr ≥0.3 mg/dL within 48 h; or a percentage increase sCr ≥50% from Baseline which is known, or presumed, to have occurred within the prior 7 d
Staging of AKI	Stage 1: increase in sCr ≥0.3 mg/dL or an increase in sCr ≥1.5-fold to 2-fold from baseline Stage 2: increase in sCr >2 to 3-fold from baseline Stage 3: increase of sCr >3-fold from baseline or sCr ≥4.0 mg/dL with an acute increase ≥0.3 mg/dL or initiation of renal replacement therapy
Baseline sCr	A value of sCr obtained in the previous 3 mo, when available, can be used as baseline sCr In patients with >1 value within the previous 3 mo, the value closest to the admission time to the hospital should be used In patients without a previous sCr value, the sCr on admission should be used as baseline
HRS-AKI (previously HRS-1)	Diagnosis of cirrhosis and ascites Diagnosis of AKI according (as defined above) No response after 2 consecutive days of diuretic withdrawal and plasma volume Expansion with albumin 1 g/kg bodyweight Absence of shock No current or recent use of nephrotoxic drugs (NSAIDs, aminoglycosides, iodinated contrast media, etc) No macroscopic signs of structural kidney injury, defined as: Absence of proteinuria (>500 mg/d) Absence of microhematuria (>50 RBCs per high power field) Normal findings on renal ultrasound examination
HRS-AKD (previously HRS-2)	Estimated GFR <60 mL/min per 1.73 m² for <3 mo in the absence of other (structural) causes Percent increase in sCr <50% using the last available value of outpatient sCr within 3 mo as the baseline value
HRS-CKD (HRS-2)	Estimated GFR <60 mL/min per 1.73 m² for ≥3 mo in the absence of other (structural) causes

Abbreviations: NSAIDs, nonsteroidal anti-inflammatory Drugs; RBCs, Red Blood Cells; sCr, serum creatinine.

transplant survival time among SLKT recipients who were not on dialysis at the time of transplantation.[5]

In an elegant review and analysis of OPTN data, investigators demonstrated that 37% of SLKT recipients were not on any renal replacement therapy before transplantation.[11] Of those who were not on renal replacement therapy, 40% had a sCr of less than 2.5 mg/dL at the time of SLKT. Those with a pretransplant renal replacement therapy duration of greater than 2 months or a sCr of greater than 2.5 mg/dL benefited from SLKT compared with LT alone. However, the outcomes with SLKT were inferior when compared with recipients of LT alone without renal dysfunction. The authors further concluded that out of the 494 and 557 SLKT performed in 2014 and 2015, respectively, 19% would not be eligible for SLKT under the current medical eligibility criteria.[11] The quality of kidneys used for SLKT is usually significantly better than those used for kidney transplantation alone.[4,5,11]

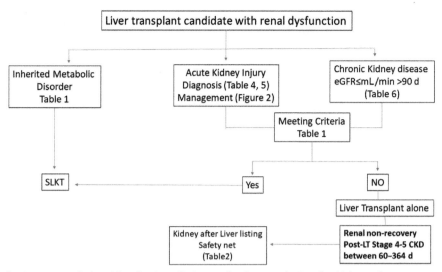

Fig. 2. Proposed algorithm for SLKT listing and safety net listing for kidney after LT.

Immunologic Considerations and Graft Survival

Historical data and clinical experience suggest that liver allograft has some protective effect against hyperacute antibody mediated kidney rejection in patients with high titers of donor-specific antibodies undergoing SLKT[39,40] and affect long-term kidney outcomes.[41,42] Compared with kidney alone transplant (n = 28), SLKT recipients (n = 14) had a significantly lower rate of the development of acute antibody-mediated rejection (46% vs 7%) and transplant glomerulopathy (54% vs 0%). The

Table 6		
Staging for CKD based on GFR and diagnostic work up		
Stage	**Terms**	**GFR (mL/min/1.73 m²)**
Grade 1	Normal or high	≥90
Grade 2	Mildly decreased	60–89
Grade 3a	Mildly to moderately decreased	45–59
Grade 3b	Moderately to severely decreased	30–44
Grade 4	Severely decreased	15–29
Grade 5	Kidney failure (add D if treated with renal replacement therapy)	<15

Workup for CKD
  Urinalysis and microscopy
  Spot urine protein/creatinine and microalbumin/creatinine ratio
  24-h urine collection for protein
  Urine protein electrophoresis (if indicated based on initial testing)
  Imaging (ultrasound examination, CT scan, MRI)
  Renal biopsy (if indicated based on initial testing)		

Abbreviations: CT, computed tomography; MRI, magnetic resonance imaging.
Data from Kidney Disease: Improving Global Outcomes (KDIGO) Acute Kidney Injury Work Group. KDIGO clinical practice guideline for acute kidney injury. Kidney International 2012;2(Suppl):1-138.

5-year renal allograft loss or a more than 50% decrease in the estimated GFR were also lower in the SLKT group (20% vs 7%).[43] In a follow-up study, the authors demonstrated that molecular markers of inflammation and T-cell activation were significantly less common in kidney biopsies of SLKT recipients compared with kidney alone recipients with similar immunologic risk profiles.[44] Transplanted liver exerts its effect by reducing preformed lymphocytotoxic antibodies and neutralizing antibodies through the release of soluble class I antigens.[45,46] In contrast, other studies have suggested a limited role of liver protection against antibody-mediated kidney rejection and renal dysfunction in SLKT recipients.[47,48] Although levels of class I donor-specific antibodies decrease significantly after SLKT, levels of class II donor-specific antibodies titers can stay high.[49,50] Under current clinical practices, desensitization of a highly sensitized transplant candidate, to lower the risk of hyperacute kidney rejection and allograft dysfunction is rarely considered for SLKT candidates; this practice is common for kidney alone transplant candidates.

Role of Recipient Age and Body Mass Index in Simultaneous Liver-Kidney Transplantation Outcomes

Over the last decade, the proportion of older aged LT candidates ($\geq$65 years) continues to increase. In 2018, 24% of the adult waitlist population was age 65 years or older, almost twice the proportion 10 years earlier.[51] Although majority of the transplant centers in United States do not have a strict age cut-off for LT or SLKT, age is usually considered along with other comorbidities when deciding for transplant candidacy. For SLKT recipients receiving pretransplant dialysis, the 1-year survival rate was significantly lower in patients older than 65 compared with their younger counterparts (67.0% vs 82.5%).[52] Another study reported that age 70 years or older was indicative of poor outcomes after SLKT compared with those aged 65 to 69 years.[53] At 1 year after SLKT, the absolute difference in adjusted survival between cohort with best survival (nondiabetics ages 40–49 years) and the cohort with the worst survival (patients without diabetes $\geq$70 years of age) was 10.3%, which increased over time: from 19.9% at 3 years, to 25.0% at 5 years, and 31.5% at 10 years.[53] It is likely that, with the aging population, the ongoing use of the MELD score for organ allocation and increasing number of candidates with nonalcoholic steatohepatitis, SLKT candidates with advanced age will continue to increase, highlighting the importance of optimization of outcomes in this age group.

Although recipients of kidney transplant with obesity are at increased risk for adverse outcomes, including delayed graft function, the literature is conflicted regarding the effect of obesity on LT outcomes with some studies suggesting that low body mass index is more deleterious than high body mass index.[54,55] Data on the effect of body mass index in SLKT are scarce. A recent report reviewing OPTN data of 7205 SLK recipients identified diagnosis of hepatitis C, donor age, diabetes mellitus, and delayed kidney graft function, but not body mass index, as risk factors for poor patient as well as liver and kidney graft survival.[56]

SUMMARY

SLKT comprises only 8% to 10% of all LT per year; however, it remained an important option for patient with CKD, sustained AKI and those with inherited metabolic disorders. SLKT policy has evolved significantly over last 15 years and the current policy is based on medical eligibility criteria. It also provides an option of safety net with 1 year of liver transplant alone to avoid the futile SLKT. With the increase in aging population and obesity epidemic, one should be careful in patient selection and consider optimization before transplant to improve post-SLKT outcomes.

CLINICS CARE POINTS

- Renal dysfunction among patients with decompensated cirrhosis is common.
- It is very difficult to predict renal recovery after liver transplant alone in those who had acute kidney injury at the time of transplant.
- Current SLKT policy will promote judicious use of kidney allograft under "safety net" option.

DISCLOSURES

The authors have nothing to disclose.

REFERENCES

1. OPTN. Organ procurement and transplantation Network policies. 2007. Available at: https://optn.transplant.hrsa.gov/media/1200/optn_policies.pdf.
2. Nadim MK, Sung RS, Davis CL, et al. Simultaneous liver-kidney transplantation summit: current state and future directions. Am J Transplant 2012;12(11):2901–8.
3. Sharma P. Liver-kidney: indications, patient selection, and allocation policy. Clin Liver Dis (Hoboken) 2019;13:165–9.
4. Reese PP, Veatch RM, Abt PL, et al. Revisiting multi-organ transplantation in the setting of scarcity. Am J Transplant 2014;14:21–6.
5. Sharma P, Shu X, Schaubel DE, et al. Propensity score-based survival benefit of simultaneous liver-kidney transplant over liver transplant alone for recipients with pretransplant renal dysfunction. Liver Transpl 2016;22:71–9.
6. Nadim MK, Davis CL, Sung R, et al. Simultaneous liver-kidney transplantation: a survey of US transplant centers. Am J Transplant 2012;12:3119–27.
7. Davis CL. Impact of pretransplant renal failure: when is listing for kidney-liver indicated? Liver Transpl 2005;(11 Suppl 2):S35–44.
8. Eason JD, Gonwa TA, Davis CL, et al. Proceedings of consensus conference on simultaneous liver kidney transplantation (SLK). Am J Transplant 2008;8:2243–51.
9. Davis CL, Feng S, Sung R, et al. Simultaneous liver-kidney transplantation: evaluation to decision making. Am J Transplant 2007;7:1702–9.
10. Formica RN Jr. Simultaneous liver-kidney allocation: let's not make perfect the enemy of good. Am J Transplant 2016;16:2765.
11. Formica RN, Aeder M, Boyle G, et al. Simultaneous liver-kidney allocation policy: a proposal to optimize appropriate utilization of scarce resources. Am J Transplant 2016;16:758–66.
12. Wiseman A, Wilk AR. Simultaneous liver-kidney (SLK): one year post-implementation monitoring. Boston (MA): American Transplant Congress; 2019.
13. Cholongitas E, Shusang V, Marelli L, et al. Review article: renal function assessment in cirrhosis - difficulties and alternative measurements. Aliment Pharmacol Ther 2007;26:969–78.
14. Francoz C, Prie D, Abdelrazek W, et al. Inaccuracies of creatinine and creatinine-based equations in candidates for liver transplantation with low creatinine: impact on the model for end-stage liver disease score. Liver Transpl 2010;16:1169–77.
15. Inker LA, Schmid CH, Tighiouart H, et al. Estimating glomerular filtration rate from serum creatinine and cystatin C. N Engl J Med 2012;367:20–9.

16. Cockcroft DW, Gault MH. Prediction of creatinine clearance from serum creatinine. Nephron 1976;16:31–41.
17. Levey AS, Bosch JP, Lewis JB, et al. A more accurate method to estimate glomerular filtration rate from serum creatinine: a new prediction equation. Modification of diet in renal disease study group. Ann Intern Med 1999;130:461–70.
18. Francoz C, Nadim MK, Baron A, et al. Glomerular filtration rate equations for liver-kidney transplantation in patients with cirrhosis: validation of current recommendations. Hepatology 2014;59:1514–21.
19. Gonwa TA, Jennings L, Mai ML, et al. Estimation of glomerular filtration rates before and after orthotopic liver transplantation: evaluation of current equations. Liver Transpl 2004;10:301–9.
20. Belcher JM, Sanyal AJ, Peixoto AJ, et al. Kidney biomarkers and differential diagnosis of patients with cirrhosis and acute kidney injury. Hepatology 2014;60:622–32.
21. Fagundes C, Pepin MN, Guevara M, et al. Urinary neutrophil gelatinase-associated lipocalin as biomarker in the differential diagnosis of impairment of kidney function in cirrhosis. J Hepatol 2012;57:267–73.
22. Barreto R, Elia C, Sola E, et al. Urinary neutrophil gelatinase-associated lipocalin predicts kidney outcome and death in patients with cirrhosis and bacterial infections. J Hepatol 2014;61:35–42.
23. Verna EC, Brown RS, Farrand E, et al. Urinary neutrophil gelatinase-associated lipocalin predicts mortality and identifies acute kidney injury in cirrhosis. Dig Dis Sci 2012;57:2362–70.
24. Otto GP, Busch M, Sossdorf M, et al. Impact of sepsis-associated cytokine storm on plasma NGAL during acute kidney injury in a model of polymicrobial sepsis. Crit Care 2013;17:419.
25. Ariza X, Sola E, Elia C, et al. Analysis of a urinary biomarker panel for clinical outcomes assessment in cirrhosis. PLoS One 2015;10:e0128145.
26. Sharma P, Goodrich NP, Zhang M, et al. Short-term pretransplant renal replacement therapy and renal nonrecovery after liver transplantation alone. Clin J Am Soc Nephrol 2013;8:1135–42.
27. Northup PG, Argo CK, Bakhru MR, et al. Pretransplant predictors of recovery of renal function after liver transplantation. Liver Transpl 2010;16:440–6.
28. Wong F, Leung W, Al Beshir M, et al. Outcomes of patients with cirrhosis and hepatorenal syndrome type 1 treated with liver transplantation. Liver Transpl 2015;21:300–7.
29. Arroyo V, Gines P, Gerbes AL, et al. Definition and diagnostic criteria of refractory ascites and hepatorenal syndrome in cirrhosis. International ascites club. Hepatology 1996;23:164–76.
30. Bellomo R, Ronco C, Kellum JA, et al. Acute dialysis quality initiative w. Acute renal failure - definition, outcome measures, animal models, fluid therapy and information technology needs: the second international consensus conference of the acute dialysis quality initiative (ADQI) group. Crit Care 2004;8:R204–12.
31. Mehta RL, Kellum JA, Shah SV, et al. Acute kidney injury network: report of an initiative to improve outcomes in acute kidney injury. Crit Care 2007;11:R31.
32. Kidney Disease: Improving Global Outcomes (KDIGO) Acute Kidney Injury Work Group. KDIGO clinical practice guideline for acute kidney injury. Kidney Int 2012;2(Suppl):1–138.
33. Angeli P, Gines P, Wong F, et al. Diagnosis and management of acute kidney injury in patients with cirrhosis: revised consensus recommendations of the international club of ascites. Gut 2015;64:531–7.

34. Piano S, Rosi S, Maresio G, et al. Evaluation of the acute kidney injury network criteria in hospitalized patients with cirrhosis and ascites. J Hepatol 2013;59: 482–9.

35. Angeli P, Garcia-Tsao G, Nadim MK, et al. News in pathophysiology, definition and classification of hepatorenal syndrome: a step beyond the international club of ascites (ICA) consensus document. J Hepatol 2019;71:811–22.

36. Cannon RM, Jones CM, Davis EG, et al. Effect of renal diagnosis on survival in simultaneous liver-kidney transplantation. J Am Coll Surg 2019;228:536–44.e3.

37. Gonwa TA, McBride MA, Anderson K, et al. Continued influence of preoperative renal function on outcome of orthotopic liver transplant (OLTX) in the US: where will MELD lead us? Am J Transplant 2006;6:2651–9.

38. Locke JE, Warren DS, Singer AL, et al. Declining outcomes in simultaneous liver-kidney transplantation in the MELD era: ineffective usage of renal allografts. Transplantation 2008;85:935–42.

39. Fung J, Makowka L, Tzakis A, et al. Combined liver-kidney transplantation: analysis of patients with preformed lymphocytotoxic antibodies. Transplant Proc 1988;20:88–91.

40. Rasmussen A, Davies HF, Jamieson NV, et al. Combined transplantation of liver and kidney from the same donor protects the kidney from rejection and improves kidney graft survival. Transplantation 1995;59:919–21.

41. Fong TL, Bunnapradist S, Jordan SC, et al. Analysis of the united network for organ sharing database comparing renal allografts and patient survival in combined liver-kidney transplantation with the contralateral allografts in kidney alone or kidney-pancreas transplantation. Transplantation 2003;76:348–53.

42. Simpson N, Cho YW, Cicciarelli JC, et al. Comparison of renal allograft outcomes in combined liver-kidney transplantation versus subsequent kidney transplantation in liver transplant recipients: analysis of UNOS Database. Transplantation 2006;82:1298–303.

43. Taner T, Heimbach JK, Rosen CB, et al. Decreased chronic cellular and antibody-mediated injury in the kidney following simultaneous liver-kidney transplantation. Kidney Int 2016;89:909–17.

44. Taner T, Park WD, Stegall MD. Unique molecular changes in kidney allografts after simultaneous liver-kidney compared with solitary kidney transplantation. Kidney Int 2017;91:1193–202.

45. Gugenheim J, Amorosa L, Gigou M, et al. Specific absorption of lymphocytotoxic alloantibodies by the liver in inbred rats. Transplantation 1990;50:309–13.

46. Sumimoto R, Kamada N. Specific suppression of allograft rejection by soluble class I antigen and complexes with monoclonal antibody. Transplantation 1990; 50:678–82.

47. Askar M, Schold JD, Eghtesad B, et al. Combined liver-kidney transplants: allosensitization and recipient outcomes. Transplantation 2011;91:1286–92.

48. Katznelson S, Cecka JM. The liver neither protects the kidney from rejection nor improves kidney graft survival after combined liver and kidney transplantation from the same donor. Transplantation 1996;61:1403–5.

49. O'Leary JG, Gebel HM, Ruiz R, et al. Class II alloantibody and mortality in simultaneous liver-kidney transplantation. Am J Transplant 2013;13:954–60.

50. Dar W, Agarwal A, Watkins C, et al. Donor-directed MHC class I antibody is preferentially cleared from sensitized recipients of combined liver/kidney transplants. Am J Transplant 2011;11:841–7.

51. Kwong A, Kim WR, Lake JR, et al. OPTN/SRTR 2018 annual data report: liver. Am J Transplant 2020;20(Suppl s1):193–299.

52. Croome KP, Lee DD, Burns JM, et al. Simultaneous liver and kidney transplantation in elderly patients: outcomes and validation of a clinical risk score for patient selection. Ann Hepatol 2016;15:870–80.
53. Goldberg DV, Vianna RM, Martin EF, et al. Simultaneous liver kidney transplant in elderly patients with chronic kidney disease. Is there an appropriate upper age cutoff? Transplantation 2020. https://doi.org/10.1097/TP.0000000000003147.
54. Bambha KM, Dodge JL, Gralla J, et al. Low, rather than high, body mass index confers increased risk for post-liver transplant death and graft loss: risk modulated by model for end-stage liver disease. Liver Transpl 2015;21:1286–94.
55. Bari K, Sharma P. Impact of body mass index on posttransplant outcomes reexamined. Liver Transpl 2015;21:1238–40.
56. Yu JW, Gupta G, Kang L, et al. Obesity does not significantly impact outcomes following simultaneous liver kidney transplantation: review of the UNOS database - a retrospective study. Transpl Int 2019;32:206–17.

Keeping Patients with End-Stage Liver Disease Alive While Awaiting Transplant

Management of Complications of Portal Hypertension

Andres F. Carrion, MD[a],*, Paul Martin, MD, FRCP, FRCPI[b]

KEYWORDS

- Cirrhosis • Varices • Ascites • Renal dysfunction • Hepatorenal syndrome
- Portopulmonary hypertension • Hepatopulmonary syndrome • Hepatic hydrothorax

KEY POINTS

- Portal hypertension is a key element in the natural history of cirrhosis and end-stage liver disease, regardless of the underlying cause.
- Complications of portal hypertension negatively affect patients' quality of life and survival. Furthermore, excessive morbidity resulting from these complications may result in delisting of candidates from liver transplant (LT) waiting lists.
- Medical care of LT candidates must be centered on prompt identification and appropriate management of complications of portal hypertension, such as gastroesophageal varices, ascites, hepatorenal syndrome, and pulmonary complications.

Liver transplant (LT) remains definitive treatment of end-stage liver disease (ESLD), regardless of cause. Current post-LT survival rates (80%–90% after 1 year and 60%–75% after 5 years) reflect major advances in surgical techniques, postoperative intensive care, immunosuppression, as well as better selection of potential candidates.[1] However, because of increasing waiting times for LT, a sizable proportion of candidates drop off the waiting list for various reasons, including clinical deterioration, often related to complications of portal hypertension.

Portal hypertension is a defining element in the natural history of cirrhosis.[2] Clinically significant portal hypertension typically occurs when the hepatic venous pressure gradient (HVPG) is greater than or equal to 10 mm Hg, the threshold for development

[a] Division of Digestive Health and Liver Diseases, University of Miami Miller School of Medicine, 1120 Northwest 14th Street, Office 1189, Miami, FL 33136, USA; [b] Division of Digestive Health and Liver Diseases, University of Miami Miller School of Medicine, 1120 Northwest 14th #1115, Miami, FL 33136, USA
* Corresponding author.
E-mail address: acarrionmonsalve@med.miami.edu

Clin Liver Dis 25 (2021) 103–120
https://doi.org/10.1016/j.cld.2020.08.007
1089-3261/21/© 2020 Elsevier Inc. All rights reserved.

of complications such as gastroesophageal varices (GOV) and ascites.[3] Other mani-festations of portal hypertension include hepatorenal syndrome, hepatopulmonary syndrome, portopulmonary hypertension (POPH), and hepatic hydrothorax. Mitigation of these complications is critical to avoid additional morbidity and transplant list drop-off in cirrhotic patients.

GASTROESOPHAGEAL VARICES

Portal hypertension leads to formation of multiple portosystemic collaterals, including GOV when the HVPG is greater than or equal to 10 mm Hg, with the risk for variceal hemorrhage increasing significantly once HVPG is greater than 12 mm Hg.[4] Gastro-esophageal varices are present in approximately 50% of patients with cirrhosis and are twice as common in patients with hepatic decompensation (Child-Turcotte-Pugh [CTP] classes B and C).[5] Variceal hemorrhage is the most dramatic complication of cirrhosis and occurs at a rate of 5% to 15% per year; risk factors include larger var-iceal size, more advanced hepatic decompensation (CTP class C>B), and presence of vascular red-wale signs during endoscopic evaluation.[6] Screening for GOV with esophagogastroduodenoscopy (EGD) is recommended if cirrhosis is suspected. Endoscopic evaluation permits risk stratification based on the size of the varices (small for those ≤5 mm vs large for those >5 mm) and presence of red-wale signs.[7] Further-more, endoscopic variceal ligation (EVL) remains an important intervention for primary and secondary prophylaxis of variceal hemorrhage. Strategies for primary prophylaxis of variceal hemorrhage are summarized in **Table 1**.

Management of esophageal varices that have previously bled (secondary prophy-laxis) includes a combination of a nonselective β-blocker with EVL, which has proved more effective than either intervention alone.[8] The dose of the nonselective β-blocker should be titrated to a resting heart rate of 55 to 60 beats/min (or 25% decrease from baseline) and EVL should be repeated frequently (every 2–4 weeks) until complete var-iceal obliteration. Recurrence of esophageal varices may occur following EVL; there-fore, surveillance is recommended: first EGD performed 3 to 6 months after variceal obliteration and then at 6-month to 12-month intervals.[7] The safety of β-blockers in pa-tients with ESLD has been questioned based on results from some individual studies suggesting increased mortality[9,10]; however, more recent meta-analyses have not confirmed increased mortality associated with these agents in this population, even in the setting of refractory ascites.[11–13]

Gastric varices are classified according to their relationship with esophageal varices and anatomic location. Management of GOV types 1 and 2 is similar to that of esoph-ageal varices, because EVL at the esophageal junction also interrupts blood supply to the gastric varices; however, isolated gastric varices are usually not amenable to EVL (**Table 2**). Although not performed at all centers, endoscopic variceal obturation by in-jection of cyanoacrylate seems to be more effective than nonselective β-blockers for primary prophylaxis of high-risk gastric varices.[14] Similarly, some data suggest that cyanoacrylate injection is more effective than β-blockers for secondary prophylaxis of gastric variceal bleeding and may also improve survival at 26-month follow-up.[15] Endovascular interventions such as transjugular intrahepatic portosystemic shunt (TIPS) and retrograde transvenous obliteration techniques (ie, balloon-occluded trans-venous obliteration [BRTO], plug-assisted retrograde transvenous obliteration, coil-assisted retrograde transvenous obliteration) are nowadays available at most centers with experienced interventional radiologists. TIPS is more effective than cyanoacrylate injection for prevention of gastric variceal rebleeding; however, survival seems to be similar after a median 33-month follow-up.[16]

Table 1
Recommendations for primary prophylaxis against esophageal variceal hemorrhage

Size of Varices	Risk of Hemorrhage	Surveillance Interval	Primary Prophylaxis
No varices	CTP class A	EGD every 2 y if ongoing liver injury (ie, obesity or alcohol abuse), or every 3 y if liver injury is quiescent (ie, viral eradication or alcohol abstinence)	None
	CTP class B/C	EGD yearly	None
Small esophageal varices	CTP class A	EGD yearly if ongoing liver injury (ie, obesity or alcohol abuse), or every 2 y if liver injury is quiescent (ie, viral eradication or alcohol abstinence)	BB may be used
	CTP class B/C	EGD yearly; if BB are used, repeat EGD unnecessary	BB recommended
Large esophageal varices	CTP class A/B/C	If BB are used, repeat EGD unnecessary; if no BB, repeat EGD for EVL every 2–8 wk until variceal eradication, then once in 3–6 mo, and regularly every 6–12 mo	Either BB or EVL recommended

Abbreviation: BB, β-blocker.

Acute variceal hemorrhage occurs at an annual rate of 5% to 15% and is associated with high mortality (at least 20% at 6 weeks).[7] Adequate resuscitation is crucial in acute variceal hemorrhage with some additional precautions; however, overly aggressive expansion of blood volume should be avoided because it may result in increased portal venous pressure. A target hemoglobin level between 7 and 9 g/dL is appropriate.[17] Current guidelines recommend against correcting the international normalized ratio by use of fresh frozen plasma or recombinant factor VIIa, because this has not shown a clear benefit in individuals with acute variceal hemorrhage.[7] There

Table 2
Classification of gastroesophageal and gastric varices and recommendations for primary prophylaxis

Type of Varices	Characteristics	Primary Prophylaxis
GOV1	Extension of esophageal varices along the lesser curvature into the gastric cardia	Similar to esophageal varices
GOV2	Extension of the esophageal varices along the greater curvature into the gastric fundus	BB can be used, although data not as strong as for esophageal varices
IGV1	Gastric varices localized in the fundus	If high risk, consider BB or cyanoacrylate injection
IGV2	Gastric varices localized in the antrum	No data, consider BB if high risk

are no data to support or recommend transfusion of platelets. Prophylactic broad-spectrum antibiotics (ie, intravenous ceftriaxone) reduce bacterial infections, risk of rebleeding, and mortality.[18,19] Administration of vasoactive drugs such as octreotide or terlipressin results in increased rates of initial endoscopic control of bleeding, reduced 7-day mortality, and lower transfusion requirements.[20] Patients with variceal hemorrhage are at high risk for aspiration, particularly if the presentation is with hematemesis, and endotracheal intubation for airway protection should be considered before endoscopy; however, an increased frequency of cardiopulmonary events has been reported following prophylactic endotracheal intubation in critically ill patients with upper gastrointestinal hemorrhage.[21] EGD is recommended within 12 hours, with EVL being the endoscopic intervention of choice.[22] Variceal sclerotherapy with injection of ethanolamine or morrhuate sodium is similarly effective in controlling the acute bleeding episode compared with EVL; however, EVL is superior to sclerotherapy because of lower risk of rebleeding, death, and stricture formation.[22,23] Balloon tamponade (ie, Sengstaken Blakemore, Minnesota, or Linton-Nachlas tubes) or temporary esophageal stenting are effective rescue therapies when variceal hemorrhage cannot be controlled endoscopically.[24] The role of TIPS has expanded from a salvage intervention for recurrent variceal hemorrhage to an early preemptive strategy in carefully selected individuals at high risk for endoscopic treatment failure following EVL (CTP classes B and C but with model for end-stage liver disease [MELD] scores ≤13), in which case it seems to be superior to nonselective β-blocker plus EVL.[25] Patients who survive an episode of esophageal variceal hemorrhage should receive secondary prophylaxis with a combination of a nonselective β-blocker and repeated EVL until complete obliteration of the varices is achieved.[7]

Cyanoacrylate injection, if available, and TIPS are the treatments of choice for management of acute gastric variceal hemorrhage. TIPS seems to be associated with lower rebleeding rate compared with cyanoacrylate injection for treatment of acute gastric variceal hemorrhage but results in higher incidence of encephalopathy, and no survival benefit has been reported.[16] BRTO (or other endovascular retrograde obliteration techniques) may be better suited for patients with severe hepatic dysfunction, because it does not divert portal blood inflow from the liver (TIPS does, and it may be associated with worsening hepatic dysfunction and even liver failure); however, it might result in increased portal pressure, which might worsen ascites or result in esophageal variceal hemorrhage.

Although concerns have been raised about increased complexity of transplant surgery in patients with TIPS, some data suggest similar surgical time and transfusion requirements for patients undergoing LT with and without TIPS.[26]

ASCITES

Portal hypertension is required for development of cirrhotic ascites, because it does not develop if the HVPG is less than 12 mm Hg.[27] Importantly, sinusoidal hypertension seems to be a requirement for development of ascites because prehepatic portal hypertension does not typically result in its development. Other contributory mechanisms include splanchnic vasodilatation and its consequences, including sodium retention and diminished free water excretion by the kidneys, hypoproteinemia and reduced oncotic pressure, and disruption of normal lymphatic drainage in the liver caused by extensive fibrosis.

A diagnostic paracentesis is mandatory in the following settings: new-onset ascites; change in clinical status, including hospitalization of a patient with previously diagnosed ascites; and suggestion of spontaneous bacterial peritonitis (SBP). The following tests on the fluid are indicated: leukocyte count with differential, culture (on 2 blood culture bottles inoculated at the bedside), total protein, and albumin. The appearance of the ascitic fluid may yield important clinical clues (**Table 3**). The serum/ascites albumin gradient (SAAG) helps to distinguish transudative and exudative ascites. A gradient of greater than or equal to 1.1 g/dL confirms portal hypertension as the cause of ascites, whereas a value less than 1.1 g/dL suggests causes other than portal hypertension. The presence of absolute number of polymorphonuclear (PMN) cells greater than or equal to 250 μL suggests SBP.

Cirrhotic ascites is unlikely to resolve without specific therapeutic intervention. Management of ascites is centered on sodium restriction rather than free water restriction; total dietary intake of sodium should be less than 2000 mg (88 mmol) per day and compliance with this intervention can be documented by monitoring urinary sodium concentrations.[28] A sodium/potassium concentration ratio of greater than 1 on a random urine sample correlates well with a 24-hour sodium excretion greater than 78 mmol/d and implies compliance with sodium restriction.[29] However, dietary restriction of sodium by itself is efficacious in only 10% of patients, and enhanced natriuresis is typically necessary to adequately control ascites. Combining diuretics that work at different sites in the nephron is more effective than using a single agent. Aldosterone production is upregulated in cirrhosis and ESLD owing to diminished effective arterial blood volume that stimulates increased renin and angiotensin activity, resulting in enhanced renal sodium and free water retention. Spironolactone competitively inhibits aldosterone-dependent sodium-potassium exchange in the distal convoluted renal tubule and the collecting ducts. The recommended initial dose of spironolactone for patients with ascites caused by portal hypertension is 100 mg orally daily. Administration of a loop-acting diuretic such as furosemide is recommended in addition to spironolactone because it potentiates natriuresis. The recommended initial dose for furosemide is 40 mg orally daily. Further increases in doses of diuretics should be made maintaining this 100:40 ratio to a maximum dose of 400 mg orally daily of spironolactone and 160 mg orally daily of furosemide, because it prevents hypokalemia or hyperkalemia. Renal function and electrolytes must be monitored regularly, particularly after dose modifications. Tender gynecomastia is an unpleasant side effect of spironolactone, and some patients may need to discontinue it, in which case amiloride (10–40 mg orally daily) or eplerenone (25–100 mg orally daily) can be used.[30] Two outcomes may occur in patients with ascites that is not adequately controlled with diuretics: (1) refractory ascites to maximum diuretic doses and sodium restriction, which typically recurs rapidly following large-volume paracentesis (LVP); and (2) inability to increase diuretic doses owing to symptomatic hypotension or deterioration in renal function.

Repeated LVP with removal of more than 5 L of ascitic fluid per session is a safe and effective intervention to treat refractory ascites; however, mortality within 6 months is 20% once this develops, reflecting the severity of the underlying liver disease.[31] Continued dietary restriction of sodium is necessary to avoid overly frequent LVP, and continuation of diuretics should be assessed on a case-by-case basis taking into consideration potential benefits and adverse reactions. Expansion of plasma volume for patients undergoing LVP is endorsed by current guidelines and supported by data showing reduced postparacentesis circulatory dysfunction and improved survival.[32] Plasma volume should be expanded with infusion of intravenous albumin at a dose of 6 to 8 g/L of ascitic fluid removed during or immediately after LVP.[31] Results from a recent small randomized pilot study suggest that oral midodrine for 30 days post-LVP is as effective as intravenous albumin infusion in reducing morbidity and mortality among patients with refractory ascites undergoing LVP; however, these results must be corroborated by larger clinical trials.[33]

Table 3
Characteristics of ascitic fluid and differential diagnosis

Fluid Appearance	Differential Diagnosis	Biochemical Hints on Fluid Analysis
Clear	Uncomplicated transudative ascites caused by cirrhosis	WBC<500 cells/μL, PMN <250 cells/μL, SAAG ≥1.1
Turbid/cloudy	Infection	PMN ≥ 250 cells/μL
Bloody	Traumatic paracentesis, hemoperitoneum	RBC>10,000 cells/μL
Milky	Chylous ascites caused by obstruction or trauma of lymphatic vessels or thoracic duct	Triglycerides>200 md/dL

Abbreviations: PMN, polymorphonuclear cells; SAAG, serum/ascites albumin gradient; WBC, white blood cell.

Insertion of TIPS corrects portal hypertension and offers an attractive alternative for amelioration of refractory ascites in selected patients, and has replaced surgical shunts. Transplant-free survival is superior with TIPS compared with repeated LVP.[34,35] Assessment of systolic and diastolic heart function as well as exclusion of aortic stenosis by transthoracic echocardiography is recommended before TIPS insertion because significant hemodynamic changes occur following the creation of the portosystemic shunt that can result in post-TIPS heart failure.[36] Patients with MELD scores greater than 14 are at high risk of death post-TIPS; thus, TIPS should be considered on an individual basis and after carefully discussing risks and benefits with patients.[37] TIPS results in frequent hepatic encephalopathy, and, although it typically responds to therapy with lactulose and/or rifaximin, reduction of the TIPS diameter may be required if it does not improve.[38]

SPONTANEOUS BACTERIAL PERITONITIS

Cirrhosis and portal hypertension are associated with abnormal intestinal permeability leading to bacterial translocation resulting in SBP.[39,40] The most commonly isolated microorganisms responsible for SBP are *Escherichia coli* (43%), *Klebsiella pneumoniae* (11%), *Streptococcus pneumoniae* (9%), other streptococcal species (19%), Enterobacteriaceae (4%), *Staphylococcus* (3%), and miscellaneous organisms depending on the region of the world (10%).[40] A small-volume diagnostic paracentesis (30–60 mL) rather than LVP (which can increase the risk of hepatorenal syndrome in SBP) is mandatory for confirmation of SBP and should be performed before antibiotic therapy. Diagnosis of SBP is supported by the presence of greater than or equal to 250 PMN/μL in the ascitic fluid without an obvious source of infection.[41] Based on the PMN count and the microbiologic analysis of the ascitic fluid, the 4 clinical scenarios summarized in **Table 4** may be encountered.

Treatment of SBP is with intravenous broad-spectrum antibiotics with bactericidal activity against the likely infecting bacteria. Third-generation cephalosporins such as cefotaxime or ceftriaxone offer appropriate antimicrobial coverage for treatment of community-acquired SBP. For patients allergic to β-lactams, alternatives include fluoroquinolones such as ciprofloxacin or levofloxacin, although these agents show less penetration into the ascitic fluid compared with third-generation cephalosporins. Health care–associated SBP should be treated with either piperacillin/tazobactam (for areas with low prevalence of infections caused by multidrug-resistant organisms

Table 4
Spontaneous bacterial peritonitis and associated conditions based on characteristics of the ascitic fluid

Clinical Entity	Polymorphonuclear Cell Count	Culture Results	Antibiotics Recommended
Spontaneous bacterial peritonitis	$\geq$250 cells/μL	Positive, single organism	Yes
Culture-negative neutrocytic ascites	$\geq$250 cells/μL	Negative	Yes
Monomicrobial nonneutrocytic bacterascites	<250 cells/μL	Positive, single organism	Yes
Polymicrobial bacterascites	<250 cells/μL	Positive, multiple organisms	Yes

[MDROs]) or carbapenems or daptomycin (for areas with high prevalence of MDROs and nosocomial SBP).[42] Current guidelines do not recommend routine repeat paracentesis in patients with a typical initial presentation of SBP and when antibiotic therapy results in rapid clinical improvement. It is indicated to document a reduction of at least 25% in the PMN count after 48 hours of empiric antibiotic therapy in patients with a slow or absent clinical response or in those with atypical microorganisms on initial culture results.[42]

Plasma volume expansion with albumin is an important adjunct to antibiotic therapy in patients with SBP because it decreases the incidence of acute kidney injury (AKI) and reduces mortality.[43] The physiologic effects of intravenous infusion of albumin include increased oncotic pressure with consequential expansion of the effective arterial blood volume, as well as its ability to bind a wide range of endogenous and exogenous ligands, including bacterial lipopolysaccharides, reactive oxygen species, nitric oxide and other nitrogen reactive species, and prostaglandins, thus modulating the inflammatory response.[44] Current guidelines recommend a selective approach for administration of intravenous albumin to patients with SBP. Specifically, this therapy should be reserved for patients at high risk, including those with serum creatinine level greater than 1 mg/dL, blood urea nitrogen level greater than 30 mL/dL, or total serum bilirubin level greater than 4 mg/dL.[31] The recommended dose of albumin is 1.5 g/kg of body weight within 6 hours of establishing the diagnosis of SBP and a second dose of 1 g/kg on day 3.

Following an initial episode of SBP, further infection occurs in 69% of individuals within 1 year; therefore, secondary prophylaxis is indicated, with current guidelines recommending long-term oral antibiotics such as trimethoprim/sulfamethoxazole.[31] Risk factors for recurrent SBP include ascitic fluid total protein concentration less than 1 g/dL and gastroesophageal variceal hemorrhage.[45] Importantly, some data suggest an increased risk for SBP in patients with cirrhosis and ascites taking proton pump inhibitors; therefore, unnecessary use of these agents should be avoided.[46]

HEPATORENAL SYNDROME

Renal dysfunction is commonly encountered in patients with cirrhosis, particularly in those with ESLD and hepatic decompensation.[47] AKI frequently complicates the course of up to 70% of patients with cirrhosis admitted to a hospital for other complications of their liver disease.[48] Worsening renal impairment is also frequent in hospitalized patients with cirrhosis and concomitant chronic kidney disease (CKD).[48] AKI is a frequent complication of intercurrent clinical events in ESLD, such as critical illness requiring intensive care support (40%–49%), spontaneous bacterial peritonitis (34%), bacterial infections other than SBP (27%), and acute upper gastrointestinal hemorrhage (11%).[49,50] The 1-year probability of developing renal dysfunction in patients with cirrhosis and ascites is 24% with advanced age, CTP class (C>B>A), and increased baseline serum creatinine level being independent risk factors.[51]

Several definitions for AKI have been proposed, the most recent by Kidney Disease Improving Global Outcomes (KDIGO) and subsequently modified by the International Club of Ascites (ICA): increase in serum creatinine level by greater than or equal to 0.3 mg/dL within 48 hours, or increase in serum creatinine level to greater than or equal to 1.5 times baseline within 7 days.[52] AKI is classified in 3 stages (**Table 5**) and distinguishing between stages 1-A and 1-B within AKI stage 1 may offer additional prognostic information (higher mortality for patients with AKI stage 1-B).[42,53,54] CKD is defined as diminished renal function for greater than or equal to 3 months, irrespective of the cause, and is classified into stages depending on the glomerular filtration rate (**Table 6**).[55]

The differential diagnosis of AKI in patients with cirrhosis is broad and includes common causes such as acute tubular necrosis and nephrotoxicity, but specific glomerulopathies associated with hepatitis B virus and hepatitis C virus must be considered (ie, membranous and membranoproliferative glomerulonephritides) because prompt initiation of antiviral therapy may improve renal function.[56] Hepatorenal syndrome (HRS) is only one of several potential causes of AKI in patients with cirrhosis and portal hypertension. Recent changes in the nomenclature of HRS need to be highlighted: HRS-AKI and HRS-CKD replaced the previous terminology of HRS type 1 and HRS type 2, respectively.[57,58] The most recent diagnostic criteria for HRS-AKI are summarized in **Box 1**. HRS-CKD is more indolent and is associated with less severe renal impairment, typically resulting in ascites resistant to diuretics. Prognosis also differs significantly for both types of HRS, with the median survival in the absence of LT being 1 month for HRS-AKI and 6 months for HRS-CKD.[59]

Discontinuation of all diuretics and nephrotoxic agents is critical in patients with HRS. Plasma volume expansion with administration of intravenous albumin at a dose of 1 g/kg of body weight (up to a maximum of 100 g/day) to augment renal

Table 5 Stages of acute kidney injury	
Stage	Change in Serum Creatinine Level
1	Increase ≥0.3 mg/dL or ≥1.5-fold to 2-fold from baseline
1-A	Peak serum creatinine <1.5 mg/dL
1B	Peak serum creatinine ≥1.5 mg/dL
2	Increase >2-fold to 3-fold from baseline
3	Increase >3-fold from baseline or ≥4.0 mg/dL with an acute increase of ≥0.3 mg/dL or initiation of renal replacement therapy

Data from European Association for the Study of the Liver. Electronic address eee, European Association for the Study of the L. EASL Clinical Practice Guidelines for the management of patients with decompensated cirrhosis. Journal of hepatology 2018;69(2):406-460 and Angeli P, Gines P, Wong F, et al. Diagnosis and management of acute kidney injury in patients with cirrhosis: revised consensus recommendations of the International Club of Ascites. Journal of hepatology 2015;62(4):968-974; with permission.

Table 6
Stages of chronic kidney disease

CKD Stage	eGFR
Stage 1	>90 mL/min/1.73 m^2
Stage 2	60–89 mL/min/1.73 m^2
Stage 3a	45–59 mL/min/1.73 m^2
Stage 3b	30–44 mL/min/1.73 m^2
Stage 4	15–29 mL/min/1.73 m^2
Stage 5	<15 mL/min/1.73 m^2

Abbreviation: eGFR, estimated glomerular filtration rate.

perfusion is recommended. The combination of intravenous albumin and vasoconstrictors reduces short-term mortality in patients with HRS-AKI compared with albumin alone.[60] Most experts agree with reserving vasoconstrictors for patients with at least AKI stage 1-B (serum creatinine level ≥1.5 mg/dL), because of concerns about overuse of these drugs.[57] The choice of vasoconstrictor depends on availability of these agents, familiarity, and the level of care: midodrine and octreotide are commonly used in non–intensive care settings, whereas norepinephrine infusion typically requires intensive care monitoring and central venous access. Some evidence suggests that albumin in combination with norepinephrine may be superior to albumin plus midodrine and octreotide in reversing HRS-AKI.[60] Although not licensed in the United States, the vasopressin analogue terlipressin seems to be more effective in reversing HRS-AKI when used in combination with albumin compared with the combination of midodrine and octreotide.[61,62] The role of terlipressin in treatment of HRS-CKD is less well defined.

Renal replacement therapy (RRT), usually in the form of continuous venovenous hemofiltration (CVVH) or dialysis, may be considered for selected patients with HRS-AKI who fail to respond to medical therapy and are candidates for LT or for those expected to recover from a reversible form of liver injury. RRT is usually only indicated

Box 1
Criteria for diagnosis of hepatorenal syndrome–acute kidney injury

Cirrhosis with ascites

Diagnosis of AKI according to ICA AKI criteria

Absence of shock

No sustained improvement of renal function (sCr level <1.5 mg/dL) following at least 2 days of diuretic withdrawal, and volume expansion with albumin at 1 g/kg/d up to a maximum of 100 g/day

No current or recent exposure to nephrotoxic agents

Absence of parenchymal renal disease as defined by proteinuria less than 0.5 g/day, no microhematuria (<50 red cells/high-power field), and normal renal ultrasonography

Abbreviation: sCr, serum creatinine.

Adapted from Angeli P, Gines P, Wong F, et al. Diagnosis and management of acute kidney injury in patients with cirrhosis: revised consensus recommendations of the International Club of Ascites. Journal of hepatology 2015;62(4):968-974; with permission.

as a bridge to either isolated LT or simultaneous liver-kidney transplant in patients with HRS-AKI. Indications for RRT in patients with ESLD are similar to those for the general population: severe hyperkalemia refractory to medical therapy, metabolic acidosis not responding to medical therapy, and volume overload. CVVH is the preferred modality, because hypotension frequently occurs during hemodialysis. Additional complications include catheter-related infections and bleeding.

TIPS may improve renal function in patients with HRS and data from a recent observational study also suggest decreased inpatient mortality compared with dialysis.[63] TIPS placement is contraindicated in patients with severe hepatic dysfunction, which is common in patients with HRS-AKI.

PORTOPULMONARY HYPERTENSION

Pulmonary arterial hypertension in a patient with established portal hypertension indicates POPH, but other causes of pulmonary hypertension must be excluded before establishing this diagnosis.[64] The prevalence of POPH varies depending on the severity of liver disease; POPH has been reported in 0.7% of patients with cirrhosis but prevalence can be as high as 12.5% in patients with ESLD undergoing evaluation for LT.[65]

Most patients with POPH remain largely asymptomatic for extended periods of time; therefore, a high index of suspicion is needed for early diagnosis. Symptoms associated with POPH are similar to those of other types of pulmonary hypertension and include dyspnea on exertion, syncope, atypical chest pain, fatigue, hemoptysis, and orthopnea.[66] Physical examination may show jugular venous distention and lower extremity edema, the latter typically being out of proportion to the severity of ascites. Cardiopulmonary auscultation usually reveals normal clear breath sounds throughout both lung fields, an accentuated pulmonic component of the second heart sound, and a systolic murmur located along the left sternal border that is accentuated with inspiration (tricuspid regurgitation). Chest radiographs may show right ventricular enlargement and a prominent pulmonary artery.[67]

Diagnostic work-up for POPH should begin with transthoracic echocardiography, which provides an estimate of right ventricular and pulmonary arterial pressures and rules out left ventricular dysfunction.[68] An estimated right ventricular systolic pressure greater than 50 mm Hg or peak tricuspid regurgitant velocity greater than 2.8 m/s are commonly used echocardiographic thresholds to obtain more accurate direct hemodynamic measurements through right heart catheterization.[69] Hemodynamic criteria used to diagnose POPH include mean pulmonary artery pressure (mPAP) greater than 25 mm Hg, pulmonary capillary wedge pressure less than or equal to 15 mm Hg, and pulmonary vascular resistance greater than or equal to 240 dyn s cm^{-5} ($\geq$3 Wood units) on right heart catheterization.[70]

Pharmacologic therapy has been extrapolated from studies in idiopathic pulmonary hypertension, including endothelin receptor antagonists (bosentan, ambrisentan, and macitentan), phosphodiesterase inhibitors (sildenafil and tadalafil), and prostacyclin analogues (epoprostenol and iloprost).[71] Calcium channel blockers, commonly used to treat idiopathic pulmonary hypertension, are not recommended for treatment of POPH because of lesser vasoactive response and side effects including hypotension and systemic vasodilatation.[72] Nonselective β-blockers used for prophylaxis of gastroesophageal variceal hemorrhage should be avoided because they may exacerbate right heart failure.[73] In general, TIPS is contraindicated in patients with POPH, because it increases right heart preload. The cardiac hemodynamic effects of BRTO remain unknown.

Survival in POPH correlates with the severity of right ventricular dysfunction. The safety and efficacy of LT in patients with POPH are determined by the severity of pulmonary arterial hypertension. LT may be offered to selected patients with POPH but is typically contraindicated in those with mPAP greater than or equal to 35 mm Hg despite medical management, particularly if right ventricular dysfunction is present, because of considerable perioperative mortality.[74]

Waiting-list mortality in patients with POPH is determined by the severity of both liver and pulmonary dysfunction (assessed by peripheral vascular resistance); therefore, it is considered a MELD exception by the United Network for Organ Sharing (UNOS).[75] Patients listed for LT with POPH who have an adequate hemodynamic response to medical therapy (defined as mPAP <35 mm Hg and PVR <240 dyn s cm^{-5} by right heart catheterization) are eligible for a MELD exception score of 22 and accrue additional points (10% mortality equivalent) if sustained hemodynamic response is documented with repeat right heart catheterization every 3 months.

POPH can worsen during the immediate postoperative period in up to 20% of LT recipients, resulting in right heart dysfunction that requires escalation of pharmacotherapy.[76] Pulmonary pressures stabilize and even normalize in most LT recipients with POPH after 6 months (with continued pharmacotherapy).[77]

HEPATOPULMONARY SYNDROME

Hepatopulmonary syndrome (HPS) is characterized by hypoxemia caused by intrapulmonary vascular dilatations with right-to-left shunting in the presence of cirrhosis and portal hypertension. Although intrapulmonary vasodilatation can be found in more than 50% of patients with cirrhosis undergoing evaluation for LT, only 15% to 30% have hypoxemia and true HPS.[78] As with POPH, most patients with HPS are largely asymptomatic and screening relies on point-of-care oximetry indicating peripheral arterial oxygen saturation (Spo_2) less than 96% at rest and at sea level.[79] Hypoxemia must be confirmed by arterial blood gas analysis showing an arterial partial pressure of oxygen (Pao_2) less than 70 mm Hg and a widened alveolar-arterial oxygen gradient greater than or equal to 15 mm Hg ($\geq$20 mm Hg for patients 65 years of age or older).[80] Importantly, blood for arterial gas analysis should be obtained with the patient sitting upright, at rest, and breathing ambient air. After establishing a diagnosis of hypoxemia, documentation of pulmonary vascular dilatations with right-to-left blood shunting is necessary. Two-dimensional contrast-enhanced transthoracic echocardiography offers high sensitivity.[80] In patients with HPS, the presence of intrapulmonary right-to-left shunting caused by vascular dilatations results in the presence of microbubbles opacifying the left heart chambers after 3 or more heartbeats after being seen in the right ventricle. Intracardiac right-to-left blood shunting (ie, atrial or ventricular septal defects, patent foramen ovale) should be suspected if contrast is seen in the left heart within 3 heartbeats. Radionuclide lung perfusion scintigraphy using technetium-labeled macroaggregated albumin particles is less sensitive than contrast-enhanced echocardiography for diagnosis of HPS but is more specific and permits accurate quantification of the intrapulmonary shunt fraction, even in the presence of coexisting intrinsic lung disorders. Shunt fractions greater than 6% confirm the diagnosis of HPS in the appropriate clinical setting.[81,82]

HPS is associated with increased mortality and diminished quality of life compared with patients with cirrhosis but no HPS. Following the diagnosis of HPS, median survival is 10.6 months; thus, patients with HPS should undergo prompt evaluation for LT.[83] Under current organ allocation policies by UNOS, patients with HPS and Pao_2

less than 60 mm Hg are eligible for standard MELD exception scores regardless of their calculated (biological) MELD score. LT remains the definitive therapy for HPS based on marked improvement or even resolution of hypoxemia in more than 85% of transplant recipients; however, clinically meaningful changes may be slow and take up to 1 year following transplant.[84–87]

HEPATIC HYDROTHORAX

Hepatic hydrothorax is a transudative process leading to accumulation of greater than 500 mL of fluid in the pleural space in patients with cirrhosis and portal hypertension in the absence of a cardiac or pulmonary cause.[88] Fluid analysis shows similar chemical characteristics to ascites: high serum-to-pleural fluid albumin gradient (>1.1 g/dL) and low total protein concentration (<2.5 g/dL).[89]

Management of noninfected hepatic hydrothorax follows the same principles as for ascites: sodium restriction, diuretics, repeated thoracentesis, and placement of TIPS for refractory cases.[90] Importantly, indwelling pleural catheters should be avoided because of the high risk for complications, including infection, that may jeopardize candidacy for LT.

In patients with fevers and worsening pleuritic chest pain, spontaneous bacterial empyema (SBEM) must to be excluded. Similar to the diagnostic criteria for SBP, a diagnosis of SBEM is established by a PMN count greater than or equal to 250 cells/μL and a positive bacterial culture in the absence of a parapneumonic effusion. In cases in which bacterial cultures are negative, a PMN count threshold of greater than 500 cells/μL should be used to diagnose SBEM. Microorganisms involved are also similar to those responsible for SBP; therefore, third-generation cephalosporins remain the antibacterial agents of choice for empiric therapy.[91]

SUMMARY

Complications related to portal hypertension commonly occur in patients with ESLD and result in increased morbidity and mortality. Efforts should be directed at prompt identification and appropriate treatment to improve quality of life, diminish additional morbidity, reduce the potential risk of delisting from LT waiting list, and increase survival.

CLINICS CARE POINTS

- Screening for gastroesophageal varices with esophagogastroduodenoscopy is recommended if cirrhosis is suspected.
- A diagnostic paracentesis is mandatory in patients with new-onset ascites, change in clinical status including hospitalization of a patient with previously diagnosed ascites, and suggestion of spontaneous bacterial peritonitis.
- Diagnosis of spontaneous bacterial peritonitis is supported by the presence of $\geq$ 250 PMN/μL in the ascitic fluid without an obvious source of infection.
- Management of hepatorenal syndrome is centered on discontinuation of all diuretics and nephrotoxic agents, plasma volume expansion with administration of intravenous albumin, and vasoconstrictors.
- Liver transplant may be offered to selected patients with portopulmonary hypertension but is typically contraindicated in those with mPAP $\geq$ 35 mmHg despite medical management, particularly if right ventricular dysfunction is present, due to high perioperative mortality.

- Liver transplant is the definitive therapy for hepatopulmonary syndrome and results in marked improvement or even resolution of hypoxemia in more than 85% of transplant recipients.

DISCLOSURE

The authors have no conflicts of interest to disclose.

REFERENCES

1. Carrion AF, Aye L, Martin P. Patient selection for liver transplantation. Expert Rev Gastroenterol Hepatol 2013;7(6):571–9.

2. de Franchis R, Baveno VF. Revising consensus in portal hypertension: report of the Baveno V consensus workshop on methodology of diagnosis and therapy in portal hypertension. J Hepatol 2010;53(4):762–8.

3. Groszmann RJ, Wongcharatrawee S. The hepatic venous pressure gradient: anything worth doing should be done right. Hepatology 2004;39(2):280–2.

4. Groszmann RJ, Garcia-Tsao G, Bosch J, et al. Beta-blockers to prevent gastroesophageal varices in patients with cirrhosis. N Engl J Med 2005;353(21): 2254–61.

5. Kovalak M, Lake J, Mattek N, et al. Endoscopic screening for varices in cirrhotic patients: data from a national endoscopic database. Gastrointest Endosc 2007; 65(1):82–8.

6. North Italian Endoscopic Club for the Study Treatment of Esophageal Varices. Prediction of the first variceal hemorrhage in patients with cirrhosis of the liver and esophageal varices. A prospective multicenter study. N Engl J Med 1988; 319(15):983–9.

7. Garcia-Tsao G, Abraldes JG, Berzigotti A, et al. Portal hypertensive bleeding in cirrhosis: risk stratification, diagnosis, and management: 2016 practice guidance by the American Association for the study of liver diseases. Hepatology 2017; 65(1):310–35.

8. Puente A, Hernandez-Gea V, Graupera I, et al. Drugs plus ligation to prevent rebleeding in cirrhosis: an updated systematic review. Liver Int 2014;34(6):823–33.

9. Serste T, Melot C, Francoz C, et al. Deleterious effects of beta-blockers on survival in patients with cirrhosis and refractory ascites. Hepatology 2010;52(3): 1017–22.

10. Serste T, Francoz C, Durand F, et al. Beta-blockers cause paracentesis-induced circulatory dysfunction in patients with cirrhosis and refractory ascites: a crossover study. J Hepatol 2011;55(4):794–9.

11. Chirapongsathorn S, Valentin N, Alahdab F, et al. Nonselective beta-blockers and survival in patients with cirrhosis and ascites: a systematic review and meta-analysis. Clin Gastroenterol Hepatol 2016;14(8):1096–104.e9.

12. Facciorusso A, Roy S, Livadas S, et al. Nonselective beta-blockers do not affect survival in cirrhotic patients with ascites. Dig Dis Sci 2018;63(7):1737–46.

13. Wong RJ, Robinson A, Ginzberg D, et al. Assessing the safety of beta-blocker therapy in cirrhosis patients with ascites: a meta-analysis. Liver Int 2019;39(6): 1080–8.

14. Mishra SR, Sharma BC, Kumar A, et al. Primary prophylaxis of gastric variceal bleeding comparing cyanoacrylate injection and beta-blockers: a randomized controlled trial. J Hepatol 2011;54(6):1161–7.

15. Mishra SR, Chander Sharma B, Kumar A, et al. Endoscopic cyanoacrylate injection versus beta-blocker for secondary prophylaxis of gastric variceal bleed: a randomised controlled trial. Gut 2010;59(6):729–35.
16. Lo GH, Liang HL, Chen WC, et al. A prospective, randomized controlled trial of transjugular intrahepatic portosystemic shunt versus cyanoacrylate injection in the prevention of gastric variceal rebleeding. Endoscopy 2007;39(8):679–85.
17. Villanueva C, Colomo A, Bosch A, et al. Transfusion strategies for acute upper gastrointestinal bleeding. N Engl J Med 2013;368(1):11–21.
18. Bernard B, Grange JD, Khac EN, et al. Antibiotic prophylaxis for the prevention of bacterial infections in cirrhotic patients with gastrointestinal bleeding: a meta-analysis. Hepatology 1999;29(6):1655–61.
19. Chavez-Tapia NC, Barrientos-Gutierrez T, Tellez-Avila F, et al. Meta-analysis: antibiotic prophylaxis for cirrhotic patients with upper gastrointestinal bleeding - an updated Cochrane review. Aliment Pharmacol Ther 2011;34(5):509–18.
20. Wells M, Chande N, Adams P, et al. Meta-analysis: vasoactive medications for the management of acute variceal bleeds. Aliment Pharmacol Ther 2012;35(11):1267–78.
21. Hayat U, Lee PJ, Ullah H, et al. Association of prophylactic endotracheal intubation in critically ill patients with upper GI bleeding and cardiopulmonary unplanned events. Gastrointest Endosc 2017;86(3):500–9.e1.
22. Dai C, Liu WX, Jiang M, et al. Endoscopic variceal ligation compared with endoscopic injection sclerotherapy for treatment of esophageal variceal hemorrhage: a meta-analysis. World J Gastroenterol 2015;21(8):2534–41.
23. Laine L, Cook D. Endoscopic ligation compared with sclerotherapy for treatment of esophageal variceal bleeding. A meta-analysis. Ann Intern Med 1995;123(4):280–7.
24. Escorsell A, Pavel O, Cardenas A, et al. Esophageal balloon tamponade versus esophageal stent in controlling acute refractory variceal bleeding: a multicenter randomized, controlled trial. Hepatology 2016;63(6):1957–67.
25. Garcia-Pagan JC, Caca K, Bureau C, et al. Early use of TIPS in patients with cirrhosis and variceal bleeding. N Engl J Med 2010;362(25):2370–9.
26. Unger LW, Stork T, Bucsics T, et al. The role of TIPS in the management of liver transplant candidates. United European Gastroenterol J 2017;5(8):1100–7.
27. Gines P, Fernandez-Esparrach G, Arroyo V, et al. Pathogenesis of ascites in cirrhosis. Semin Liver Dis 1997;17(3):175–89.
28. Runyon BA. Care of patients with ascites. N Engl J Med 1994;330(5):337–42.
29. El-Bokl MA, Senousy BE, El-Karmouty KZ, et al. Spot urinary sodium for assessing dietary sodium restriction in cirrhotic ascites. World J Gastroenterol 2009;15(29):3631–5.
30. Sehgal R, Singh H, Singh IP. Comparative study of spironolactone and eplerenone in management of ascites in patients of cirrhosis of liver. Eur J Gastroenterol Hepatol 2020;32(4):535–9.
31. Runyon BA, Committee APG. Management of adult patients with ascites due to cirrhosis: an update. Hepatology 2009;49(6):2087–107.
32. Bernardi M, Caraceni P, Navickis RJ, et al. Albumin infusion in patients undergoing large-volume paracentesis: a meta-analysis of randomized trials. Hepatology 2012;55(4):1172–81.
33. Yosry A, Soliman ZA, Eletreby R, et al. Oral midodrine is comparable to albumin infusion in cirrhotic patients with refractory ascites undergoing large-volume paracentesis: results of a pilot study. Eur J Gastroenterol Hepatol 2019;31(3):345–51.

34. Salerno F, Merli M, Riggio O, et al. Randomized controlled study of TIPS versus paracentesis plus albumin in cirrhosis with severe ascites. Hepatology 2004; 40(3):629–35.

35. Bureau C, Thabut D, Oberti F, et al. Transjugular intrahepatic portosystemic shunts with covered stents increase transplant-free survival of patients with cirrhosis and recurrent ascites. Gastroenterology 2017;152(1):157–63.

36. Billey C, Billet S, Robic MA, et al. A prospective study identifying predictive factors of cardiac decompensation after transjugular intrahepatic portosystemic shunt: the toulouse algorithm. Hepatology 2019;70(6):1928–41.

37. Kim HK, Kim YJ, Chung WJ, et al. Clinical outcomes of transjugular intrahepatic portosystemic shunt for portal hypertension: Korean multicenter real-practice data. Clin Mol Hepatol 2014;20(1):18–27.

38. Pereira K, Carrion AF, Martin P, et al. Current diagnosis and management of post-transjugular intrahepatic portosystemic shunt refractory hepatic encephalopathy. Liver Int 2015;35(12):2487–94.

39. Llovet JM, Bartoli R, Planas R, et al. Bacterial translocation in cirrhotic rats. Its role in the development of spontaneous bacterial peritonitis. Gut 1994;35(11): 1648–52.

40. Runyon BA, Squier S, Borzio M. Translocation of gut bacteria in rats with cirrhosis to mesenteric lymph nodes partially explains the pathogenesis of spontaneous bacterial peritonitis. J Hepatol 1994;21(5):792–6.

41. Hoefs JC, Canawati HN, Sapico FL, et al. Spontaneous bacterial peritonitis. Hepatology 1982;2(4):399–407.

42. European Association for the Study of the Liver. EASL Clinical Practice Guidelines for the management of patients with decompensated cirrhosis. J Hepatol 2018; 69(2):406–60.

43. Sort P, Navasa M, Arroyo V, et al. Effect of intravenous albumin on renal impairment and mortality in patients with cirrhosis and spontaneous bacterial peritonitis. N Engl J Med 1999;341(6):403–9.

44. Arroyo V, Garcia-Martinez R, Salvatella X. Human serum albumin, systemic inflammation, and cirrhosis. J Hepatol 2014;61(2):396–407.

45. Saab S, Hernandez JC, Chi AC, et al. Oral antibiotic prophylaxis reduces spontaneous bacterial peritonitis occurrence and improves short-term survival in cirrhosis: a meta-analysis. Am J Gastroenterol 2009;104(4):993–1001 [quiz: 1002].

46. Goel GA, Deshpande A, Lopez R, et al. Increased rate of spontaneous bacterial peritonitis among cirrhotic patients receiving pharmacologic acid suppression. Clin Gastroenterol Hepatol 2012;10(4):422–7.

47. Choi YJ, Kim JH, Koo JK, et al. Prevalence of renal dysfunction in patients with cirrhosis according to ADQI-IAC working party proposal. Clin Mol Hepatol 2014;20(2):185–91.

48. Warner NS, Cuthbert JA, Bhore R, et al. Acute kidney injury and chronic kidney disease in hospitalized patients with cirrhosis. J Invest Med 2011;59(8):1244–51.

49. Cardenas A, Gines P, Uriz J, et al. Renal failure after upper gastrointestinal bleeding in cirrhosis: incidence, clinical course, predictive factors, and short-term prognosis. Hepatology 2001;34(4 Pt 1):671–6.

50. Carvalho GC, Regis Cde A, Kalil JR, et al. Causes of renal failure in patients with decompensated cirrhosis and its impact in hospital mortality. Ann Hepatol 2012; 11(1):90–5.

51. Montoliu S, Balleste B, Planas R, et al. Incidence and prognosis of different types of functional renal failure in cirrhotic patients with ascites. Clin Gastroenterol Hepatol 2010;8(7):616–22 [quiz: e680].
52. Palevsky PM, Liu KD, Brophy PD, et al. KDOQI US commentary on the 2012 KDIGO clinical practice guideline for acute kidney injury. Am J Kidney Dis 2013;61(5):649–72.
53. Fagundes C, Barreto R, Guevara M, et al. A modified acute kidney injury classification for diagnosis and risk stratification of impairment of kidney function in cirrhosis. J Hepatol 2013;59(3):474–81.
54. Huelin P, Piano S, Sola E, et al. Validation of a staging system for acute kidney injury in patients with cirrhosis and association with acute-on-chronic liver failure. Clin Gastroenterol Hepatol 2017;15(3):438–45.e5.
55. Levey AS, Eckardt KU, Tsukamoto Y, et al. Definition and classification of chronic kidney disease: a position statement from Kidney Disease: Improving Global Outcomes (KDIGO). Kidney Int 2005;67(6):2089–100.
56. Fabrizi F, Martin P, Messa P. Hepatitis B and hepatitis C virus and chronic kidney disease. Acta Gastroenterol Belg 2010;73(4):465–71.
57. Angeli P, Gines P, Wong F, et al. Diagnosis and management of acute kidney injury in patients with cirrhosis: revised consensus recommendations of the International Club of Ascites. J Hepatol 2015;62(4):968–74.
58. Angeli P, Garcia-Tsao G, Nadim MK, et al. News in pathophysiology, definition and classification of hepatorenal syndrome: a step beyond the International Club of Ascites (ICA) consensus document. J Hepatol 2019;71(4):811–22.
59. Alessandria C, Ozdogan O, Guevara M, et al. MELD score and clinical type predict prognosis in hepatorenal syndrome: relevance to liver transplantation. Hepatology 2005;41(6):1282–9.
60. Facciorusso A, Chandar AK, Murad MH, et al. Comparative efficacy of pharmacological strategies for management of type 1 hepatorenal syndrome: a systematic review and network meta-analysis. Lancet Gastroenterol Hepatol 2017;2(2):94–102.
61. Cavallin M, Kamath PS, Merli M, et al. Terlipressin plus albumin versus midodrine and octreotide plus albumin in the treatment of hepatorenal syndrome: a randomized trial. Hepatology 2015;62(2):567–74.
62. Nanda A, Reddy R, Safraz H, et al. Pharmacological therapies for hepatorenal syndrome: a systematic review and meta-analysis. J Clin Gastroenterol 2018;52(4):360–7.
63. Charilaou P, Devani K, Petrosyan R, et al. Inpatient mortality benefit with transjugular intrahepatic portosystemic shunt for hospitalized hepatorenal syndrome patients. Dig Dis Sci 2020. https://doi.org/10.1007/s10620-020-06136-2.
64. Kochar R, Fallon MB. Pulmonary diseases and the liver. Clin Liver Dis 2011;15(1):21–37.
65. Machicao VI, Balakrishnan M, Fallon MB. Pulmonary complications in chronic liver disease. Hepatology 2014;59(4):1627–37.
66. Hadengue A, Benhayoun MK, Lebrec D, et al. Pulmonary hypertension complicating portal hypertension: prevalence and relation to splanchnic hemodynamics. Gastroenterology 1991;100(2):520–8.
67. Robalino BD, Moodie DS. Association between primary pulmonary hypertension and portal hypertension: analysis of its pathophysiology and clinical, laboratory and hemodynamic manifestations. J Am Coll Cardiol 1991;17(2):492–8.
68. Galie N, Humbert M, Vachiery JL, et al. 2015 ESC/ERS guidelines for the diagnosis and treatment of pulmonary hypertension: the Joint Task Force for the

diagnosis and treatment of pulmonary hypertension of the European Society of Cardiology (ESC) and the European Respiratory Society (ERS): endorsed by: association for European Paediatric and Congenital Cardiology (AEPC), International Society for Heart and Lung Transplantation (ISHLT). Eur Respir J 2015; 46(4):903–75.

69. Krowka MJ, Swanson KL, Frantz RP, et al. Portopulmonary hypertension: results from a 10-year screening algorithm. Hepatology 2006;44(6):1502–10.

70. Goldberg DS, Fallon MB. The art and science of diagnosing and treating lung and heart disease secondary to liver disease. Clin Gastroenterol Hepatol 2015; 13(12):2118–27.

71. Raevens S, De Pauw M, Reyntjens K, et al. Oral vasodilator therapy in patients with moderate to severe portopulmonary hypertension as a bridge to liver transplantation. Eur J Gastroenterol Hepatol 2013;25(4):495–502.

72. Montani D, Savale L, Natali D, et al. Long-term response to calcium-channel blockers in non-idiopathic pulmonary arterial hypertension. Eur Heart J 2010; 31(15):1898–907.

73. Provencher S, Herve P, Jais X, et al. Deleterious effects of beta-blockers on exercise capacity and hemodynamics in patients with portopulmonary hypertension. Gastroenterology 2006;130(1):120–6.

74. Krowka MJ, Plevak DJ, Findlay JY, et al. Pulmonary hemodynamics and perioperative cardiopulmonary-related mortality in patients with portopulmonary hypertension undergoing liver transplantation. Liver Transplant 2000;6(4):443–50.

75. DuBrock HM, Goldberg DS, Sussman NL, et al. Predictors of waitlist mortality in portopulmonary hypertension. Transplantation 2017;101(7):1609–15.

76. Acosta F, Sansano T, Palenciano CG, et al. Portopulmonary hypertension and liver transplantation: hemodynamic consequences at reperfusion. Transplant Proc 2005;37(9):3865–6.

77. Reymond M, Barbier L, Salame E, et al. Does portopulmonary hypertension impede liver transplantation in cirrhotic patients? a French multicentric retrospective study. Transplantation 2018;102(4):616–22.

78. Koch DG, Fallon MB. Hepatopulmonary syndrome. Clin Liver Dis 2014;18(2): 407–20.

79. Arguedas MR, Singh H, Faulk DK, et al. Utility of pulse oximetry screening for hepatopulmonary syndrome. Clin Gastroenterol Hepatol 2007;5(6):749–54.

80. Rodriguez-Roisin R, Krowka MJ. Hepatopulmonary syndrome–a liver-induced lung vascular disorder. N Engl J Med 2008;358(22):2378–87.

81. Lange PA, Stoller JK. The hepatopulmonary syndrome. Ann Intern Med 1995; 122(7):521–9.

82. Krowka MJ. Management of pulmonary complications in pretransplant patients. Clin Liver Dis 2011;15(4):765–77.

83. Schenk P, Schoniger-Hekele M, Fuhrmann V, et al. Prognostic significance of the hepatopulmonary syndrome in patients with cirrhosis. Gastroenterology 2003; 125(4):1042–52.

84. Swanson KL, Wiesner RH, Krowka MJ. Natural history of hepatopulmonary syndrome: impact of liver transplantation. Hepatology 2005;41(5):1122–9.

85. Arguedas MR, Abrams GA, Krowka MJ, et al. Prospective evaluation of outcomes and predictors of mortality in patients with hepatopulmonary syndrome undergoing liver transplantation. Hepatology 2003;37(1):192–7.

86. Krowka MJ, Mandell MS, Ramsay MA, et al. Hepatopulmonary syndrome and portopulmonary hypertension: a report of the multicenter liver transplant database. Liver Transplant 2004;10(2):174–82.

87. Gupta S, Castel H, Rao RV, et al. Improved survival after liver transplantation in patients with hepatopulmonary syndrome. Am J Transplant 2010;10(2):354–63.
88. Cardenas A, Kelleher T, Chopra S. Review article: hepatic hydrothorax. Aliment Pharmacol Ther 2004;20(3):271–9.
89. Badillo R, Rockey DC. Hepatic hydrothorax: clinical features, management, and outcomes in 77 patients and review of the literature. Medicine 2014;93(3):135–42.
90. Dhanasekaran R, West JK, Gonzales PC, et al. Transjugular intrahepatic porto-systemic shunt for symptomatic refractory hepatic hydrothorax in patients with cirrhosis. Am J Gastroenterol 2010;105(3):635–41.
91. Xiol X, Castellvi JM, Guardiola J, et al. Spontaneous bacterial empyema in cirrhotic patients: a prospective study. Hepatology 1996;23(4):719–23.

Expanding Donor Selection and Recipient Indications for Living Donor Liver Transplantation

Akshata Moghe, MD, PhD[a], Swaytha Ganesh, MD[b],
Abhinav Humar, MD[c], Michele Molinari, MD, MSc[d],
Naudia Jonassaint, MD, MHS[e],*

KEYWORDS

- Living donor • Liver transplant • Extended criteria • Transplant oncology

KEY POINTS

- Living donor liver transplantation (LDLT) can play a significant role in increasing the national donor pool.
- Donor selection criteria are being expanded with the help of surgical innovation, increasing technical expertise, and novel outcomes data.
- Donor organ pool expansion requires a structured and robust initiative promoting public awareness and education.
- The growth of LDLT programs nationally will help meet the organ demand created by expansion of recipient indications (eg, HCC outside of Milan, cholangiocarcinoma, metastatic colorectal cancer).

[a] Division of Gastroenterology, Hepatology and Nutrition, Department of Medicine, University of Pittsburgh Medical Center, Mezzanine Level, C-Wing, PUH 200 Lothrop Street, Pittsburgh, PA 15213, USA; [b] Living Donor Liver Transplantation Program, Department of Medicine, University of Pittsburgh Medical Center, Center for Liver Diseases, 3471 Fifth Avenue, 900 Kaufmann Building, Pittsburgh, PA 15213, USA; [c] Division of Abdominal Transplantation Surgery, Thomas E. Starzl Transplantation Institute, University of Pittsburgh Medical Center, UPMC Montefiore, Seventh Floor – N723, 3459 Fifth Avenue, Pittsburgh, PA 15213, USA; [d] Department of Surgery, University of Pittsburgh Medical Center, UPMC Montefiore, N761, 3459 Fifth Avenue, Pittsburgh, PA 15213, USA; [e] Division of Gastroenterology, Hepatology, and Nutrition, Department of Medicine, University of Pittsburgh Medical Center, Center for Liver Diseases, 3471 Fifth Avenue, 900 Kaufmann Building, Pittsburgh, PA 15213, USA
* Corresponding author.
E-mail address: jonassaintnl@upmc.edu
Twitter: @AkshataMoghe (A.M.); @nljonassaint (N.J.)

Clin Liver Dis 25 (2021) 121–135
https://doi.org/10.1016/j.cld.2020.08.011
1089-3261/21/© 2020 Elsevier Inc. All rights reserved.

liver.theclinics.com

INTRODUCTION

Each year in the United States, only about 8000 of the 14,000 patients awaiting transplantation receive a liver transplant.[1] Nearly 25% of patients die while awaiting liver transplantation and another 10% get delisted[2] because of disease progression. A significant shortage of deceased donor organs is the prime reason for waitlisted patients not receiving a transplant. The shortfall between the number of patients listed for liver transplantation and the available grafts can potentially be addressed by living donor liver transplantation (LDLT). LDLT is an effective and safe method that increases the donor pool, improves the likelihood of timely transplants, and extends the survival of patients. Despite the proven benefits of LDLT,[3] uptake in the United States has been slow,[4] and widespread implementation of LDLT has been limited, because of concerns about donor risk. In addition, there is a perception that healthy individuals will not be willing to donate and therefore many programs are challenged with identifying and enrolling living donors.

However, some programs in the United States and globally have successfully adopted LDLT.[3,4] Growth in LDLT volume has led to an increase in LDLT surgical expertise, which in turn has paved the path for technical innovation in LDLT at these centers.[4] Success, in the form of decreased transplant list waiting time and waitlist mortality, has prompted expansion of recipient indications for LDLT. Now, traditional donor selection criteria are also being challenged and expanded, while trying to balance donor safety with recipient and graft survival.

In this article, we present the current knowledge of donor selection criteria and recipient indications for LDLT, and describe the recent advances made on these fronts. We also present a comprehensive patient support program that may serve as a model for programs trying to expand LDLT, by supporting recipients in identifying their own donor.

EXPANDING DONOR SELECTION CRITERIA
Donor Body Mass Index and Hepatic Graft Steatosis

With the rising prevalence of obesity, increasing body mass index (BMI) of potential donors has become a real obstacle to LDLT. A higher BMI frequently, but not always, correlates with hepatic steatosis. In a 2001 study with 33 potential live donors, no donor with a BMI less than 25 had histologic evidence of hepatic steatosis, but 76% of the donors with a BMI greater than 28 had steatosis on liver biopsy.[5] At some transplant centers, potential donors who are obese (BMI >30), or those who have hepatic steatosis on imaging, might undergo a liver biopsy as part of the donor evaluation. Donors with BMI greater than 35 are frequently excluded at the outset. Potential donors with macrovesicular steatosis of greater than 10% on biopsy are also excluded, whereas microvesicular steatosis is less of a concern.[6,7]

The reason for this practice is the body of literature that has demonstrated that moderate to severe steatosis in the graft can lead to primary nonfunction, reduced graft survival, ischemia-reperfusion injury, and biliary strictures.[8,9] However, a more recent systematic review of 3226 recipients demonstrated that even though short-term outcomes were unfavorable, longer-term outcomes, such as 1-year mortality, were similar to control subjects without moderate-severe hepatic steatosis.[10] Another recent study in recipients of right-lobe grafts showed that after matching for age, Model for End-Stage Liver Disease (MELD), and graft recipient weight ratio (GRWR), the short-term outcomes of graft function, postoperative morbidity, hospital stay, and 30-day mortality were similar for grafts with less than 10% steatosis and grafts with 10% to 20% steatosis.[11]

Knaak and colleagues[12] from Toronto, asked the important question of whether donor obesity without hepatic steatosis has an independent impact on transplant outcomes. They found that right-lobe donation from donors with a BMI greater than or equal to 30 but with hepatic steatosis of less than 10% and no other comorbidity had similar donor and recipient outcomes including recipient graft function, surgical complications, and hospital stay.[12] Overall, it has become clear that there is a complex interplay of multiple donor and recipient factors in the decision to use a graft from an obese donor. Even so, the key factors that are pushing the boundaries of donor BMI are the growing surgical expertise in LDLT and the rapidly advancing science of medical management of LDLT donors and recipients.

Donor Age

Donor age is a well-known prognosticator of outcomes in liver transplantation. The impact of donor age on recipient survival in adult-to-adult LDLT has been studied. In a study by Kubota and colleagues,[13] donors from age 20 to 67 years were studied. Donor age was divided into five groups: 20s, 30s, 40s, 50s, and 60s. Not surprisingly, this study demonstrated that recipient survival is the best with the youngest group of donors (20s). However, what this study does not answer one might argue is the more critical question: Does recipient survival differ between those with a donor in their 50s versus 60s? In extrapolating from this study, at 1 year, 67 of 94 (71%) recipients were alive when they received a graft from a donor in their 50s, whereas 25 of 32 (78%) recipients were alive at 1 year when they received a graft from a donor in their 60s.[13] The clinical significance of these numbers is unclear but suggest that pushing the age limits for donor may be one safe way to increase the donor pool.

Although most of the focus has largely been on the appropriateness of older recipients, some have pushed the envelope in terms of accepting younger donors. The hesitation in accepting younger donors for centers focuses on the concern that the young donors (age <18) lack a deep understanding of the possible complications that may arise and their long-term implications. Nonetheless, a standard age cutoff might be deemed somewhat arbitrary because maturity is starkly different in two persons of the same age. Teenagers are allowed to drive at the age of 16, knowing that there is a significant risk of fatal car crashes in this group, nearly 1.5 times higher than in those just 2 years older.[14] The University of Toronto has tested this idea after getting to know a 16-year-old son and allowing him to donate to his mother at the age of 17; and now has the policy that persons older than the age of 16 can be evaluated as donors.[15]

Although we acknowledge the importance of center guidelines for age limits, we believe that each potential donor deserves individual consideration. The level of maturity of young donors should be rigorously assessed by members of the multidisciplinary transplant team before arriving at a consensus. In addition, when considering older donors, protocols need to be developed for performing a sound physiologic assessment rather than simply a chronologic one. The age limits for LDLT require continued exploration as ways to increase the donor pool are examined.

Graft Recipient Weight Ratio

Compared with the full-size grafts of deceased donors, the smaller volume of single-lobe grafts from live donors has frequently garnered concern regarding outcomes, especially during LDLT in sicker recipients. A GRWR of at least 0.8 has been generally considered a prerequisite for right lobe LDLT, based on initial LDLT literature from Asia. Several transplant centers still use this cutoff, even though subsequent research has shown good outcomes with smaller grafts.[16] A 2009 study from Toronto compared outcomes in LDLT recipients with a GRWR of 0.59 to 0.79, LDLT recipients with a GRWR of greater than or equal to 0.8, and deceased donor liver transplant recipients with full-sized grafts. The study demonstrated similar patient outcomes of reperfusion injury (peak aspartate aminotransferase and alanine aminotransferase), graft function, complications, and graft and patient survival across all three groups. This study challenged the safe lower limit of GRWR for LDLT.[16] A more recent study investigated the use of absolute graft weight rather than a GRWR of 0.8. The study found that a cutoff value of 643 g for the right lobe provided the highest positive predictive value (94%) for a good outcome in recipients with GRWR less than 0.8; with 15 (19.4%) deaths in the group with absolute graft weight less than 643 g and only 5 (7.1%) deaths in the group with absolute graft weight greater than or equal to 643 g.[17]

Wong and colleagues[18] published a study in 2020 that concluded that the incidence of small-for-size-syndrome (SFSS; defined as GRWR <0.8) could be kept low even with a GRWR of 0.6, if meticulous care was taken with recipient selection, surgical technique including the use of portal flow modulation, and perioperative management. Their findings were in agreement with a meta-analysis of 1821 LDLT recipients that showed inferior medium-term (3-year) but comparable long-term (5-year) graft survival with SFSS, with the use of appropriate flow modulatory measures,[19] once again highlighting the importance of scrupulous surgical protocols for improving patient outcomes.

ABO Incompatibility

ABO incompatibility is usually thought of as a relative contraindication to transplantation because of a fear of humoral or antibody-mediated rejection. The susceptibility to rejection is thought to be driven by antigens expressed on the vascular endothelium and bile ducts driving hyperacute rejection and biliary complications.[20,21] Although the early outcomes for ABO-incompatible (ABOi) transplant were poor,[22,23] ABOi liver transplantation was not abandoned.[24] The need to expand the donor pool, particularly in Asian centers, drove the improvement of clinical protocols.[24,25]

To overcome the initial poor outcomes in ABOi transplants, high-dose immunosuppression, splenectomy, and plasmapheresis were instituted with little change in the initial outcomes.[26,27] With the addition of rituximab to the surgical conditioning regimen, the outcomes of ABOi LDLT have shown similar survival rates to ABO-compatible LDLT.[28] In a study by Egawa and colleagues,[28] 381 ABOi LDLT in the prerituximab and postrituximab era were studied and an increase in 3-year survival from 30% to 80% from the prerituximab era and the postrituximab era. A meta-analysis by Yadav and colleagues[29] suggests that there is no significant difference in 1-, 3-, and 5-year survival in ABO-compatible versus ABOi liver transplants with rituximab prophylaxis. However, increased rates of cytomegalovirus infection, antibody-mediated rejection, and biliary complications emphasize the importance of a formal desensitization protocol and careful consideration of the donor characteristics when selecting recipients for ABOi LDLT.[29,30] Another consideration to overcome the issue of ABO-incompatibility is the possibility of a paired organ exchange or swap, which allows for recipients to swap donors for compatibility.[31] If such a swap negating the issue of ABO incompatibility is available, it is preferred. If a swap is not available, ABOi LDLT remains a viable option in selected recipients.

Dual-Graft Adult Living Donor Liver Transplantation

A novel surgical technique that was developed to overcome the issue of SFSS while ensuring donor safety is the dual-graft technique, first described by Lee and colleagues[32] in 2001. This technique uses smaller grafts from two living donors into one recipient, thus ensuring adequate residual liver in the donor while avoiding SFSS in the recipient; and has been successfully adopted in selected cases of LDLT, especially in Asia in the past few years.[33–35] As rising obesity in the recipient population is balanced with optimal BMI donors, the dual-graft technique is expected to gain popularity in the western world.

In summary, it is fair to say that this is an exciting time where the boundaries for selection of living donors are being pushed more than ever before. The limits of donor BMI, age, and graft steatosis are expanding not only because of vigorous outcomes research, but also because of major advances in technical innovation and increasing expertise in LDLT surgery. In the next several years, the driving forces for donor criteria expansion will be the multidisciplinary teams supporting the LDLT enterprise, including but not limited to transplant hepatology, transplant infectious disease, psychiatry, and physical therapy.[36]

EXPANDING THE DONOR ORGAN POOL
Living Donor Champion Program

LDLT is a lifesaving option for many patients but finding a living donor can serve as a significant barrier to surgery. To overcome the challenge of finding a donor, Johns Hopkins created a Live Donor Champion Program for kidney transplantation in 2010[37] that has subsequently been adapted across the country. Expanding this model to liver transplantation, the University of Pittsburgh created the Living Donor Champion Program in June 2017.[3,38] Recognizing that much of the burden for finding a donor typically falls on the patient, the program attempts to alleviate that burden.

The first step in the program asks the patient to identify a surrogate (champion) to advocate for them. The champion is the recipient's primary advocate in identifying a living donor using the program's multipronged strategy and resources. This allows the patient to concentrate on the management of their liver disease while their surrogate champions their cause. The next part of the process is raising public awareness regarding live donation through public education efforts, such as town hall style meetings, our program Web site, social media outreach via Twitter and a Facebook support group, and radio and television commercials. Lastly, we provide an additional level of personal support to the recipient and their champion by providing one-on-one support of a transplant team member we call the Live Donor Ambassador. All of these efforts together (**Fig. 1**) have created successful and sustained growth in the LDLT program at the University of Pittsburgh (**Fig. 2**).

Anonymous Live Donation

Unrelated LDLT has been considered over the last two decades as a response to the national organ shortage. This involves donation to a recipient from someone with no biologic connection or prior relationship.[39] The donation may be directed (preidentified) or nondirected, often referred to as altruistic donation. This form of transplantation is allowed in some countries including the United States, Canada, Saudi Arabia, and the Netherlands and prohibited in other countries, such as Poland, Italy, and France suggesting that controversies surrounding the ethics of unrelated donation still persist.[39] In a recent study, the Toronto group led by Goldaracena and colleagues[40] described their 12-year experience with anonymous donation. The group explored anonymous donor characteristics, drivers for donation, and patient outcomes. Most donors in this study reported feeling compelled to perform a kind act or good deed after an appeal from potential recipients. In addition, this study suggested that anonymous donation can have a sustainable impact on the growth of the donor pool,

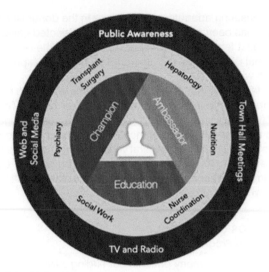

Fig. 1. Elements of the Living Donor Champion program.

representing 6.7% (50/743) of the total number of LDLTs performed by the Toronto group over the 12 years, and 2.5% (50/2037) of the total number of liver transplants. The overall donor and recipient outcomes were excellent, with 1-year recipient survival of 91% for adult recipients and 98% for children, no donor deaths, and only one Dindo-Clavien grade 3 donor complication with complete resolution.[40] The possible impact of anonymous live donation is summarized best by the authors when they point out that if 1 in every 17,000 US citizens between the ages of 18 and 65 years anonymously donated there would be no liver transplant waiting list.[40] The controversies

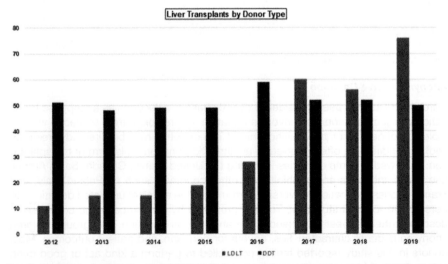

Fig. 2. Number of adult-to-adult LDLT and deceased donor liver transplants (DDT) at the University of Pittsburgh (2012–2019).

surrounding anonymous live donation will continue but this study helps to understand the possible impact of anonymous donation on increasing the size of the donor pool.

EXPANDING RECIPIENT INDICATIONS

LDLT helps all patients that may benefit from liver transplantation but more notably, presents a unique opportunity to offer timely liver transplants to patients who fall outside of the conventional United Network for Organ Sharing criteria. In this section, we explore some of the extended recipient indications that have a reasonable chance of success with LDLT. LDLT is the avenue to test the outcomes of liver transplantation in this population where drawing organs from the limited deceased donor pool cannot be currently justified. Over time, if LDLT proves successful, new vistas of management for these patients will have been opened.

Metastatic Colorectal Carcinoma

Transplantation as a modality for treatment of colorectal liver metastasis (CLM) was first attempted in the initial cohort of human liver transplants,[41] abandoned because of poor outcomes, and then revisited years later.[42,43] One of the seminal investigations in this area was a small prospective study (SECA trial) conducted in 2013 to assess survival in patients with CLM following liver transplantation.[44] For the 21 patients without extrahepatic disease in the SECA trial, median survival was 27 months and the 1-, 3-, and 5-year survival was 95%, 68%, and 60%, respectively.[44] Notably, this trial had no standardized protocol for the administration of neoadjuvant or adjuvant chemotherapy. The study demonstrated that median time to recurrence for patients transplanted for CLM was 6 months. However, if recurrence of disease was outside the liver, primarily pulmonary, 5-year survival was 72%.[45]

Such studies on liver transplantation for CLM have made an increasingly compelling argument for consideration of liver transplantation for patients with CLM given the improvement in patient survival compared with standard chemotherapy alone.[46] There are no prospective data on liver transplantation compared with modern chemotherapeutic agents or multimodal treatments, but trials are ongoing[47] to answer these questions. Nevertheless, the current literature clearly suggests that select patients with CLM benefit from transplantation. These patients are often disadvantaged by low MELDNa scores, making them noncompetitive on the transplant wait-list. CLM is therefore, an indication well-suited for LDLT.

Hepatocellular Carcinoma Outside Milan Criteria

The original Milan criteria for liver transplantation in patients with hepatocellular carcinoma (HCC) were published nearly 30 years ago.[48] In their 1996 *New England Journal of Medicine* paper, Mazzaferro and colleagues[49] defined the criteria that are still considered the gold standard in many transplant centers around the world. Fifteen years later, they published a meta-analysis confirming a statistically significant survival benefit with liver transplantation for patients with HCC within the Milan criteria as compared with patients with HCC exceeding the Milan criteria on explant pathology, with a hazard ratio of 1.68.

However, over time, many centers found the Milan criteria too restrictive, and attempted to use less stringent criteria for transplantation. Of these, the most well-known are the University of San Francisco criteria that were published in 2001.[50] These criteria increased the tumor size limit while maintaining comparable 1-year and 5-year survival rates to the Milan criteria. The next major advance came a decade later, with the extended Toronto Criteria.[51] Research had shown that imaging findings frequently understage or overstage HCC, and that tumor size and number did not always go hand-in-hand with tumor biology.[52–55] The Toronto group studied patients with HCC who met Milan criteria (M; n = 189) and exceeded Milan criteria (M+; n = 105) and underwent liver transplantation between 1996 and 2008. They found no difference in the 5-year overall or recurrence-free survival between the 2 groups. However, excluding patients with poorly differentiated tumors and aggressive pre-transplant bridging therapies significantly improved overall survival in the M+ group. Hence, the extended Toronto Criteria advocated for a protocol biopsy to rule out aggressive features in the largest tumor, but had no limitations on the size or number of tumors present.[51] They also noted that serum α-fetoprotein greater than or equal to 400 ng/mL associated with poorer recurrence-free survival.[51]

Several other attempts have since been made to expand transplant criteria for HCC (**Table 1**). Many of these criteria successfully captured a subset of patients outside of the Milan criteria for whom one could still expect outcomes similar to those within the Milan criteria. These criteria have pushed the limits of tumor size and number, refined patient selection by factoring in key laboratory tests, and included patients with segmental portal vein thrombosis.[56–59] Over the years, multiple studies have validated several of the criteria.[49,60–64] However, the quest for refining the criteria continues, with the ultimate aim of being most inclusive and still producing the most acceptable transplant outcomes. For a cancer where the only curative treatment today is transplantation, this quest is a noble one.

Severe Acute Alcoholic Hepatitis

After many years of US transplant programs defaulting to the 6-month rule for sobriety, the issue of transplantation in severe acute alcoholic hepatitis again gained attention with the paper by Mathurin and colleagues[65] in 2011. This study looked at the benefit of early transplantation in severe acute alcoholic hepatitis and demonstrated a survival benefit in those patients who underwent early transplantation (<2%) versus matched control subjects (77 ± 8% vs 23 ± 8%). Patients who did not undergo early transplantation were typically excluded because of "unfavorable social or familial profiles."[65]

Despite the clear survival benefit, transplantation for severe alcoholic hepatitis is still controversial. Given their acute severity of illness, these patients are immediately placed at a high priority for transplantation ahead of other waitlist candidates. This apparent inequity in transplant allocation would be less controversial if graft availability was a nonissue. Indeed, LDLT resolves the issue of organ supply and allows patients to be considered for transplantation without altering the deceased donor pool. In addition, willingness of family or friends to donate may be the best indicator of social support, an important predictor of transplant outcomes. Thus, for several reasons, LDLT may prove to be a lifesaving option for patients with severe alcoholic hepatitis.

Cholangiocarcinoma

Cholangiocarcinoma (CCA) is the second most common primary hepatobiliary malignancy following HCC. Hilar CCA represents two-thirds of the cases of CCA and has dismal overall survival. Despite the curative intent of resection, it is often achieved in only 25% to 40% of patients.[66–68] After original exploration of neoadjuvant chemoradiation by Sudan and colleagues,[69] the Mayo Clinic (2002) created a protocol that would serve as the standard of treatment before transplantation in CCA. This study along with the Nebraska study[69] supported the idea that for selected patients with early disease (stages I and II) durable long-term survival was possible with the combination for neoadjuvant chemoradiation followed by transplantation. Later in 2004, the original study was updated and reported overall 1-, 3-, and 5-year survival for

Table 1
HCC criteria for transplantation

	Name of Criterion	Criterion Characteristics
1996	Milan	Single tumor ≤5 cm in diameter, or up to 3 tumors, each ≤3 cm in diameter; plus absence of nodal or vascular tumor invasion
2001	University of San Francisco	Single tumor ≤6.5 cm in diameter, or up to 3 tumors with largest tumor ≤4.5 cm in diameter, along with total tumor diameter of ≤8 cm
2007	5–5 rule (Tokyo)	Up to 5 tumors, with a maximum tumor size ≤5 cm
2007	10–5 rule (Kyoto)	Up to 10 tumors, all ≤5 cm in diameter, and PIVKA II ≤400 mAU/mL
2008	Asan Medical Center	Up to 6 tumors, with largest tumor diameter ≤5 cm, and no gross vascular invasion
2009	Up-to-seven	Sum of the size of the largest tumor in cm and the total number of tumors ≤7
2011	Extended Toronto Criteria	Protocol biopsy to rule out aggressive features in the largest tumor No limitations on the size or number of tumors
2014	Samsung Medical Center	Maximal tumor size ≤6 cm, tumor number <7, and/or AFP levels <1000 ng/mL
2015	Hangzou	Tumor stratification as type A or B; A has better outcomes Type A = tumor burden ≤8 cm, or tumor burden >8 cm with AFP ≤100 ng/mL Type B = tumor burden >8 cm with AFP 100–400 ng/mL
2016	Seoul National University	PVTT that has not spread to the main portal vein, and a low AP score (≤20,000)
2017	Seoul St. Mary's hospital	Only segmental PVTT not lobar, plus AFP <100 ng/mL
2017	Soonchunhyang University Seoul Hospital	PVTT less than the Vp4 type per the Liver Cancer Study Group of Japan staging (Vp4 = presence of tumor thrombus in the main trunk of the portal vein or a portal vein branch contralateral to the primarily involved lobe, or both), and good biologic response to downstaging by radiotherapy
2019	5-5-500 rule	Nodule size ≤5 cm in diameter, nodule number ≤5, and AFP ≤500 ng/mL

Abbreviations: AFP, α-fetoprotein; AP score, AFP × PIVKA II score; PIVKA II, protein induced by vitamin K absence/antagonist–II; PVTT, portal vein tumor thrombus.

transplanted patients as 92%, 82%, and 82%, respectively, compared with 82%, 48%, and 21%, for those who underwent resection alone.[70]

Intrahepatic CCA (iCCA) is a contraindication to transplantation at most centers. Early studies demonstrated very poor post-transplant outcomes for patients transplanted for iCCA.[71] However, one study found that the overall 5-year survival in patients with iCCA following transplant was greater than 50%. More importantly, the study demonstrated that patients with small tumors (<2 cm) had a long-term disease-free survival of 73%, and better outcomes compared with patients with more advanced disease (either tumor >2 cm or multifocal disease).[72]

For hilar cholangiocarcinoma and iCCA, similar to CLM, the MELDNa score provides no advantage in their listing for a deceased donor organ. This raises the importance of considering early intervention with LDLT in this population who may achieve durable long survival.

Low Model for End-Stage Liver Disease and Other Considerations

The MELD score currently determines liver transplant waitlist position. However, it does not always capture the true severity of disease, especially with cholestatic diseases. Physicians must step away from objective data and weigh the benefit of transplantation for each individual patient based on what is known about the natural trajectory of their individual disease. LDLT gives this opportunity. In fact, Goldberg and colleagues[73] showed that LDLT has superior graft survival compared with deceased donor liver transplantation in autoimmune and cholestatic diseases.

SUMMARY

There is a significant organ shortage for transplantation throughout the world. LDLT is a viable option for meeting the shortfall in available organs. The process of increasing the number of living donor transplants must be thoughtful and must maintain donor safety as the top priority. To improve implementation of LDLT, we have three recommendations:

1. Educate more transplant programs on the benefits of LDLT and demonstrate that donor safety is improving with each procedure performed.

    There is an urgent need for lifesaving measures, and valuable opportunities are being missed. Transplant programs need to invest in establishing LDLT programs and health care systems. Over time, advances in transplant technology and continued improvements in LDLT protocols will progressively decrease donor risk and increase post-transplant longevity for recipients. Therefore, as the number of LDLTs is increased throughout the world, it is critical to document and disseminate longitudinal data on outcomes.

2. Encourage transplant programs to adopt the Living Donor Champion model.

    To help overcome the barriers of public perception and also take the responsibility of finding a donor out of the patient's hands, comprehensive educational and patient advocacy programs, such as the Living Donor Champion model, must be implemented. The widespread adoption of such programs will help increase the living donor pool and address the nation's unmet needs.

3. Expand LDLT access to a larger group of potential transplant recipients while continuously testing the boundaries of donor selection criteria.

    Such conditions as HCC outside of Milan, CCA, CLM, and low MELD should be considered for transplantation. This, along with safe expansion of donor criteria, will offer lifesaving treatment while simultaneously improving the transplantation process leading to new guidelines, protocols, and technologies to accelerate advancements in the effectiveness and safety of LDLT.

CLINICS CARE POINTS

- Donors with BMI >30 but with hepatic steatosis of <10% can potentially be considered for LDLT if they have no other relevant comorbidities, and there is both surgical and medical expertise for LDLT care at the center.
- Careful assessment of emotional maturity in younger donors and rigorous physiological assessment in older individuals can safely expand donor age criteria in both directions.
- Absolute graft weight of more than or equal to 643g may be a better predictor of outcomes than a GRWR of 0.8 SFSS incidence can be low even with GRWR of <0.8 with meticulous recipient selection, and well-defined surgical protocols including appropriate portal flow modulation.
- Although ABOi LDLT is a viable option in selected recipients, a paired organ exchange or swap should be considered to eliminate the issue of ABO incompatibility altogether.
- The Living Donor Champion Program allows the patient to focus on the management of their medical condition while their surrogate 'champions' their cause to help find a live donor.
- Selected patients with colorectal metastases to the liver may benefit from LDLT, however, no studies have compared survival post-LDLT with modern chemotherapeutic or multi-modal treatments.
- LDLT for severe acute alcoholic hepatitis remains controversial, but social support in the form of a friend or a family member willing to donate could receive favorable consideration.
- The combination of neoadjuvant chemoradiation and transplantation can improve survival in hilar CCA with careful consideration of the role of tumor size in long term outcomes.

DISCLOSURE

The authors have nothing to disclose.

REFERENCES

1. OPTN Database. Available at: http://optn.transplant.hrsa.gov. Accessed July 21, 2020.
2. Cullaro G, Sarkar M, Lai JC. Sex-based disparities in delisting for being "too sick" for liver transplantation. Am J Transplant 2018;18(5):1214–9.
3. Humar A, Ganesh S, Jorgensen D, et al. Adult living donor versus deceased donor liver transplant (LDLT versus DDLT) at a single center: time to change our paradigm for liver transplant. Ann Surg 2019;270(3):444–51.
4. Abu-Gazala S, Olthoff KM. Status of adult living donor liver transplantation in the United States: results from the adult-to-adult living donor liver transplantation cohort study. Gastroenterol Clin North Am 2018;47(2):297–311.
5. Rinella ME, Alonso E, Rao S, et al. Body mass index as a predictor of hepatic steatosis in living liver donors. Liver Transpl 2001;7(5):409–14.
6. Soin AS, Chaudhary RJ, Pahari H, et al. A worldwide survey of live liver donor selection policies at 24 centers with a combined experience of 19 009 adult living donor liver transplants. Transplantation 2019;103(2):e39–47.

7. Andert A, Ulmer TF, Schöning W, et al. Grade of donor liver microvesicular steatosis does not affect the postoperative outcome after liver transplantation. Hepatobiliary Pancreat Dis Int 2017;16(6):617–23.

8. Chu MJ, Dare AJ, Phillips AR, et al. Donor hepatic steatosis and outcome after liver transplantation: a systematic review. J Gastrointest Surg 2015;19(9):1713–24.

9. Frongillo F, Lirosi MC, Sganga G, et al. Graft steatosis as a risk factor of ischemic-type biliary lesions in liver transplantation. Transplant Proc 2014;46(7):2293–4.

10. Wu C, Lu C, Xu C. Short-term and long-term outcomes of liver transplantation using moderately and severely steatotic donor livers: a systematic review. Medicine (Baltimore) 2018;97(35):e12026.

11. Bhangui P, Sah J, Choudhary N, et al. Safe use of right lobe live donor livers with up to 20% macrovesicular steatosis without compromising donor safety and recipient outcome. Transplantation 2020;104(2):308–16.

12. Knaak M, Goldaracena N, Doyle A, et al. Donor BMI >30 is not a contraindication for live liver donation. Am J Transplant 2017;17(3):754–60.

13. Kubota T, Hata K, Sozu T, et al. Impact of donor age on recipient survival in adult-to-adult living-donor liver transplantation. Ann Surg 2018;267(6):1126–33.

14. Available at: https://aaafoundation.org/rates-motor-vehicle-crashes-injuries-deaths-relation-driver-age-united-states-2014-2015/.

15. Aulakh R. Too young to save his mother's life? Hospital changes policy for teen. Available at: https://www.thestar.com/life/health_wellness/news_research/2011/07/12/too_young_to_save_his_mothers_life_hospital_changes_policy_for_teen.html. Accessed July 21, 2020.

16. Selzner M, Kashfi A, Cattral MS, et al. A graft to body weight ratio less than 0.8 does not exclude adult-to-adult right-lobe living donor liver transplantation. Liver Transpl 2009;15(12):1776–82.

17. Agarwal S, Selvakumar N, Rajasekhar K, et al. Minimum absolute graft weight of 650 g predicts a good outcome in living donor liver transplant despite a graft recipient body weight ratio of less than 0.8. Clin Transplant 2019;33(10):e13705.

18. Wong TC, Fung JYY, Cui TYS, et al. The Risk of Going Small: Lowering GRWR and Overcoming Small-For-Size Syndrome in Adult Living Donor Liver Transplantation. Ann Surg 2020. [Epub ahead of print].

19. Ma KW, Wong KHC, Chan ACY, et al. Impact of small-for-size liver grafts on medium-term and long-term graft survival in living donor liver transplantation: a meta-analysis. World J Gastroenterol 2019;25(36):5559–68.

20. Kawagishi N, Satomi S. ABO-incompatible living donor liver transplantation: new insights into clinical relevance. Transplantation 2008;85(11):1523–5.

21. Egawa H, Oike F, Buhler L, et al. Impact of recipient age on outcome of ABO-incompatible living-donor liver transplantation. Transplantation 2004;77(3):403–11.

22. Pratschke J, Tullius SG. Promising recent data on ABO incompatible liver transplantation: restrictions may apply. Transpl Int 2007;20(8):647–8.

23. Stewart ZA, Locke JE, Montgomery RA, et al. ABO-incompatible deceased donor liver transplantation in the United States: a national registry analysis. Liver Transpl 2009;15(8):883–93.

24. Kim JM, Kwon CH, Joh JW, et al. ABO-incompatible living donor liver transplantation is suitable in patients without ABO-matched donor. J Hepatol 2013;59(6):1215–22.

25. Egawa H, Teramukai S, Haga H, et al. Present status of ABO-incompatible living donor liver transplantation in Japan. Hepatology 2008;47(1):143–52.

26. Gugenheim J, Samuel D, Reynes M, et al. Liver transplantation across ABO blood group barriers. Lancet 1990;336(8714):519–23.

27. Farges O, Kalil AN, Samuel D, et al. The use of ABO-incompatible grafts in liver transplantation: a life-saving procedure in highly selected patients. Transplantation 1995;59(8):1124–33.
28. Egawa H, Teramukai S, Haga H, et al. Impact of rituximab desensitization on blood-type-incompatible adult living donor liver transplantation: a Japanese multicenter study. Am J Transplant 2014;14(1):102–14.
29. Yadav DK, Hua YF, Bai X, et al. ABO-incompatible adult living donor liver transplantation in the era of rituximab: a systematic review and meta-analysis. Gastroenterol Res Pract 2019;2019:8589402.
30. Kim JM, Kwon CH, Joh JW, et al. Case-matched comparison of ABO-incompatible and ABO-compatible living donor liver transplantation. Br J Surg 2016;103(3):276–83.
31. Lo AL, Sonnenberg EM, Abt PL. Evolving swaps in transplantation: global exchange, vouchers, liver, and trans-organ paired exchange. Curr Opin Organ Transplant 2019;24(2):161–6.
32. Lee S, Hwang S, Park K, et al. An adult-to-adult living donor liver transplant using dual left lobe grafts. Surgery 2001;129(5):647–50.
33. Song GW, Lee SG, Moon DB, et al. Dual-graft adult living donor liver transplantation: an innovative surgical procedure for live liver donor pool expansion. Ann Surg 2017;266(1):10–8.
34. Jwa EK, Choi DL, Kim JD. Feasibility of dual living donor liver transplantation from donors with complex portal vein variations. Transplant Proc 2020;52(6):1791–3.
35. Vinayak N, Ravi M, Ankush G, et al. Dual graft living donor liver transplantation: a case report. BMC Surg 2019;19(1):149.
36. Rockstroh JK, Gonzalez-Scarano F. Living donor liver transplant from an HIV-positive individual to an HIV-negative individual: could this become a new reality? AIDS 2018;32(16):2423–4.
37. Garonzik-Wang JM, Berger JC, Ros RL, et al. Live donor champion: finding live kidney donors by separating the advocate from the patient. Transplantation 2012;93(11):1147–50.
38. Hughes CB, Humar A. Liver transplantation: current and future. Abdom Radiol (NY) 2020. [*Epub ahead of print*].
39. Duvoux C. Anonymous living donation in liver transplantation: squaring the circle or condemned to vanish? J Hepatol 2019;71(5):864–6.
40. Goldaracena N, Jung J, Aravinthan AD, et al. Donor outcomes in anonymous live liver donation. J Hepatol 2019;71(5):951–9.
41. Starzl TE. The saga of liver replacement, with particular reference to the reciprocal influence of liver and kidney transplantation (1955-1967). J Am Coll Surg 2002;195(5):587–610.
42. Foss A, Adam R, Dueland S. Liver transplantation for colorectal liver metastases: revisiting the concept. Transpl Int 2010;23(7):679–85.
43. Hoti E, Adam R. Liver transplantation for primary and metastatic liver cancers. Transpl Int 2008;21(12):1107–17.
44. Hagness M, Foss A, Line PD, et al. Liver transplantation for nonresectable liver metastases from colorectal cancer. Ann Surg 2013;257(5):800–6.
45. Hagness M, Foss A, Egge TS, et al. Patterns of recurrence after liver transplantation for nonresectable liver metastases from colorectal cancer. Ann Surg Oncol 2014;21(4):1323–9.
46. Glinka J, Ardiles V, Pekolj J, et al. Liver transplantation for non-resectable colorectal liver metastasis: where we are and where we are going. Langenbecks Arch Surg 2020;405(3):255–64.

47. Adam R. Curative potential of liver transplantation in patients with definitively unresectable colorectal liver metastases (CLM) treated by chemotherapy: a prospectihe multicentric randomized trial. Available at: https://clinicaltrials.gov/ct2/show/NCT02597348. Accessed July 21, 2020.

48. Mazzaferro V, Regalia E, Doci R, et al. Liver transplantation for the treatment of small hepatocellular carcinomas in patients with cirrhosis. N Engl J Med 1996; 334(11):693–9.

49. Mazzaferro V, Bhoori S, Sposito C, et al. Milan criteria in liver transplantation for hepatocellular carcinoma: an evidence-based analysis of 15 years of experience. Liver Transpl 2011;17(Suppl 2):S44–57.

50. Yao FY, Ferrell L, Bass NM, et al. Liver transplantation for hepatocellular carcinoma: expansion of the tumor size limits does not adversely impact survival. Hepatology 2001;33(6):1394–403.

51. DuBay D, Sandroussi C, Sandhu L, et al. Liver transplantation for advanced hepatocellular carcinoma using poor tumor differentiation on biopsy as an exclusion criterion. Ann Surg 2011;253(1):166–72.

52. Zavaglia C, De Carlis L, Alberti AB, et al. Predictors of long-term survival after liver transplantation for hepatocellular carcinoma. Am J Gastroenterol 2005; 100(12):2708–16.

53. Jonas S, Bechstein WO, Steinmüller T, et al. Vascular invasion and histopathologic grading determine outcome after liver transplantation for hepatocellular carcinoma in cirrhosis. Hepatology 2001;33(5):1080–6.

54. Shah SA, Tan JC, McGilvray ID, et al. Accuracy of staging as a predictor for recurrence after liver transplantation for hepatocellular carcinoma. Transplantation 2006;81(12):1633–9.

55. Sotiropoulos GC, Malagó M, Molmenti E, et al. Liver transplantation for hepatocellular carcinoma in cirrhosis: is clinical tumor classification before transplantation realistic? Transplantation 2005;79(4):483–7.

56. Sugawara Y, Tamura S, Makuuchi M. Living donor liver transplantation for hepatocellular carcinoma: Tokyo University series. Dig Dis 2007;25(4):310–2.

57. Lee KW, Suh SW, Choi Y, et al. Macrovascular invasion is not an absolute contraindication for living donor liver transplantation. Liver Transpl 2017;23(1):19–27.

58. Choi JY, Yu JI, Park HC, et al. The possibility of radiotherapy as downstaging to living donor liver transplantation for hepatocellular carcinoma with portal vein tumor thrombus. Liver Transpl 2017;23(4):545–51.

59. Choi HJ, Kim DG, Na GH, et al. The clinical outcomes of patients with portal vein tumor thrombi after living donor liver transplantation. Liver Transpl 2017;23(8):1023–31.

60. Bonadio I, Colle I, Geerts A, et al. Liver transplantation for hepatocellular carcinoma comparing the Milan, UCSF, and Asan criteria: long-term follow-up of a Western single institutional experience. Clin Transplant 2015;29(5):425–33.

61. Kaido T, Ogawa K, Mori A, et al. Usefulness of the Kyoto criteria as expanded selection criteria for liver transplantation for hepatocellular carcinoma. Surgery 2013;154(5):1053–60.

62. Patel SS, Arrington AK, McKenzie S, et al. Milan criteria and UCSF criteria: a preliminary comparative study of liver transplantation outcomes in the United States. Int J Hepatol 2012;2012:253517.

63. Unek T, Karademir S, Arslan NC, et al. Comparison of Milan and UCSF criteria for liver transplantation to treat hepatocellular carcinoma. World J Gastroenterol 2011;17(37):4206–12.

64. Sapisochin G, Goldaracena N, Laurence JM, et al. The extended Toronto criteria for liver transplantation in patients with hepatocellular carcinoma: a prospective validation study. Hepatology 2016;64(6):2077–88.
65. Mathurin P, Moreno C, Samuel D, et al. Early liver transplantation for severe alcoholic hepatitis. N Engl J Med 2011;365(19):1790–800.
66. Jarnagin WR, Fong Y, DeMatteo RP, et al. Staging, resectability, and outcome in 225 patients with hilar cholangiocarcinoma. Ann Surg 2001;234(4):507–17 [discussion: 517–9].
67. DeOliveira ML, Cunningham SC, Cameron JL, et al. Cholangiocarcinoma: thirty-one-year experience with 564 patients at a single institution. Ann Surg 2007; 245(5):755–62.
68. Kimura N, Young AL, Toyoki Y, et al. Radical operation for hilar cholangiocarcinoma in comparable Eastern and Western centers: outcome analysis and prognostic factors. Surgery 2017;162(3):500–14.
69. Sudan D, DeRoover A, Chinnakotla S, et al. Radiochemotherapy and transplantation allow long-term survival for nonresectable hilar cholangiocarcinoma. Am J Transplant 2002;2(8):774–9.
70. Rea DJ, Heimbach JK, Rosen CB, et al. Liver transplantation with neoadjuvant chemoradiation is more effective than resection for hilar cholangiocarcinoma. Ann Surg 2005;242(3):451–8 [discussion: 458–61].
71. Robles R, Figueras J, Turrión VS, et al. Liver transplantation for peripheral cholangiocarcinoma: Spanish experience. Transplant Proc 2003;35(5):1823–4.
72. Sapisochin G, Rodríguez de Lope C, Gastaca M, et al. Very early" intrahepatic cholangiocarcinoma in cirrhotic patients: should liver transplantation be reconsidered in these patients? Am J Transplant 2014;14(3):660–7.
73. Goldberg DS, French B, Abt PL, et al. Superior survival using living donors and donor-recipient matching using a novel living donor risk index. Hepatology 2014;60(5):1717–26.

The Changing Liver Transplant Recipient

From Hepatitis C to Nonalcoholic Steatohepatitis and Alcohol

Ross Vyhmeister, MD[a], C. Kristian Enestvedt, MD[b],*

KEYWORDS

- Liver transplant • Indications • Hepatitis C • Nonalcoholic steatohepatitis
- Alcoholic liver disease

KEY POINTS

- Hepatitis C virus (HCV) has historically been the leading indication for liver transplant in the United States, followed by nonalcoholic steatohepatitis (NASH) and alcoholic liver disease (ALD).
- The development of highly effective and well-tolerated direct-acting antivirals for HCV introduced a new era in 2014 and liver transplant for HCV is declining, now trailing NASH and ALD.
- ALD is an increasingly common reason for liver transplant, with increasing adoption of transplant for the indication of severe alcoholic hepatitis in the last decade.
- Prevalence of NASH and resulting cirrhosis continues to increase in the United States in conjunction with a continued increase in rates of obesity.

INTRODUCTION

The landscape of liver transplant has evolved significantly because it was first performed on humans in 1963.[1] Outcomes have improved, with better graft quality and survival, following multiple advances, including the acceptance of the concept of brain death in the United States in 1968, and the introduction of cyclosporine in the 1970s.[2] In 1989, the first successful living donor liver transplant was performed.[3] With continued advancements, both short-term and long-term graft outcomes have continued to improve, with graft survival of 91.2% at 1 year for those transplants

a Department of Medicine, Oregon Health and Science University, 3181 Southwest Sam Jackson Park Road, Portland, OR 97239, USA; b Division of Abdominal Organ Transplantation and HPB Surgery, School of Medicine, Oregon Health and Science University, 3181 Southwest Sam Jackson Park Road, Portland, OR 97239, USA
* Corresponding author.
E-mail address: ENESTVED@OHSU.EDU

Clin Liver Dis 25 (2021) 137–155
https://doi.org/10.1016/j.cld.2020.08.012
1089-3261/21/© 2020 Elsevier Inc. All rights reserved.

performed in 2017, 76.5% at 5 years for those performed in 2013, and 56.4% at 10 years for those performed in 2008.[4]

The indications for liver transplant have continued to expand to include a broad range of diagnoses, as summarized in **Box 1**.[5] Current guidelines state that liver transplant is indicated for severe acute or advanced chronic liver disease that has reached the limitation of medical therapy.[6] Over the last decade, the proportions of adults on the waiting list for liver transplant have remained highest for those with one of 3 primary diagnoses: hepatitis C virus (HCV), alcoholic liver disease (ALD), and other/unknown, which encompasses nonalcoholic steatohepatitis (NASH), with historical trends as shown in **Fig. 1** and **Table 1**. However, in recent years the proportion of candidates listed with a primary diagnosis of HCV has begun to decline, whereas the proportion with ALD and NASH have continued to increase (**Fig. 2**).[4,7–9] Within the past 5 years, ALD replaced HCV as the leading indication for liver transplant in the United States, as shown in **Fig. 3**, showing the divergent trajectory of transplant for HCV compared with ALD and NASH. These 2 causes, NASH and ALD, accounted for 51% of transplant listings by 2016.[10] This article explores these dramatic changes, examines the underlying clinical and epidemiologic causes for the changing dynamics, and discusses possible future implications for both listing practices and therapeutic strategies.

HEPATITIS C VIRUS

HCV has historically been the most common indication for liver transplant in the United States, representing more than a third of all liver transplants by 2006.[11] Demographics for patients with HCV are changing toward younger adults, likely reflective of increased injection drug use in the setting of the opioid epidemic in the United States. It is estimated that, globally, approximately 65% of people who inject drugs have a positive antibody to HCV.[12] Treatment of HCV entered into a new era in 2014 when direct-acting antivirals (DAAs) became available in the United States. In contrast with interferon, DAAs are generally well tolerated and result in cure in approximately 95% of patients following typically 8 to 12 weeks of oral therapy.

The benefit of DAAs was quickly reflected in the liver transplant waiting list. One study assessing registrants on liver transplant waiting lists in the United States from 2003 to 2015 showed a greater than 30% reduction in the rate of registration for decompensated cirrhosis in patients with HCV in the less than 2 years following approval of oral DAA regimens.[13] This trend is also reflected in data from the European Liver Transplant Registry that showed a decline in the percentage of liver transplants for HCV, decreased from 21.1% in 2014 to 10.6% 3 years later in 2017. This decline was most prominently noted in patients transplanted for decompensated cirrhosis secondary to HCV, with a decrease of 58% for this indication over these 3 years, but was also noted to a lesser extent for patients with hepatocellular carcinoma (HCC) whose numbers also declined by 41.2% over this same period.[14] This discrepancy has been thought to be related in part to bias against older patients with decompensated HCV cirrhosis as transplant candidates for multiple reasons: (1) they may be viewed as poor candidates relative to younger counterparts; (2) they may be selected against compared with similar-aged patients without decompensations; (3) they may pass predetermined transplant center age limits; (4) they may improve clinically but receive HCC priority. This fourth phenomenon suggests a possible differential effect on HCC compared with decompensation wherein the risk for HCC persists (with the subsequent exception point benefit) despite HCV cure.

Box 1
Reasons for liver transplant

Acute liver failure
    Hepatitis A, acetaminophen, autoimmune hepatitis
    Hepatitis B
    Hepatitis C
    Drugs, hepatitis D
    Wilson disease, Budd-Chiari syndrome
    Fatty infiltration

Cirrhosis from chronic liver disease
    Chronic hepatitis B infection
    Chronic hepatitis C infection
    Alcoholic liver disease
    Autoimmune hepatitis
    Cryptogenic liver disease
    Nonalcoholic fatty liver disease

Malignant diseases of the liver
    Hepatocellular carcinoma
    Hilar cholangiocarcinoma
    Carcinoid tumor
    Islet cell tumor
    Epithelioid hemangioendothelioma
    Cholangiosarcoma

Metabolic liver disease
    Wilson disease
    Hereditary hemochromatosis
    Alpha1-antitrypsin deficiency
    Glycogen storage disease
    Cystic fibrosis
    Glycogen storage disease I and IV
    Crigler-Najjar syndrome
    Galactosemia
    Type 1 hyperoxaluria
    Familial homozygous hypercholesterolemia
    Hemophilia A and B

Vascular diseases of the liver
    Budd-Chiari syndrome
    Veno-occlusive disease

Cholestatic liver disease
    Primary biliary cholangitis
    Primary sclerosing cholangitis
    Secondary biliary cirrhosis
    Biliary atresia
    Alagille syndrome
    Byler disease

Miscellaneous
    Adult polycystic liver disease
    Nodular regenerative hyperplasia
    Caroli disease
    Severe graft-versus-host disease
    Amyloidosis
    Sarcoidosis
    Hepatic trauma

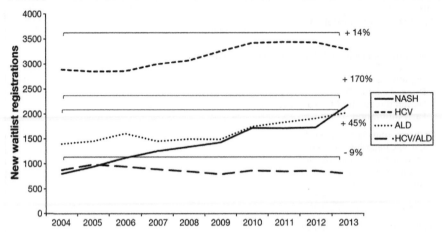

Fig. 1. Annual trends in new liver transplant waitlist registrations from 2004 to 2013. (*From* Wong RJ, Aguilar M, Cheung R, et al. Nonalcoholic steatohepatitis is the second leading etiology of liver disease among adults awaiting liver transplantation in the United States. *Gastroenterology.* 2015;148(3):547-555; with permission.)

Development of DAAs also contributed to the World Health Organization's target of eliminating HCV by 2030. However, multiple barriers to treatment and elimination persist. Substantial financial constraints remain, although costs are declining. In addition, HCV remains globally underdiagnosed and undertreated, with only an estimated 20% of cases having been diagnosed and only 7% of those diagnosed having been treated.[15] As mentioned previously, the ongoing opioid epidemic has contributed to HCV transmission and the impact of this disease on a younger cohort.

In addition to the benefit of a declining need for liver transplants for HCV, DAAs have also afforded an increase in donor availability. The opioid epidemic in the United States has resulted in an increase in the number of increased-risk donors with HCV because of intravenous drug use. Those recipients willing to accept HCV antibody–positive donor organs have benefited from good short-term outcomes with cure of HCV following liver transplant.[16]

ALCOHOLIC LIVER DISEASE

ALD represents a spectrum of disease, including steatosis, alcoholic hepatitis, and cirrhosis, and is a leading cause of preventable liver disease–associated mortality in the United States.[17] Steatosis and/or steatohepatitis develops in most individuals consuming more than 60 g/d of alcohol and can progress in a minority of patients to cirrhosis despite abstinence from alcohol. Women have been found to be approximately twice as sensitive as men to hepatotoxicity mediated by alcohol, whereas other risk factors include drinking outside of mealtimes and binge drinking.[18] However, the increase in ALD as an indication for transplant listing has been most pronounced among the male population, among whom ALD has supplanted HCV since 2013 (**Fig. 4**). For men registered for liver transplant compared by the years 2004 and 2016, ALD increased by 49%, whereas HCV decreased 67%.[19]

Treatment strategies for alcohol abuse before progression to end-stage liver disease include psychosocial and behavioral therapies such as 12-step facilitation, cognitive behavior therapy, and motivational enhancement therapy. These therapies

Table 1
Characteristics of new liver transplant waitlist registrants in the United States from 2004 to 2013

Characteristics	NASH	HCV	ALD	HCV/ALD	P Value
Male, n (%)	7631 (54.9)	21,620 (69.8)	12,338 (76.5)	7111 (83.1)	<.01
Age, mean ± SD (y)	58.0 ± 8.7	55.0 ± 7.1	54.2 ± 8.7	53.0 ± 6.2	<.001
BMI, median (range) (kg/m²)	31.6 (18.7–47.7)	28.0 (18.5–43.9)	27.6 (17.6–44.1)	28.1 (18~4–43.3)	<.001
Race/ethnicity	—	—	—	—	<.001
Non-Hispanic white, n (%)	10,796 (78.5)	21,221 (69.1)	12,501 (78.5)	6131 (72.4)	—
Black, n (%)	460 (3.3)	3598 (11.7)	528 (3.3)	735 (8.7)	—
Hispanic, n (%)	2070 (15.0)	4803 (15.7)	2674 (16.8)	1542 (18.2)	—
Asian, n (%)	433 (3.2)	1,06 (93.5)	229 (1.4)	56 (0.7)	—
HCC, n (%)	2925 (21.0)	7632 (24.6)	1212 (7.5)	1128 (13.2)	<.001
MELD, mean ± SD	16.5 ± 7.8	15.7 ± 7.6	19.1 ± 8.4	17.3 ± 8.1	<.001
Albumin, mean ± SD (g/dL)	3.1 ± 0.7	3.0 ± 0.7	3.1 ± 0.7	2.9 ± 0.7	<.001
Bilirubin, median (range) (mg/dL)	2.1 (1.0–38.0)	2.0 (1.0–38.4)	2.9 (1.0–40.4)	2.4 (1.0–40.8)	<.01
INR, mean ± SD	1.52 ± 0.80	1.51 ± 0.85	1.69 ± 0.69	1.63 ± 0.68	<.01
Creatinine, mean ± SD (mg/dL)	1.45 ± 0.90	1.38 ± 0.86	1.55 ± 1.03	1.42 ± 0.90	<.01
GFR, mean ± SD (mL/min/1.73 m²)	55.2 ± 20.0	61.6 ± 19.9	57.3 + 21.6	62.7 ± 20.5	<.02
Ascites, n (%)	10,585 (76.1)	22,338 (72.1)	13,903 (86.2)	7114 (83.1)	<.001
Hepatic encephalopathy, n (%)	8490 (61.1)	18,004 (58.2)	11,533 (71.5)	6160 (72.0)	<.001
Diabetes, n (%)	6032 (46.3)	6307 (21.3)	3008 (19.5)	8211 (17.7)	<.001

Abbreviations: BMI, body mass index; GFR, glomerular filtration rate (calculated using Modification of Diet in Renal Disease study calculations); HCC, hepatocellular carcinoma; INR, international normalized ratio; MELD, model for end-stage liver disease; SD, standard deviation.

From Wong RJ, Aguilar M, Cheung R, et al. Nonalcoholic steatohepatitis is the second leading etiology of liver disease among adults awaiting liver transplantation in the United States. *Gastroenterology.* 2015;148(3):547-555; with permission.

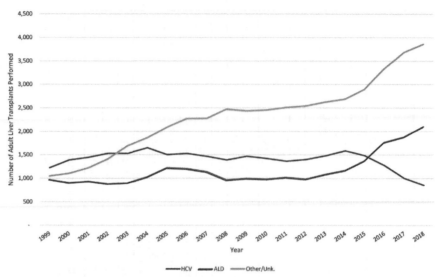

Fig. 2. Number of adult liver transplants performed per year in the United States for primary indication of HCV, ALD, and other/unknown (Unk.), which encompasses NASH. (*Data from* Kwong A, Kim WR, Lake JR, et al. OPTN/SRTR 2018 Annual Data Report: Liver. *Am J Transplant.* 2020;20 Suppl s1:193-299 and additional OPTN/SRTR Annual Data Report Archives at https://srtr.transplant.hrsa.gov/archives.aspx.)

can be implemented in conjunction with medical therapies, including acamprosate, disulfiram, and naltrexone, although notably naltrexone carries a US Food and Drug Administration (FDA) black-box warning because of hepatotoxicity, which limits its use in ALD.[20] Although treatment strategies remain limited, alcohol use in the United States continues to increase, with estimated increase in prevalence of 0.3% per year and increase in binge drinking by 0.7% per year in conservative estimates.[21]

Apart from limited pharmacologic options for treatment of severe alcoholic hepatitis, therapeutic management of ALD is focused on abstinence from alcohol and nutritional support.[17,22] Notable increased mortality among maturing generations in the United States compared with prior generations has been attributed to the problems of substance abuse. Although identification of alcohol use disorders relies heavily on appropriate screening in the primary care setting, it is estimated that only a quarter of people with the condition ever seek help.[23] Thus many patients present with more advanced disease and it is not surprising that ALD has become a fast-growing indication for liver transplant listing. Renewed interest in evaluating, listing, and transplanting patients with acute alcoholic hepatitis has further contributed to these changes in listing practices.[24–27]

Risk of recidivism is a key assessment in the consideration for liver transplant in ALD and is often a reason for declining to even refer for liver transplant evaluation. A period of abstinence from alcohol, traditionally 6 months, was historically required for consideration for liver transplant. However, because of the high mortality associated with severe alcoholic hepatitis refractory to medical management, earlier liver transplant has been studied and shown to have improved survival in recipients for this indication.[24,28]

The changing perspective on transplant in acute alcoholic hepatitis was driven by the results of the French experience reported in 2011.[24] The investigators examined outcomes for patients with acute alcoholic hepatitis who were not responders to

A

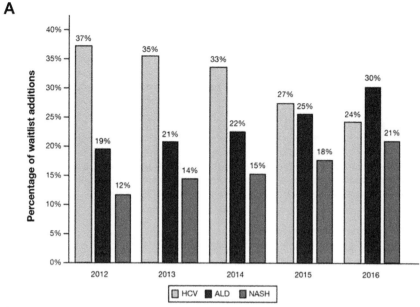

B

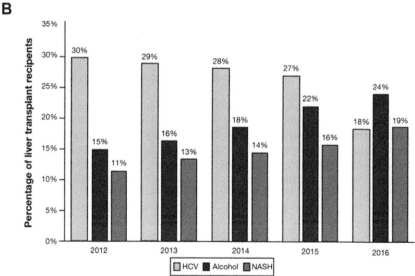

Fig. 3. Annual trends in (*A*) waitlist additions and (*B*) liver transplant recipients for the 3 leading indications for liver transplant in the United States. (*From* Cholankeril G, Ahmed A. Alcoholic Liver Disease Replaces Hepatitis C Virus Infection as the Leading Indication for Liver Transplantation in the United States. *Clin Gastroenterol Hepatol.* 2018;16(8):1356-1358; with permission.)

traditional therapy, but did not meet the traditional 6-month minimum sobriety paradigm. There was a stark, but expected, survival advantage between those transplanted and randomly matched controls (**Fig. 5**). Potential candidates were selected based on the following criteria:

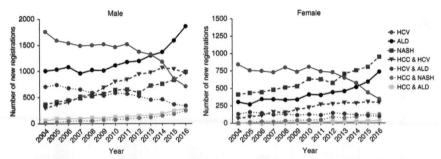

Fig. 4. Number of new waitlist registrants by disease category and gender from 2004 to 2016. (*From* Noureddin M, Vipani A, Bresee C, et al. NASH Leading Cause of Liver Transplant in Women: Updated Analysis of Indications For Liver Transplant and Ethnic and Gender Variances. *Am J Gastroenterol.* 2018;113(11):1649-1659; with permission.)

- Nonresponse to medical therapy
- Severe alcoholic hepatitis as the patient's first liver-decompensating event
- Presence of good social support
- Favorable psychosocial profile suggesting a low risk of alcohol relapse

The predictors of success identified in this study have been used in conjunction with the Mount Sinai experience to define optimal patient selection criteria for transplant in the acute ALD setting.[29] From an array of clinical variables, 8 factors were significantly associated with favorable candidate selection: (1) good insight, (2) first presentation for liver-decompensating event, (3) agreement with collaterals regarding use, (4) recent life stressor, (5) previously undiagnosed psychiatric disorder, (6) stable employment, (7) longer duration of sobriety, and (8) being a good historian (**Table 2**).[29]

Outcomes have been favorable for patients who have received transplants for acute alcoholic hepatitis. In a study including 147 liver transplant recipients across 12 US transplant centers who received transplants for severe alcoholic hepatitis between 2006 and 2017, cumulative survival was 94% at 1 year and 84% at 3 years. Cumulative incidence of sustained alcohol use following transplant was 10% at 1 year and 17% at 3 years, with younger age being the only characteristic clearly identified as a risk factor for continued alcohol use following transplant, as detailed in **Table 3**.[30] As expected, alcohol use following liver transplant increased over time and was associated with increased mortality.

NONALCOHOLIC STEATOHEPATITIS

Fatty liver disease is currently the most common liver disease in the world, affecting approximately 25% of adults in the United States.[31] Nonalcoholic fatty liver disease (NAFLD) is commonly associated with other metabolic comorbidities, including obesity, diabetes mellitus, and dyslipidemia. Histology can further categorize NAFLD as nonalcoholic fatty liver (NAFL) or nonalcoholic steatohepatitis (NASH). Although both NAFL and NASH are defined by the presence of at least 5% hepatic steatosis, NASH is distinguished from NAFL by the presence of evidence of inflammation and hepatocellular injury regardless of the presence of fibrosis. Liver biopsy remains the gold standard for the diagnosis of NASH, and this limits the ability to directly assess the incidence or prevalence of NASH in the general population. However, it is estimated that the prevalence of NASH in the general population is between 1.5% and

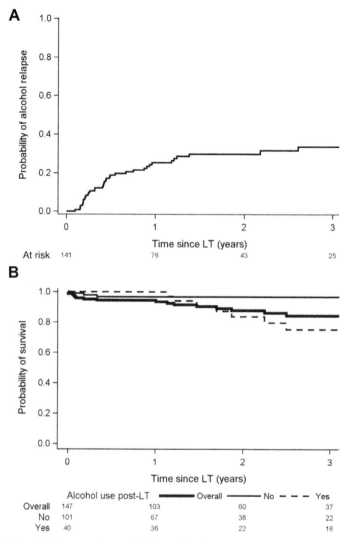

Fig. 5. (*A*) Kaplan-Meier curve for probability of alcohol use post-LT in 141 patients surviving to home discharge. The cumulative rate of alcohol use was 25%, 30%, and 34% at 1, 2, and 3 years, respectively. (*B*) Kaplan-Meier post-LT survival curve in 141 patients surviving to home discharge, stratified by no alcohol use post-LT (nonbolded solid line) versus alcohol use post-LT (dashed line). The cumulative survival at 1 and 3 years post-LT was 97% and 97% in those with no alcohol use compared with 100% and 75% in those with post-LT alcohol use (P 5 .03). The cumulative overall survival of the entire cohort (n 5 147; bolded solid line) at 1 and 3 years post-LT was 94% and 84%. (*From* Lee BP, Mehta N, Platt L, et al. Outcomes of Early Liver Transplantation for Patients With Severe Alcoholic Hepatitis. *Gastroenterology.* 2018;155(2):422-430 e421; with permission.)

6.45%.[32] In addition, obesity rates have approximately doubled worldwide since 1980, with the highest rates in the Americas and continue to rise in the United States as can be seen in **Fig. 6**. Although rates of obesity have begun to level off in more developed countries, global rates continue to increase.[33] A recent analysis, correcting

Table 2
Comparison of accepted candidates and candidates declined for poor psychosocial profiles for early liver transplant

Variables	Declined Candidates	Accepted Candidates	P Value
Number of patients (n)	59	20	—
Age, median (y)	48	44	.22
Women, n (%)	36 (61)	9 (45)	.21
Ethnicity	—	—	—
White, n (%)	28 (47)	16 (80)	.11
Hispanic, n (%)	14 (24)	1 (5)	—
African American, n (%)	9 (15)	1 (5)	—
Asian, n (%)	6 (10)	2 (10)	—
First liver-decompensating event, n (%)	21 (36)	19 (95)	<.01
Alcoholic drinks per day, median	11.9	11.5	.85
Type of Alcohol			
Liquor, n (%)	46 (78)	16 (80)	.85
Wine, n (%)	16 (27)	9 (45)	.14
Beer, n (%)	13 (22)	4 (20)	.85
Duration of alcohol use, median (y)	23.5	24	.84
Last alcohol use, mean (d)	16	33	<.01
Family history of alcoholism, n (%)	25 (42)	12 (60)	.17
Presence of life partner, n (%)	37 (63)	14 (70)	.56
Good social support, n (%)	52 (88)	20 (100)	.11
Stable employment history, n (%)	17 (29)	13 (65)	<.01
Insight into Alcoholism, n (%)			
Poor	38 (64)	1 (5)	—
Developing	17 (29)	1 (5)	—
Good	4 (68)	18 (90)	<.01
Recent life stressor, n (%)	22 (37)	16 (80)	<.01
Prior Axis 1 psychiatric diagnosis, n (%)	18 (31)	7 (35)	.71
Undiagnosed Axis 1 psychiatric disorder, n (%)	11 (19)	11 (55)	<.01
Good historian, n (%)	22 (37)	16 (80)	<.01
Agreement with collaterals on alcohol use, n (%)	39 (66)	18 (90)	.04
Illicit drug use, n (%)	6 (10)	1 (5)	.48
Cigarette smoking, n (%)	14 (24)	4 (20)	.73
Presence of children, n (%)	34 (58)	9 (45)	.33

From Im GY, Kim-Schluger L, Shenoy A, et al. Early Liver Transplantation for Severe Alcoholic Hepatitis in the United States–A Single-Center Experience. *Am J Transplant*. 2016;16(3):841-849; with permission.

for self-reporting bias in more than 6.2 million adults in the United States, has yielded results predicting a national prevalence of obesity increasing to 48.9%, and severe obesity, defined as body mass index (BMI) greater than or equal to 35, to 24.2%, by the year 2030. With noted wide variations by state, it was also able to project overall obesity of more than 50% in 29 states with no states being less than 35%.[34]

Table 3
Factors associated with alcohol use following liver transplant for severe alcoholic hepatitis

Characteristic	Univariable		Multivariable	
	OR (95% CI)	P Value	OR (95% CI)	P Value
Sex, female	1.32 (0.60–2.92)	.49	—	—
Race, nonwhite	1.66 (0.66–4.19)	.28	—	—
Age (per year)	*0.95 (0.92–0.99)*	*.01*	*0.95 (0.91–0.99)*	*.01*
No private insurance	1.29(0.60–2.78)	.51	—	—
Single/divorced/widowed	1.54(0.73–3.25)	.25	—	—
History of comorbid psychiatric disease	1.22(0.56–2.64)	.62	—	—
History of illicit substance abuse	1.31 (0.45–3.76)	.62	—	—
History of failed rehabilitation attempt	1.56(0.72–3.39)	.26	—	—
Family history of alcohol use disorder	1.33 (0.63–2.82)	.46	—	—
Unemployed immediately before hospitalization	1.22 (0.58–2.55)	.60	—	—
History of alcohol-related legal issues	*2.03(0.93–4.41)*	*.08*	2.03 (0.91–4.52)	.08
More than 10 drinks/d at presentation	1.28 (0.60–2.72)	.53	—	—
Years of heavy drinking	0.98 (0.94–1.01)	.21	—	—
Days of pretransplant abstinence	1.00(0.99–1.01)	.74	—	—

Italics indicate variables significantly associated with alcohol use after liver transplant, with $P<.05$.
Abbreviations: CI, confidence interval; OR, odds ratio.
From Lee BP, Mehta N, Platt L, et al. Outcomes of Early Liver Transplantation for Patients With Severe Alcoholic Hepatitis. *Gastroenterology.* 2018;155(2):422-430 e421; with permission.

NASH is a dynamic condition that may regress, remain constant, or progress to cirrhosis. It is estimated that approximately 25% of patients with NASH will ultimately progress to cirrhosis, resulting in approximately 2% of American adults developing cirrhosis secondary to NASH during their lifetimes.[31] In addition to cirrhosis, patients with NAFLD are also at increased risk for HCC, with estimated incidence of 6.7% to 15% at 5 to 10 years in patients with cirrhosis, and 2.3% at 10 years in patients without cirrhosis.[35]

Despite increasing prevalence of NAFLD, there are currently no FDA-approved therapies for NAFL or NASH. Weight loss remains the mainstay of treatment, with current clinical practice reflecting limited evidence of benefit from vitamin E or pioglitazone in patients with diabetes. A multitude of therapies is currently being investigated with varied targets, including modulation of bile acid synthesis, metabolic homeostasis, inflammation, and fibrosis. Although many of these therapies show early promise, investigation into long-term efficacy and safety will be crucial because of the natural history of slow progression of NAFLD.[36]

The increase in obesity and NAFLD in the setting of a paucity of effective therapies is reflected in the liver transplant waiting list. In 1 study evaluating the liver transplant waiting list in the United States from 2004 through 2013, an increase of 170% was observed in new registrants with NASH.[9] The rate of liver transplant registrations for NASH continues to increase among all age groups but particularly among younger patients, as shown in **Fig. 7**.[37] The impact of increasing obesity, NASH, and implications for transplant also reveals gender differences, with NASH the most common indication for transplant listing for women in 2016 (see **Fig. 4**, **Table 4**).[19]

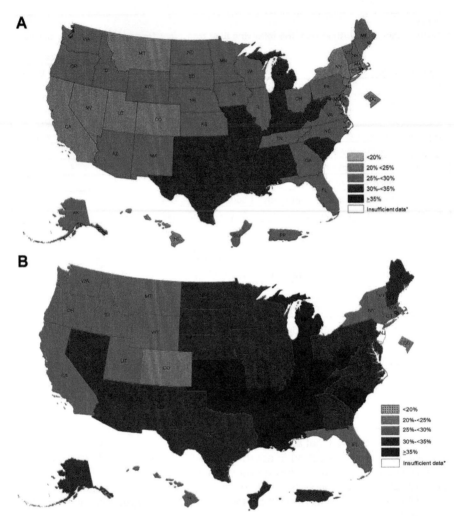

Fig. 6. Prevalence of Self-Reported Obesity Among U.S. Adults by State and Territory in (A) 2011 and (B) 2019. (*From* Centers for Disease Control and Prevention. 2020. New Adult Obesity Maps. Available at: http://www.cdc.gov/obesity/data/prevalence-maps.html, Accessed 1 September 2020.)

The continued increase in the rate of obesity not only affects the proportion of patients listed for transplant because of NASH but also introduces complexity to the transplant evaluation. Obesity is associated with increased rates of diabetes mellitus and coronary artery disease, which can affect transplant candidacy. In patients with compensated cirrhosis, lifestyle interventions and weight loss have been shown to be beneficial and, as previously discussed, are currently the mainstay of management for NASH. However, in patients with decompensated cirrhosis, BMI may be influenced by ascites and hypervolemic state. Furthermore, these patients are at higher risk for sarcopenia, frailty, and malnutrition, which may be exacerbated by restrictive diets, and, instead, frequent high-protein, high-nutrient meals are recommended.[38]

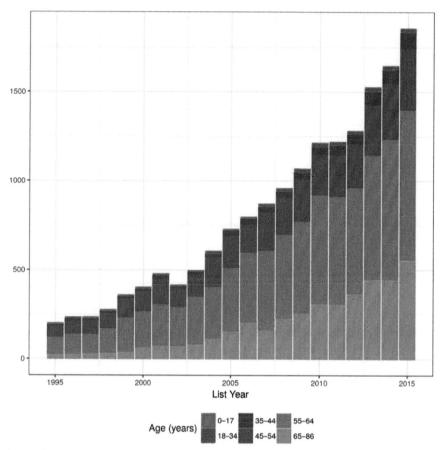

Fig. 7. Observed liver transplant registration rates among patients with NASH, by age group, among new registrants in United Network for Organ Sharing from 1995 to 2015. (*From* Shingina A, DeWitt PE, Dodge JL, et al. Future Trends in Demand for Liver Transplant: Birth Cohort Effects Among Patients With NASH and HCC. *Transplantation.* 2019;103(1):140-148.)

Bariatric surgery is finding an increasing role in the peritransplant period, although clear consensus regarding timing of surgery before transplant, simultaneous with transplant, or after transplant is still lacking.[39] The efficacy of bariatric surgery for weight loss is well established, and its benefit for NAFLD has also been shown. In a study during which 18 consecutive patients with NAFLD underwent Roux-en-Y gastric bypass with liver biopsy at the time of surgery, repeat liver biopsy 2 years later showed resolution of steatosis in 89% and resolution of fibrosis in 75%.[40] Similar benefits in NAFLD activity scores and fibrosis scores have been observed following endoscopic bariatric therapy with intragastric balloon placement.[41]

Sleeve gastrectomy before liver transplant has shown promising results, and a recent study at University of California, San Francisco, following 32 patients with sleeve gastrectomy performed before listing for liver transplant resulted in median weight loss of 52.4% excess body weight after surgery, and 88% of patients were subsequently deemed to be eligible for active listing for transplant.[42] Bariatric surgery at the time of liver transplant has also been studied; in a program at Mayo Clinic,

Table 4
Change in rates of liver transplant waitlist registration over time by gender

Cause	Male 2016 vs 2004		Male 2016 vs 2015		Female 2016 vs 2004		Female 2016 vs 2015	
	Change (%)	P Value	Change (%)	P Value	Change (%)	P Value	Change (%)	P Value
HCV	−67	<.0001	−22	<.0001	−68	<.0001	−27	<.0001
ALD	49	<.0001	10	.0957	87	<.0001	15	.0564
NASH	114	<.0001	12	.0991	80	<.0001	9	.2061
HCC and HCV	171	<.0001	−12	.0139	233	<.0m1	−11	.1576
HCV and ALD	−61	<.0001	−12	.0932	−43	.0103	−15	.2266
HCC and NASH	1172	<.0001	29	.0203	2383	<.0001	−11	.3322
HCC and ALD	273	<.0001	11	.3195	NA	<.0001	5	.8819

Percentage change computed from observed counts over time and P values computed from multinomial regression analysis within each sex; NA indicates percentage change not computed because of zero observations in divisor.
From Noureddin M, Vipani A, Bresee C, et al. NASH Leading Cause of Liver Transplant in Women: Updated Analysis of Indications For Liver Transplant and Ethnic and Gender Variances. *Am J Gastroenterol*. 2018;113(11):1649-1659; with permission.

patients who failed to reach a specified weight target, generally BMI less than 35, despite an aggressive weight management protocol then proceeded to combined liver transplant and sleeve gastrectomy. A total of 7 patients after 2006 underwent the combined surgery, and, at mean follow-up of 17 months, had significant weight loss to mean BMI of 28 and normal allograft function.[43] These benefits in weight loss following bariatric surgery have been seen without associated deleterious effects on immunosuppressive maintenance following liver transplant.[44]

HEPATOCELLULAR CARCINOMA

Prioritization for allocation of liver transplants is based on medical necessity and urgency, as measured by the Model for End-stage Liver Disease (MELD) or Pediatric End-stage Liver Disease (PELD) score, or by registration as status 1A or 1B. However, there are several circumstances in which a candidate's risk for mortality while on the waiting list may not be accurately reflected by the MELD/PELD score and an exception may be requested.[45] Standardized exceptions for which specific criteria must be met include the following:

- Cholangiocarcinoma
- Cystic fibrosis
- Familial amyloid polyneuropathy
- Hepatic artery thrombosis
- Hepatopulmonary syndrome
- Metabolic disease
- Portopulmonary hypertension
- Primary hyperoxaluria
- Hepatocellular carcinoma

In addition to standardized MELD/PELD exceptions, a transplant program can also request exceptions from the national review board for candidates who do not meet these criteria.[46] Among MELD exceptions, HCC is the most common and accounts for more liver transplants annually than all other indications combined. In 2018, a total of 1571 liver transplant recipients had an HCC exception, comprising 20.4% of all liver transplants in the United States that year, compared with 991 recipients who had a MELD exception for any other reason.[4]

In a large prospective trial following more than 900,000 US adults for a period of 16 years, the relationship between excess body weight and risk of death from multiple types of cancer, including liver cancer, was characterized. Men with a BMI greater than or equal to 35 were found to have a relative risk of death from liver cancer of 4.52, compared with those with a normal BMI.[47] The pathologic relationship between obesity and development of HCC is understood to be mediated by the development of hepatic steatosis, necroinflammatory activity, and fibrosis,[48] although NAFLD and the metabolic syndrome have been shown to be risk factors for the development of HCC in patients without cirrhosis.[49] In another study designed to estimate the incidence of HCC in patients with NASH-related cirrhosis, the yearly cumulative incidence of HCC was 2.6% in patients with NASH cirrhosis compared with 4.0% in patients with HCV cirrhosis. In addition, the risk of HCC was found to be increased in patients who consumed alcohol in both the NASH and HCV groups compared with those with no alcohol consumption.[50]

Historically, patients with HCC secondary to HCV have been more likely than those with HCC associated with NASH or ALD to receive MELD exceptions or liver transplant.[51] However, as previously discussed, the rates of liver transplant for HCC/HCV are expected to continue to decline over time, whereas those secondary to NASH are projected to increase.[37] Early evidence of this trend can be seen in **Fig. 8**, which shows the increase of liver transplant for NASH, and specifically HCC-associated NASH, over time.[14]

INNOVATIONS

As the need for liver transplant in the United States increases year after year, the liver transplant community continues to be challenged by an ongoing disparity between the need for and the shortage of donor organs.[52] Many innovative approaches are being studied to further improve the transplant process or even explore alternatives to it. Interspecies blastocyst complementation may enable human organ generation in animals to address the ongoing challenge of organ shortages.[53] Hepatocyte transplant

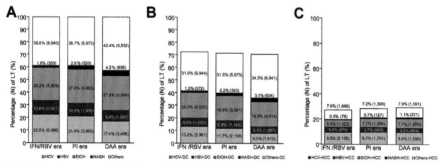

Fig. 8. Percentage and number of liver transplants over 3 eras stratified by etiology of liver disease (*A*) overall, (*B*) with decompensated cirrhosis, and (*C*) with HCC. Interferon (IFN)/ribavirin (RBV) era defined as 2007 to 2010, when only IFN and RBV were available; protease inhibitor (PI) era from 2011 to 2013, when PIs became available; and DAA era from 2014 to June 2017, when DAAs became available. (*From* Belli LS, Perricone G, Adam R, et al. Impact of DAAs on liver transplantation: Major effects on the evolution of indications and results. An ELITA study based on the ELTR registry. *J Hepatol.* 2018;69(4):810-817; with permission.)

has shown promise in small animal models of chronic liver failure. The development of bioartificial liver transplant systems using hepatoblastoma cells or hepatocytes from healthy pig donors brings hope of a dialysis-based artificial liver support device. Tissue engineered regenerated livers show potential to address both the donor shortage and the risk of rejection necessitating chronic immunosuppression.[54]

DISCUSSION

Within the last decade, the indications for listing and subsequent liver transplant have shifted dramatically. The advent of successful treatment of HCV has resulted in a sharp decline in the proportion of patients on the liver transplant waiting list for this diagnosis, whereas the proportion of adults with ALD and NASH continues to increase. The projected upward trajectory for both substance abuse and obesity ensure that this trend will endure into the foreseeable future.

Although DAAs introduced a generally well-tolerated oral HCV treatment for 8 to 12 weeks with high overall cure rates, treatment of NASH and ALD is currently much more challenging because the mainstay of treatment of both conditions is behavioral change. As rates of obesity and alcohol consumption continue to increase in the United States, the consequent need for liver transplant for these indications is expected to place increasing demand on the existing liver transplant infrastructure.

Costs related to the diagnosis and management of NAFLD are significantly higher than those associated with the metabolic syndrome alone, and screening for the general population is not yet recommended by current guidelines, although, if implemented, it would surely place additional strain on the limited number of hepatologists in the United States.[55] Upcoming pharmacologic therapies for NASH may help to alter the natural course of the disease, and wider adoption of bariatric surgery in the peritransplant setting may broaden the availability of liver transplant to this population. Although underlying disease processes such as NASH and ALD are inherently difficult to treat, it is encouraging that patients with these diagnoses have improved posttransplant outcomes compared with those transplanted for HCV.[8]

SUMMARY

The landscape of liver transplant in the United States and globally is changing, driven by continued increase in disease processes of NASH and ALD. Fortunately, HCV as an indication for liver transplant has seen a precipitous decline following the advent of highly efficacious treatment with DAAs. As obesity rates and alcohol use continue to increase in the United States, greater focus on multidisciplinary care and innovation will be necessary to combat the mounting crisis.

CLINICS CARE POINTS

- A greater than 30% reduction in the rate of registration for decompensated cirrhosis in patients with HCV was seen in the less than 2 years following approval of oral DAA regimens, and HCV is no longer the leading indication for liver transplant.
- Outcomes have been favorable for patients who have received transplants for alcoholic hepatitis, with cumulative survival of 94% at 1 year and 84% at 3 years.
- It is predicted that, in the United States, prevalence of obesity will increase to 48.9% and severe obesity, defined as BMI greater than or equal to 35, to 24.2% by the year 2030.

- Bariatric surgery has been shown to improve steatosis and fibrosis in patients with NASH and has also been successfully used in the peritransplant period.

DISCLOSURE

The authors have nothing to disclose.

REFERENCES

1. Starzl TE, Marchioro TL, Vonkaulla KN, et al. Homotransplantation of the liver in humans. Surg Gynecol Obstet 1963;117:659–76.
2. Song AT, Avelino-Silva VI, Pecora RA, et al. Liver transplantation: fifty years of experience. World J Gastroenterol 2014;20(18):5363–74.
3. Strong RW, Lynch SV, Ong TH, et al. Successful liver transplantation from a living donor to her son. N Engl J Med 1990;322(21):1505–7.
4. Kwong A, Kim WR, Lake JR, et al. OPTN/SRTR 2018 annual data Report: liver. Am J Transplant 2020;20(Suppl s1):193–299.
5. Varma V, Mehta N, Kumaran V, et al. Indications and contraindications for liver transplantation. Int J Hepatol 2011;2011:121862.
6. Martin P, DiMartini A, Feng S, et al. Evaluation for liver transplantation in adults: 2013 practice guideline by the American Association for the Study of Liver Diseases and the American Society of Transplantation. Hepatology 2014;59(3): 1144–65.
7. Terrault NA, Pageaux GP. A changing landscape of liver transplantation: King HCV is dethroned, ALD and NAFLD take over! J Hepatol 2018;69(4):767–8.
8. Cholankeril G, Wong RJ, Hu M, et al. Liver transplantation for nonalcoholic steatohepatitis in the US: temporal trends and outcomes. Dig Dis Sci 2017;62(10): 2915–22.
9. Wong RJ, Aguilar M, Cheung R, et al. Nonalcoholic steatohepatitis is the second leading etiology of liver disease among adults awaiting liver transplantation in the United States. Gastroenterology 2015;148(3):547–55.
10. Cholankeril G, Ahmed A. Alcoholic liver disease Replaces hepatitis C virus infection as the leading indication for liver transplantation in the United States. Clin Gastroenterol Hepatol 2018;16(8):1356–8.
11. Thuluvath PJ, Guidinger MK, Fung JJ, et al. Liver transplantation in the United States, 1999-2008. Am J Transplant 2010;10(4 Pt 2):1003–19.
12. Wu T, Konyn PG, Cattaneo AW, et al. New face of hepatitis C. Dig Dis Sci 2019; 64(7):1782–8.
13. Flemming JA, Kim WR, Brosgart CL, et al. Reduction in liver transplant wait-listing in the era of direct-acting antiviral therapy. Hepatology 2017;65(3):804–12.
14. Belli LS, Perricone G, Adam R, et al. Impact of DAAs on liver transplantation: Major effects on the evolution of indications and results. An ELITA study based on the ELTR registry. J Hepatol 2018;69(4):810–7.
15. Ward JW, Hinman AR. What is needed to eliminate hepatitis B virus and hepatitis C virus as global Health threats. Gastroenterology 2019;156(2):297–310.
16. Ting PS, Hamilton JP, Gurakar A, et al. Hepatitis C-positive donor liver transplantation for hepatitis C seronegative recipients. Transpl Infect Dis 2019;21(6): e13194.
17. Singal AK, Bataller R, Ahn J, et al. ACG clinical guideline: alcoholic liver disease. Am J Gastroenterol 2018;113(2):175–94.
18. O'Shea RS, Dasarathy S, McCullough AJ. Practice guideline Committee of the American Association for the Study of Liver D, Practice Parameters Committee

of the American College of G. Alcoholic liver disease. Hepatology 2010;51(1): 307–28.

19. Noureddin M, Vipani A, Bresee C, et al. NASH leading cause of liver transplant in women: updated analysis of indications for liver transplant and ethnic and gender variances. Am J Gastroenterol 2018;113(11):1649–59.

20. Leggio L, Lee MR. Treatment of alcohol use disorder in patients with alcoholic liver disease. Am J Med 2017;130(2):124–34.

21. Grucza RA, Sher KJ, Kerr WC, et al. Trends in adult alcohol use and binge drinking in the early 21st-Century United States: a meta-analysis of 6 National Survey Series. Alcohol Clin Exp Res 2018;42(10):1939–50.

22. Im GY. Acute alcoholic hepatitis. Clin Liver Dis 2019;23(1):81–98.

23. Schuckit MA. Alcohol-use disorders. Lancet 2009;373(9662):492–501.

24. Mathurin P, Moreno C, Samuel D, et al. Early liver transplantation for severe alcoholic hepatitis. N Engl J Med 2011;365(19):1790–800.

25. Stroh G, Rosell T, Dong F, et al. Early liver transplantation for patients with acute alcoholic hepatitis: public views and the effects on organ donation. Am J Transplant 2015;15(6):1598–604.

26. Leong J, Im GY. Evaluation and selection of the patient with alcoholic liver disease for liver transplant. Clin Liver Dis 2012;16(4):851–63.

27. Dom G, Wojnar M, Crunelle CL, et al. Assessing and treating alcohol relapse risk in liver transplantation candidates. Alcohol Alcohol 2015;50(2):164–72.

28. Lee BP, Terrault NA. Early liver transplantation for severe alcoholic hepatitis: moving from controversy to consensus. Curr Opin Organ Transplant 2018;23(2): 229–36.

29. Im GY, Kim-Schluger L, Shenoy A, et al. Early liver transplantation for severe alcoholic hepatitis in the United States–A single-center experience. Am J Transplant 2016;16(3):841–9.

30. Lee BP, Mehta N, Platt L, et al. Outcomes of early liver transplantation for patients with severe alcoholic hepatitis. Gastroenterology 2018;155(2):422–30.e1.

31. Diehl AM, Day C. Cause, pathogenesis, and treatment of nonalcoholic steatohepatitis. N Engl J Med 2017;377(21):2063–72.

32. Chalasani N, Younossi Z, Lavine JE, et al. The diagnosis and management of nonalcoholic fatty liver disease: practice guidance from the American Association for the Study of Liver Diseases. Hepatology 2018;67(1):328–57.

33. Chooi YC, Ding C, Magkos F. The epidemiology of obesity. Metabolism 2019; 92:6–10.

34. Ward ZJ, Bleich SN, Cradock AL, et al. Projected U.S. State-level prevalence of adult obesity and severe obesity. N Engl J Med 2019;381(25):2440–50.

35. Reig M, Gambato M, Man NK, et al. Should patients with NAFLD/NASH Be surveyed for HCC? Transplantation 2019;103(1):39–44.

36. Konerman MA, Jones JC, Harrison SA. Pharmacotherapy for NASH: current and emerging. J Hepatol 2018;68(2):362–75.

37. Shingina A, DeWitt PE, Dodge JL, et al. Future trends in demand for liver transplant: Birth cohort effects among patients with NASH and HCC. Transplantation 2019;103(1):140–8.

38. Spengler EK, O'Leary JG, Te HS, et al. Liver transplantation in the obese Cirrhotic patient. Transplantation 2017;101(10):2288–96.

39. Diwan TS, Rice TC, Heimbach JK, et al. Liver transplantation and bariatric surgery: timing and outcomes. Liver Transpl 2018;24(9):1280–7.

40. Furuya CK Jr, de Oliveira CP, de Mello ES, et al. Effects of bariatric surgery on nonalcoholic fatty liver disease: preliminary findings after 2 years. J Gastroenterol Hepatol 2007;22(4):510–4.
41. Bazerbachi F, Vargas EJ, Rizk M, et al. Intragastric balloon placement induces significant metabolic and histologic improvement in patients with nonalcoholic steatohepatitis. Clin Gastroenterol Hepatol 2020. S1542-3565(20)30613-3.
42. Sharpton SR, Terrault NA, Posselt AM. Outcomes of sleeve gastrectomy in obese liver transplant candidates. Liver Transpl 2019;25(4):538–44.
43. Heimbach JK, Watt KD, Poterucha JJ, et al. Combined liver transplantation and gastric sleeve resection for patients with medically complicated obesity and end-stage liver disease. Am J Transplant 2013;13(2):363–8.
44. Yemini R, Nesher E, Winkler J, et al. Bariatric surgery in solid organ transplant patients: long-term follow-up results of outcome, safety, and effect on immunosuppression. Am J Transplant 2018;18(11):2772–80.
45. Guidance to Liver Transplant Programs and the National Liver Review Board for: Adult MELD Exception Review. Organ Procurement and Transplantation Network. Available at: https://optn.transplant.hrsa.gov/media/3939/20200804_nlrb_adult_other_guidance.pdf.
46. Organ Procurement and Transplantation Network (OPTN) Policies. Organ Procurement and Transplantation Network. Available at: https://optn.transplant.hrsa.gov/media/1200/optn_policies.pdf.
47. Calle EE, Rodriguez C, Walker-Thurmond K, et al. Overweight, obesity, and mortality from cancer in a prospectively studied cohort of U.S. adults. N Engl J Med 2003;348(17):1625–38.
48. El-Serag HB, Rudolph KL. Hepatocellular carcinoma: epidemiology and molecular carcinogenesis. Gastroenterology 2007;132(7):2557–76.
49. Mittal S, El-Serag HB, Sada YH, et al. Hepatocellular carcinoma in the absence of cirrhosis in United States veterans is associated with nonalcoholic fatty liver disease. Clin Gastroenterol Hepatol 2016;14(1):124–31.e1.
50. Ascha MS, Hanouneh IA, Lopez R, et al. The incidence and risk factors of hepatocellular carcinoma in patients with nonalcoholic steatohepatitis. Hepatology 2010;51(6):1972–8.
51. Young K, Aguilar M, Gish R, et al. Lower rates of receiving model for end-stage liver disease exception and longer time to transplant among nonalcoholic steatohepatitis hepatocellular carcinoma. Liver Transpl 2016;22(10):1356–66.
52. Bodzin AS, Baker TB. Liver transplantation today: where we are now and where we are going. Liver Transpl 2018;24(10):1470–5.
53. Wu J, Platero-Luengo A, Sakurai M, et al. Interspecies Chimerism with mammalian pluripotent stem cells. Cell 2017;168(3):473–86.e15.
54. Nicolas CT, Hickey RD, Chen HS, et al. Concise review: liver regenerative medicine: from hepatocyte transplantation to bioartificial livers and bioengineered grafts. Stem Cells 2017;35(1):42–50.
55. Paul S, Charlton M. Liver transplantation for nonalcoholic steatohepatitis: new evidence of a profound increase across age cohorts. Transplantation 2019;103(1):1–2.

Cardiac and Pulmonary Vascular Risk Stratification in Liver Transplantation

Blessing Aghaulor, MD, MPH[a], Lisa B. VanWagner, MD, MSc, FAST[a,b],*

KEYWORDS

- Cardiovascular • Stratification • Liver • Transplant • Risk factors
- Early complications

KEY POINTS

- Cardiovascular disease complications are the leading cause of early mortality among liver transplant recipients.
- Traditional cardiac risk factors, such as diabetes, hypertension, and hyperlipidemia, are increasing in prevalence among liver transplant candidates and are highly associated with post–liver transplant cardiac events.
- Most cardiovascular disease complications after liver transplant are nonischemic.
- Atrial fibrillation has been shown to be the most common cause of early (within 90 days) major cardiovascular events among liver transplant recipients.
- The Cardiovascular Risk in Orthotopic Liver Transplantation score is a cardiovascular disease risk prediction model that uses pretransplant demographic, social, and clinical variables to estimate the risk of a major cardiovascular events in the first year after transplant.

INTRODUCTION

Approximately 8000 liver transplants (LTs) are performed in the United States every year for patients with fulminant liver failure or end-stage liver disease (ESLD).[1] The survival rates are greater than 90% and 70% for LT recipients (LTRs) at 1 year and 5 year posttransplant, respectively.[2] Advancements in organ preservation techniques, antiviral agents, immunosuppression, and screening protocols will likely further improve survival rates by decreasing rates of hepatic disease and malignancy, which previously were common causes of death in LTRs.[3,4] However, despite the improvement

Financial disclosures: Dr L.B. VanWagner is currently supported by the National Institutes of Health's National Heart, Lung, and Blood Institute, grant number K23HL136891.
[a] Division of Gastroenterology and Hepatology, Department of Medicine, Northwestern University Feinberg School of Medicine, 676 North St Clair Street, Suite 1400, Chicago, IL 60611, USA; [b] Division of Epidemiology, Department of Preventive Medicine, Northwestern University Feinberg School of Medicine, Chicago, IL, USA
* Corresponding author. 676 North St Clair Street, Suite 1400, Chicago, IL 60611.
E-mail address: lvw@northwestern.edu

in short-term and long-term survival after LT, there has been a marked increase in chronic disease burden and morbidity in this population.[5] Complications caused by cardiac and pulmonary vascular diseases are a leading cause of morbidity and mortality after LT. Cardiovascular disease (CVD) complications, defined in the literature to include arrhythmias, cardiac arrest, heart failure (HF), stroke, myocardial infarction, and thromboembolism, are now the leading cause of early (<1 year) mortality and the third leading cause of late (>1 year) mortality in LTRs.[6-8] CVD mortality after LT has increased by 50% since 2002,[9] and LTRs have a 64% increased risk of having a cardiovascular event (CVE) over 10 years compared with the general population.[10] Impressively, 1 in 3 LTRs experience a CVE within 1 year of transplant.[7,8]

Reasons for the observed increased CVD risk in LT candidates are multifactorial. First, traditional cardiac risk factors such as hypertension, diabetes, and hyperlipidemia[7,11,12] are all increasing in prevalence among LT candidates and are highly associated with post-LT CVEs both short and long term after transplant.[8] For example, 1 study showed that postoperative ischemic complications are 40% higher in patients with pre-LT insulin-dependent diabetes or known coronary artery disease (CAD) than in those without.[12] Second, liver-specific risk factors have also been associated with high rates of post-LT CVEs. Nonalcoholic steatohepatitis (NASH) and alcohol-induced liver disease have both been shown to have an increased association with early major CVEs compared with other causes of ESLD.[8] This finding is particularly relevant because NASH cirrhosis is now the second most common and quickest-growing indication for LT,[13] and is projected to become the number 1 indication for LT within the next decade.[13,14] Patients with NASH cirrhosis in particular have been shown to have a 4 times higher risk of CVE after LT compared with patients with other causes of cirrhosis, such as cholestatic liver disease.[7] Third, the use of the Model for End-stage Liver Disease (MELD) score to prioritize donor livers to the sickest patients generates a candidate pool with a high burden of critical illnesses and, as a result, a high prevalence of subclinical and clinical CVD.[15] Fourth, an aging candidate pool has resulted in a high burden of comorbid medical conditions, including CVD, at the time of LT.[8] Fifth, the LT operation itself is associated with significant stress on the cardiac and pulmonary vascular system, which can unmask subclinical CVD.[16] In addition, posttransplant chronic immunosuppression can accelerate or contribute to de novo CVD.[17] All of these things in concert contribute to the high burden of CVD in LT candidates and recipients, and the incidence of CVD and its associated complications are expected to continue to increase over the next decade.

This article discusses the approach to cardiac and pulmonary vascular disease risk stratification in LT candidates, with a specific focus on perioperative and short-term (<1 year) CVE risk.[7,8] It addresses the epidemiology and available data supporting risk assessment for underlying arrhythmia, HF, stroke, coronary heart disease, valvular heart disease, and portopulmonary hypertension in LT candidates. This article also explores the prognostic tools available to risk stratify candidates based on their global risk for CVEs, which can be used to improve the candidate selection process and potentially improve allocation of scarce donor organs. In addition, although not the primary focus of this article, the emerging data on long-term CVD risk factors and complications are also briefly discussed.

Arrhythmias

Arrhythmias are the most common CVD complication among LTRs within 30 days of LT.[18] Arrhythmias present before LT indicate underlying cardiac disorder that increases the risk of CVD complications following LT.[19,20] The primary screening modality for underlying arrhythmia is an electrocardiogram (ECG). Current American

Association for the Study of Liver Diseases (AASLD)/American Society of Transplantation (AST) guidelines recommend that all LT candidates be screened with an ECG to assess for prevalent arrhythmia, and, if identified, investigation into underlying causes and consultation with a cardiologist is recommended.[21]

Atrial fibrillation, a common marker of underlying hypertension and cirrhotic cardiomyopathy (CCM),[16] is the most common preexisting arrhythmia, and is present in 1% to 6% of LT candidates,[8,22] in contrast with 0.95% to 2.3% among the general population.[8] Although conflicting data exist about the association between preexisting atrial fibrillation and liver graft dysfunction and mortality,[8,22] several studies have shown that preexisting atrial fibrillation confers a higher risk of cardiovascular (CV) complications both intraoperatively and postoperatively.[8,19,22] For example, Van-Wagner and colleagues[8] showed that preexisting atrial fibrillation was present in 33% of patients with major CVE within 90 days of LT compared with 7% of patients without a CVE.

Intraoperative electrolyte imbalances are common during LT and can instigate cardiac dysfunction and arrhythmias. For example, the donor graft is commonly preserved in a high-potassium solution, which contributes to arrhythmias and cardiac arrest, during reperfusion. In a retrospective study of 146 patients who underwent LT, Dec and colleagues[23] found that either ventricular tachycardia or fibrillation was the most common intraoperative cardiac complication (3.4%), but the fourth most common postoperative complication (2.7%). Donovan and colleagues[24] found that, among 71 patients who underwent LT, 10 patients (14%) developed perioperative arrhythmias, with 5 patients developing atrial fibrillation and 2 developing ventricular arrhythmias. Postoperatively, atrial fibrillation occurs in up to 43% of LTRs and is the most common contributing cause to rehospitalization within 90 days of LT.[8] In the same study, cardiac arrest occurred in 6% of recipients and was the fifth most common complication in this early 90-day period.[8]

One potential risk factor for development of arrhythmia post-LT is corrected QT (QTc) prolongation, which is present in 30% to 60% of patients with ESLD.[25] QTc prolongation is a disorder of myocardial depolarization and occurs when a QT interval is greater than 0.45 seconds in men and 0.47 seconds in women.[16,18] When QTc prolongation is present, the incidence of sudden cardiac death in patients with ESLD is the same as that in patients without ESLD.[24] However, QTc prolongation may predispose LT candidates to ventricular arrhythmias.[24] Some studies have shown that QTc prolongation is not associated with increased mortality and it is not a contraindication for LT,[12] whereas others conclude that the risk of post-LT CVEs and mortality is increased.[18,24,26] Current clinical practice guidance from the AST recommends that patients with a prolonged QTc should be evaluated for reversible causes, such as electrolyte derangements and medications.[21] In addition, in patients with known dysrhythmias, perioperative hemodynamic monitoring is recommended, with anticipated treatment readily available, including antiarrhythmic medications, transcutaneous or transvenous pacing, electrical cardioversion, or defibrillation.[21] Family history should be obtained and the patient should be referred to a cardiologist if there is a positive family history of sudden cardiac death.[21] In most patients with ESLD, QTc prolongation resolves on its own following LT.[27]

Heart Failure and Cardiomyopathy

Studies have shown that HF is the second most common early CVD complication post-LT, occurring in 28% of patients within 90 days of LT, and contributing to a quarter of all hospital admissions within the same time frame.[8] Both HF and arrhythmias make up 50% of CVD complications within 1 year of LT,[20] and postoperative

HF is associated with mortalities as high as 15%.[28] In the general population, the definition of HF with preserved ejection fraction (HFpEF) requires an ejection fraction (EF) greater than 50%, whereas that of HF with reduced ejection fraction (HFrEF) requires an EF less than or equal to 40%.[29] Notably, based on published clinical practice guidance from the AST, the absolute and relative contraindications to LT are EFs less than 40% and less than 50%, respectively.[21] However, there are few data to support these EF thresholds beyond clinical experience and center-specific risk tolerance. Pretransplant left ventricle dysfunction has been shown to predispose LTRs to increased risk of CV complications.[6,8] Diastolic dysfunction before LT, specifically, has been associated with an increased risk of graft rejection and failure, post-LT systolic dysfunction, and mortality.[30]

Postoperative HFpEF is more common than HFrEF in LTRs, and ranges from 3% to 43% depending on which echocardiographic consensus guidelines are used for the definition of diastolic dysfunction,[9,22,31] with the 2016 American Society of Echocardiography (ASE) and European Association of Cardiac Imaging (EACI) guidelines being the most up to date.[25,32] The prevalence of HFrEF post-LT is much lower, at just 2% to 7%,[9,22,32] likely because of the exclusion of patients with ESLD with prevalent HFrEF from LT as discussed earlier.

LT candidates are screened for HF preoperatively using echocardiography, which can detect both HFpEF, which corresponds to diastolic dysfunction, and HFrEF, which corresponds to systolic dysfunction.[33,34] The preoperative risk assessment also includes an assessment for left ventricular outflow tract obstruction (LVOTO), which is inducible on dobutamine stress echocardiography in more than 40% of patients.[35] LVOTO can occur as a result of concurrent left ventricular hypertrophy and hyperdynamic systolic function resulting in a significant outflow gradient. One study showed that a gradient of greater than 36 mm Hg is significantly associated with intraoperative hypotension in transplant candidates and is a contraindication to transplant in some centers.[35] Cardiac magnetic resonance (CMR) imaging can also be used to screen for or diagnose structural or functional cardiac abnormalities in patients with ESLD. CMR provides markers of abnormal cardiac structure and function that cannot be assessed with echocardiography. For example, CMR T1 and T2 tissue mapping can detect subendocardial edema and myocardial fibrosis, which are markers of myocardial remodeling described in patients with ESLD.[36-38] Functional testing, including the 6-minute walk test (6MWT) and cardiopulmonary exercise testing (CPET), may also be used preoperatively to assess cardiopulmonary reserve in LT candidates.[39] In the 6MWT, the distance an LT candidate is able to walk in the allotted 6-minute period correlates with overall cardiopulmonary fitness. One study found that a distance of less than 250 m was associated with a higher waitlist mortality; however, the correlation with posttransplant outcomes was not investigated.[40] CPET measures a participant's anaerobic threshold during a progressive exercise regimen.[39] An aerobic threshold greater than 9 mL/kg/min is an accurate predictor of early (90-day) posttransplant survival.[41] Of note, functional testing in LT candidates is often limited by the high prevalence of malnutrition, sarcopenia, and severe deconditioning, which may prohibit patient participation in this type of testing.[39]

If guideline-directed medical therapy for HF is initiated before LT, it should be continued postoperatively. However, angiotensin-converting enzyme inhibitors may need to be dose reduced for kidney dysfunction or electrolyte abnormalities that may be caused by calcineurin inhibitors or aldosterone antagonists.[12] In addition, although carvedilol is often the optimal β-blocker in patients with ESLD,[42] it should be used with caution post-LT because of its ability to reduce portal pressures, which can lead to graft ischemia.[42]

An important contributor to HF prevalence in LT candidates is the presence of cirrhotic cardiomyopathy (CCM). CCM is the most common risk factor for post-LT HF and is found in 40% to 50% of patients with ESLD.[43,44] CCM has long been characterized as hyperdynamic cardiac function caused by low systemic vascular resistance and high cardiac output in the absence of known causes of cardiac disease (eg, prior myocardial infarction).[38] The diagnostic criteria for CCM based on echocardiography have recently been updated to require:

1. Left ventricular EF (LVEF) less than or equal to 50%, or
2. Absolute global longitudinal strain of less than 18%

And 3 or more of the following:

1. Septal e' velocity less than 7 cm/s
2. E/e' ratio greater than 15
3. Left atrial volume index greater than 34 mL/m^2
4. Tricuspid regurgitant (TR) velocity greater than 2.8 m/s[38]

CCM is thought to be caused by myocardial hypertrophy, myocardial fibrosis, and subendocardial edema.[16,45] The risk of developing CCM depends in part on the cause of the ESLD, and is highest with cirrhosis caused by NASH, alcohol, hepatitis C virus, and hemochromatosis.[21] CCM has been shown to increase the risk of intraoperative complications and of developing HF postoperatively.[46] Given the demonstration of poor CV outcomes in patients with HF before LT, and that most patients with ESLD have some component of CCM,[43,44] appropriate screening of LT candidates and close monitoring with repeated echocardiography post-LT are important. Based on recommendation from the Cirrhotic Cardiomyopathy Consortium, the recommended screening interval for CCM using echocardiogram in LT candidates is, at minimum, every 6 months before transplant and at intervals of 6, 12, and 24 months posttransplant in all patients with any degree of pretransplant systolic or diastolic dysfunction based on the aforementioned criteria.[38]

Stroke

Stroke is a CVD complication that is not well studied in LT. Few data exists on the prevalence of ischemic and hemorrhagic stroke in candidates before LT; however, hemorrhagic stroke may be more prevalent in patients with alcohol-related cirrhosis compared with other causes.[47] In a multivariable analysis of 32,810 LTRs, VanWagner and colleagues[8] reported that pretransplant stroke increased the likelihood of 30-day and 90-day major CVEs with an incidence risk ratio of 6.3 and 4.8, respectively. The same study found that stroke occurred in 9% of those hospitalized within 90 days of transplant.

The risk of post-LT stroke is highest in recipients of older age and those with pretransplant diabetes, hypertension, hyperlipidemia.[48] Hypertension is a potentially modifiable risk factor for stroke and is present in up to 53.7% of LT candidates.[49] Hypertension prevalence increases after LT, with up to 92% of LTRs having hypertension by 6 years posttransplant.[49] This finding is a result of several factors, including direct calcineurin inhibition, nephrotoxicity from calcineurin inhibitors (particularly with the combination of cyclosporine and mammalian target of rapamycin inhibitors), steroid use, preexisting hypertension, older age, and both renal and systemic vasoconstriction.[7,49] Adherence to blood pressure management guidelines has been shown to be inversely related to CVD complication rates and CVD mortality; however, patients at highest risk for poor CV outcomes are less likely to have appropriate blood pressure management.[49] In addition to improved blood pressure control before and after LT, smoking cessation, statin use, and anticoagulation, if indicated, can also reduce the risk of stroke.[8] There is currently no guideline recommendation to perform routine imaging screening in LT waitlist candidates for stroke. However, in LT candidates and recipients who present with cognitive, sensory, or motor dysfunction, a high index of suspicion for possible stroke is required and diagnostic imaging should be pursued.

Coronary Artery Disease

Surgical and pharmacologic advancements in the management of CAD have significantly decreased the burden of CV morbidity and mortality in the general public.[50] The prevalence of CAD among patients with ESLD is the same or greater than for the general population,[51] ranging from 2.5% to 27%.[49,50] LT candidates with known CAD are at greater risk for intraoperative complications during LT surgery.[5] Roughly 25% of LT candidates with traditional CAD risk factors (such as hypertension, hyperlipidemia, and diabetes) have moderate CAD stenosis,[51] defined as greater than 50% stenosis, and those with 2 or more traditional CAD risk factors are more likely to have obstructive CAD.[52–54] Those with severe stenosis had a higher risk of mortality despite coronary revascularization.[55] Even in the absence of severe stenosis, multivessel CAD is associated with increased mortality and postoperative hemodynamic instability.[55] LT candidates with NASH cirrhosis are more likely to have traditional risk factors for CAD,[56] and both NASH and renal dysfunction predispose to critical coronary stenosis.[56,57] Conflicting data exist about whether NASH cirrhosis is an CAD risk factor independent of traditional CAD risk factors.[57–59]

The utility of stress testing as a means of CAD risk stratification in LT waitlist candidates is debated.[60] Exercise stress testing has poor predictive value in the ESLD population because patients are often too debilitated to reach their target heart rates,[23] and, therefore, pharmacologic stress testing using dobutamine, dipyridamole, or adenosine is often used. Plevak[61] suggested that the stress imaging modality of choice should be dobutamine stress echocardiography (DSE). However, studies have shown that subsequent cardiac catheterization does not correlate with imaged wall motion abnormalities.[62] Williams and colleagues[63] showed a lack of correlation between positive DSE and intraoperative CVEs, and another study showed that stress echocardiography failed to identify LT candidates at high cardiac risk for LT surgery.[55,60] Thus, DSE has very poor sensitivity, as low as 13%, and low negative predictive value (75%) for the detection of obstructive CAD.[23,63–65] Furthermore, other studies have shown pre-LT DSE to have a positive predictive value of only 27% and a specificity of 87% for determining adverse CVEs within 30 days post-LT.[55] Therefore, DSE is not useful for risk stratification for obstructive CAD or CVEs in patients with ESLD.[62] The chronic vasodilatory state of patients with ESLD makes pharmacologic vasodilator testing unreliable as well,[65] with 1 study showing that even high-risk patients were identified as low risk in a myocardial perfusion study (MPS).[60] A meta-analysis explored the utility of DSE and MPS in CAD detection compared with the gold standard of coronary catheterization among LT candidates.[66] The pooled sensitivity was 28% and 61% and specificity was 82% and 74% for DSE and MPS, respectively.

Given the poor performance of noninvasive stress testing in the detection of CAD among patients with ESLD,[12] coronary angiography, either invasive or noninvasive, is the gold standard for detecting CAD in this population.[21] Several studies have proposed that patients more than 45 years of age and with 2 or more traditional CAD risk factors undergo invasive coronary catheterization (**Fig. 1**).[12,67] However, computed tomography angiography (CTA) is emerging as a noninvasive alternative to invasive coronary catheterization.[12] Anatomic coronary assessment with coronary CTA is not limited by the hemodynamic abnormalities of ESLD, and computed tomography

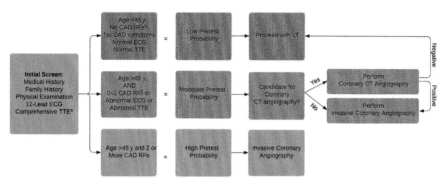

Fig. 1. Proposed screening algorithm for coronary artery disease risk. [a] Tissue Doppler echocardiography with myocardial deformation imaging according to American Society for Echocardiography guidelines. [b] CAD risk factors include hypercholesterolemia, hypertension, diabetes, current/prior tobacco use, prior CVD, or left ventricular hypertrophy. CT, computed tomography; RFs, risk factors; TTE, transthoracic echocardiogram.

provides the additional advantage of simultaneously obtaining a coronary artery calcium score (CACS), which in itself adds prognostic information.[68,69] CACS greater than 400 is associated with increased risk for underlying obstructive CAD in LT.[70] Furthermore, coronary artery calcium scoring has been shown to be predictive of CAD requiring revascularization and 1-month post-LT complications.[70] In addition, coronary CTA recently showed superior sensitivity for evaluation of obstructive CAD compared with other noninvasive modalities before kidney transplant.[71]

When examining how best to mitigate the risk of atherosclerotic CVD (ASCVD) complications post-LT, it is important to recognize 3 facts. First, not all candidates undergo coronary angiography and, therefore, some may have undetected subclinical CAD going into LT surgery. Second, LTRs are at risk of accelerated atherosclerosis following transplant, as shown in several studies,[72–74] and are therefore less likely to form collaterals, leading to an increased long-term risk of CAD mortality. Third, LTRs are at an increased risk of developing dyslipidemia post-LT as a result of immunosuppressive agents (**Fig. 2**). Therefore, more studies are needed to determine the degree to which LTRs' risk of CAD-related mortality is a result of undiagnosed subclinical CAD versus post-LT risk factors.[75]

As a result of improved ASCVD screening, interventions, and medical management for LT candidates before LT, CAD is increasingly becoming a later-term (>1 year) CVD complication,[76] constituting up to 39.8% of CV complications among patients over roughly a 10-year period post-LT.[26] Management of traditional risk factors (eg, hypertension, diabetes mellitus, and hyperlipidemia), exacerbated by immunosuppressive agents, is necessary to secure the long-term health of LTRs. In addition to traditional risk factors, posttransplant metabolic syndrome and renal dysfunction, both influenced by chronic immunosuppressive agents, also need to be continually addressed in the posttransplant period in order to reduce long-term ASCVD complications.

Valvular Heart Disease

Aortic stenosis (AS) is the most common stenotic valvular lesion in adults, although the specific prevalence in LT candidates is unknown.[39] AS can result in systemic hypoperfusion, and the associated left ventricular hypertrophy can be arrhythmogenic.[77] Mitral regurgitation, TR, or both have been found in 28% of all LTRs.[78] The effect of these

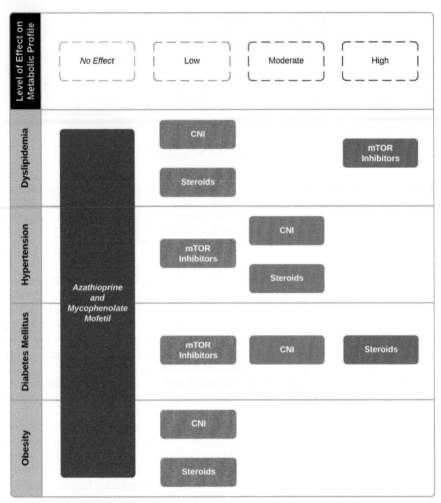

Fig. 2. Effects of immunosuppressive classes on components of the metabolic profile. CNI, calcineurin inhibitors (e, tacrolimus, cyclosporine); mTOR inhibitors, mammalian target of rapamycin inhibitors (eg, everolimus).

valvular disorders on post-LT CV outcomes remains unclear; however they seem to be of greatest significance intraoperatively and perioperatively. For example, TR can result in venous congestion and lead to right ventricular HF, thereby causing hypoperfusion to the new graft.[39] For this reason, LT candidates should be screened preoperatively for valvular dysfunction, and pretransplant repair in appropriate candidates is recommended in severe cases.[39]

The treatment options for AS, in particular, have been well studied. These options include surgical aortic valve repair (SAVR) and transcatheter aortic valve replacement (TAVR). A retrospective cohort study performed by Peeraphatdit and colleagues[79] showed comparable in-hospital (1.8% vs 2%) and 30-day mortality (3.2% vs 4.6%) among 105 cirrhotic patients undergoing TAVR and SAVR respectively. However, when stratified by MELD scores, the SAVR group showed improved median survival among patients with a MELD less than 12 compared with the TAVR group (4.4 years vs 2.8 years). There was no difference in survival between TAVR and SAVR in patients with MELD greater than or equal to 12.[79]

Severe valvular disease in LT candidates necessitates close hemodynamic monitoring, and repair is recommended in severe cases before transplant. MELD scores, shown to be an independent predictor of survival in the repair of aortic valves,[79] may be of utility in determining optimal management of tricuspid and mitral valve disorders as well.

Portopulmonary Hypertension

Portopulmonary hypertension (PoPH) is a disorder that occurs in 5% to 10% of LT candidates, where pulmonary vasculature constriction leads to remodeling.[80] By definition, patients with PoPH also have pulmonary hypertension, which can lead to right-sided HF, resulting in adverse CV outcomes.[21]

Findings of increased pulmonary artery systolic pressure (PASP) on echocardiography may indicate PoPH. Although no consensus has been reached on a cutoff value for PASP that should trigger further invasive testing, a threshold of PASP greater than 45 mm Hg has been suggested.[81] If PASP is greater than 45 mm Hg, right heart catheterization findings diagnostic for primary pulmonary hypertension are:

1. Increased mean pulmonary arterial pressure (mPAP) greater than or equal to 25 mm Hg
2. Pulmonary vascular resistance (PVR) of greater than 240 dyn·s cm^{-5}
3. Low pulmonary capillary wedge pressure (PCWP) less than or equal to 15 mm Hg[12,21]

mPAP of 25 to 34 mm Hg is consistent with mild PoPH, whereas mPAP greater than or equal to 35 mm Hg is consistent with moderate to severe PoPH. One study showed that LT candidates with PoPH and mPAP greater than or equal to 35 mm Hg had a 50% mortality, which increased to 100% for those with mPAP of 50 mm Hg or greater.[82] If left untreated, the median survival for all patients with PoPH approaches 15 months, with a 5-year survival of just 14%.[83] In contrast, for those treated with pulmonary vasodilators, median survival increases to 46 months and 5-year mortality increases to 45%.[83]

LT is possible in patients with mild PoPH; however, those with moderate to severe PoPH must undergo a trial of vasodilator therapy with prostaglandins, phosphodiesterase inhibitors, or endothelin receptor antagonists in an attempt to decrease pulmonary pressures before LT.[84] If mPAP is successfully decreased to less than 35 mm Hg and PVR less than 400 dyn·s cm^{-5}, MELD exception points can be granted to the LT candidates.[85] A study was done on outcomes after LT among 11 patients with moderate-severe PoPH, in whom adequate mPAP reduction was achieved with vasodilator therapy before LT. Interestingly, the 1-year and 5-year survivals following LT were 91% and 67%, respectively, and 9 of the 11 patients were off vasodilator therapy at 9.2 months post-LT.[86] In another, smaller study, 4 patients with PoPH who responded to vasodilator therapy with epoprostenol were successfully transplanted. Of the 4, 2 were weaned off epoprostenol within 8 months post-LT, whereas 2 remained on oral vasodilators at the time of publication, corresponding with 9 to 18 months posttransplant.[87] These studies show that pharmacologic therapy can permit safe LT in patients with PoPH. However, intraoperative challenges exist with PoPH, and cardiac output, which is a surrogate marker of right ventricle function, is a predictor of operative survival.[83,88] Therefore, inotropes and prostacyclins may need to be administered during the procedure, and consultation with pulmonary hypertension specialists is recommended.[21] Importantly, there are no data to support the concept that PoPH (treated or untreated) should be an indication for LT.[89]

Risk Scores for Prediction of Global Cardiovascular Risk in Liver Transplant Recipients

Risk prediction for cardiac complications can be divided between general risk assessment tools and surgical cardiac risk calculators (**Fig. 3**).

General risk assessment tools

The Framingham Risk Score (FRS) predicts the 10-year risk of fatal or nonfatal coronary events using a multivariable risk prediction algorithm.[90] This score has been evaluated in LT candidates and studies show an inverse relationship between candidates with high FRS (FRS>20) and median survival at 1, 3, and 5 years post-LT.[91] The C-statistic for FRS ranges from 0.76 to 0.79, and shows moderate discrimination for CVEs and mortality among LT candidates.[91]

The Reynold Risk Score (RRS) builds on the traditional CV risk factors used in the FRS by also adding high-sensitivity C-reactive protein and parental family history of premature CHD.[92] Although this risk score has been shown to be more predictive of CVD than FRS in the general population,[92] it has not been applied to LT candidates and so its utility in this population has yet to be verified.

The American College of Cardiology (ACC) and American Heart Association (AHA) developed the pooled cohort equations (PCE) risk calculator to estimate the 10-year and lifetime risk of atherosclerotic CV disease (ASCVD) events.[93] The purpose of this calculator is to guide therapeutic interventions (eg, statins, antihypertensive medications) to decrease the risk of CVEs. However, patients with cirrhosis and LTRs were not included in the studies used to derive these equations and, thus, the predictive ability of the PCE in our patient population is unknown. Other risk assessment tools include the European Systemic Coronary Risk Evaluation Project (SCORE) and the German Prospective Cardiovascular Munster Study (PROCAM), which have limited predictive power in waitlist candidates.[94]

The utility of standard risk algorithms as a predictive tool is limited in the LT population, particularly in patients with subclinical disease.[20] Most CVD complications post-LT are noncoronary[6]; however, these risk scores are intended to identify the risk of events related to CAD. These tools are also yet to be calibrated to LT candidates[12,81] and may be inaccurate in patients with subclinical CVD. Troponin levels, a marker of cardiac myocyte injury and death, have been shown to correlate with risk of post-LT CV events in subclinical or asymptomatic patients regardless of concomitant comorbidities. One study showed that an increase in pretransplant

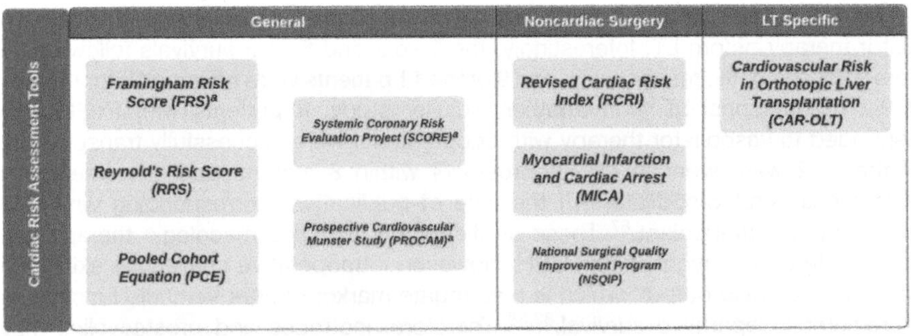

Cardiac Risk Assessment Tools	General		Noncardiac Surgery	LT Specific
	Framingham Risk Score (FRS)[a]		Revised Cardiac Risk Index (RCRI)	Cardiovascular Risk in Orthotopic Liver Transplantation (CAR-OLT)
		Systemic Coronary Risk Evaluation Project (SCORE)[a]		
	Reynold's Risk Score (RRS)		Myocardial Infarction and Cardiac Arrest (MICA)	
		Prospective Cardiovascular Munster Study (PROCAM)[a]		
	Pooled Cohort Equation (PCE)		National Surgical Quality Improvement Program (NSQIP)	

Fig. 3. Available cardiac risk assessment tools. [a] Studied in the LT population.

troponin I level (>0.07 ng/mL) was associated with de novo CVD in posttransplant patients,[76] whereas another showed that troponin level increase (>0.1 ng/mL) was associated with higher 30-day post-LT mortality.[95] The I isoform has been shown to be more reliable in patients with renal dysfunction than the T isotope and may be a useful risk stratification tool in patients with ESLD.[95]

Surgical cardiac risk calculators

Perioperative cardiac events are a leading cause of death following noncardiac surgery.[96] As such, risk stratification before surgery allows cardiac optimization and is an important part of the informed consent process.[97]

The Revised Cardiac Risk Index (RCRI) is a cardiac risk tool that uses 6 variables (history of ischemic heart disease, HF, stroke, insulin-dependent diabetes, CKD, high-risk surgery) to risk stratify patients into either low-risk, medium-risk, or high-risk categories for perioperative cardiac complications in noncardiac surgeries. This risk calculator was incorporated into the ACC/AHA and European Society of Cardiology (ESC) guidelines for perioperative cardiac risk assessment and management.[98] Park and colleagues[99] investigated the combined predictive ability of the RCRI and MELD and found that patients with both higher MELD and RCRI scores had higher rate of cumulative cardiac events. Predictive ability was increased in models that used both RCRI and MELD compared with models using MELD alone, suggesting significant potential utility if adapted to the ESLD population.[99]

Despite its popularity, the RCRI was validated on just 4315 patients.[20] In contrast, the MICA (myocardial infarction and cardiac arrest) risk calculator developed by Gupta and colleagues[98] was validated on a cohort of more than 400,000 patients. MICA is an interactive risk calculator and uses 5 predictors (type of surgery, dependent functional status, abnormal creatinine, American Society of Anesthesiologists class, and increasing age) to provide a probability estimate of MICA.[98] With a C-statistic of 0.88, MICA has superior discriminative and predictive abilities compared with the RCRI, although neither have been studied in the LT population.[98]

The American College of Surgeons (ACS) National Surgical Quality Improvement Program (NSQIP) developed a nationally validated, risk-adjusted, outcomes-based program that aims to improve the quality of surgical care. The ACS NSQIP developed a risk calculator to predict 30-day postoperative risks using 21 variables, including American Society of Anesthesiology class and functional status.[100] The C-statistic for this calculator ranges from 0.806 to 0.99 and was 0.895 for cardiac complications. Despite its good discriminative ability, it has questionable validity among LT candidates given the likely small proportion of LT candidates among the national sample.[100]

The Cardiovascular Risk in Orthotopic Liver Transplantation (CAR-OLT) score is a CVD risk prediction model that was derived in LT candidates and uses pretransplant demographic, social, and clinical variables to estimate the risk of a major CVEs in the first year posttransplant.[9] The model uses a point-based system for 12 weighted covariates, namely preoperative recipient age, sex, race, employment status, education status, history of hepatocellular carcinoma, diabetes, HF, atrial fibrillation, pulmonary or systemic hypertension, and respiratory failure (available at www.carolt.us).[9] The model defines major CVEs as myocardial infarction, cardiac revascularization, HF, atrial fibrillation, cardiac arrest, pulmonary embolism, or stroke within 1 year after LT.[9] This score has a good discriminative ability with a C-statistic of 0.78 and is unique in that it estimates risk of CVD complications specifically after LT.[101] Therefore, it is a potential prognostic tool in assessing a patient's risk of a CVE after LT and informing risk-based discussions. However, it has not been prospectively validated in LT, and whether closer monitoring or risk factor optimization in patients with high CAR-OLT risk alters post-LT outcomes is unknown.

Risk Factors for Long-Term (>1 Year) Cardiovascular Disease Complications in Liver Transplant Recipients

Traditional cardiac risk factors, namely hypertension, diabetes, and hyperlipidemia, play an important role in the development of long-term CVD complications,[8] which are the third leading cause of long-term mortality in LTRs, as previously stated. Posttransplant diabetes mellitus has been shown to confer the greatest long-term risk for major CVEs in LTRs, with cumulative incidences of 13% and 27% at 5 and 10 years respectively.[102] In addition, studies have shown that hypertension can develop in 65% to 80% of previously normotensive LTRs.[103] Hypertension is often missed in LTRs when assessed solely by in-office blood pressure checks, which detected 2.5 times fewer cases compared with 24-hour ambulatory blood pressure monitoring, in part because of loss of normal nocturnal decrease in blood pressure following organ transplant.[103] This failure to capture hypertensive patients prevents providers from managing CV risk factors appropriately among LTRs. In addition, in a single-center retrospective cohort of 495 LTRs, Patel and colleagues[104] showed the accelerated development and progression of traditional CVD risk factors after orthotopic liver transplant (OLT). In particular, they found that the prevalence of dyslipidemia before LT was 20% and increased to 55% at 5 years post-LT.

Hypertension, diabetes, and hypertriglyceridemia (>150 mg/dL) are 3 of 5 components of posttransplant metabolic syndrome (PTMS), a significant risk factor for long-term CVD complications. The remaining 2 components of PTMS are high-density lipoprotein level (<40 mg/dL) and body mass index greater than 30 kg/m^2; however, only 3 are required to make the diagnosis.[7] The prevalence of PTMS following OLT is 2 to 3 times higher than the rates of metabolic syndrome in the general population, and ranges from 40% to 58%.[105] Among LTRs, the risk of having a CVE is 3 to 4 times higher in those with PTMS compared with those without, although there is no difference in all-cause mortality.[10] Immunosuppressive agents also contribute to PTMS given their tendency to cause metabolic derangements.[7,10] By identifying and managing traditional risk factors early in the posttransplant course, the prevalence of PTMS, and therefore the prevalence of CVD events, can be significantly reduced.[10]

Overall, there is a small amount of data on the risk factors for long-term CVD complications compared with perioperative and early CVEs in LTRs. However, application of evidence-based guideline-directed medical therapy has been shown to reduce CVEs and long-term mortality in LTRs. For example, among 602 LTRs at a large tertiary care network, achieving a blood pressure less than 140/90 mm Hg within the first year following LT was associated with a 35% lower hazard of CVEs and a 42% lower hazard of mortality compared with LTRs with BP greater than or equal to 140/90 mm Hg.[49] In another retrospective study, Patel and colleagues[75] showed that statin use for secondary prevention of ASCVD was both safe and associated with a 75% lower hazard of mortality compared with non–statin use in LTRs. Although more research studies are needed to better characterize long-term CVD morbidity and mortality in LTRs, these studies highlight an important practice gap between actual and optimal medical management for CVD in LTRs.[72] Future prospective studies that use mixed-methods approaches in which the underlying reasons for a lack of guideline adherence are elucidated and that focus on primary prevention of ASCVD are needed in order to optimize care for LTRs.

Table 1
Cardiovascular outcomes, modalities for screening and their limitations, and areas for future research

CV Outcome	Screening Modalities	Thresholds for Increased CV Risk	Limitations	Research Gaps
Arrhythmias	• 12-lead ECG	• Any abnormal heart rhythm • QTc prolongation: >0.45 s in men, >0.47 s in women	• Abnormalities may not be captured during single ECG	• Rate vs rhythm control and anticoagulation management in atrial fibrillation and associations with clinical outcomes
HF and cardiomyopathy	• Functional testing (6MWT, CPET) • 12-lead ECG • 2D echocardiography • DSE • CMR	• 6MWD <250 m • Anaerobic threshold <9 mL/min/kg • Decreased exercise tolerance • Systolic dysfunction • Global longitudinal strain < −18% • Diastolic dysfunction • Inducible LVOTO • Chamber enlargement • Myocardial edema or fibrosis	• Functional testing may be limited to ambulatory patients • Renal dysfunction may preclude gadolinium administration in CMR	• Clinical significance of impaired excitation contraction coupling on ECG • Role of CMR for screening
Stroke	—	—	• No modality recommended for stroke screening - imaging with CT/MRI recommended only for diagnosis	• Prevalence of ischemic and hemorrhagic stroke in LT candidates and recipients
CAD	• Noninvasive stress testing (DSE, MPS) • Noninvasive coronary evaluation (CCTA, CACS) • Invasive coronary evaluation (coronary catheterization)	• Wall motion abnormalities • Perfusion defects • CACS>400 HU	• Patients may not achieve maximum chronotropy with pharmacologic stress testing • MPS of limited utility given chronic vasodilatory state in ESLD	• The impact of subclinical CVD vs accelerated ASCVD development on post-LT CVD complications

(continued on next page)

Table 1
(continued)

CV Outcome	Screening Modalities	Thresholds for Increased CV Risk	Limitations	Research Gaps
			• CCTA, CACS limited in obese patients and those unable to stay still or following required breathing maneuvers • Risk of contrast-induced nephropathy with CCTA, CACS, and coronary catheterization	
Valvular heart disease	• 2D echocardiography	• Valvular stenosis or insufficiency	• Visualization may be limited with 2D echocardiography, and may require TEE	• Outcomes following valvular repair in mitral and tricuspid regurgitation • Effects of valvular disorders on CV outcomes, beyond perioperative period • Role of MELD in selection of appropriate therapy
PoPH	• 2D echocardiography	• Increased RVSP/PASP >45 mm Hg	• Volume optimization important before echocardiography	—

Abbreviations: 2D, two-dimensional; 6MWD, 6-minute walk distance; CCTA, coronary CT angiography; RFs, risk factors; RVSP, right ventricular systolic pressure; TEE, transesophageal echocardiography.

SUMMARY

Because of the scarcity of donor organs, LTRs should be appropriately selected and their CV risk factors appropriately monitored and managed because CVD represents a major contributor to short-term and long-term adverse outcomes in this population **(Table 1)**. Preoperative cardiac assessments are intended to (1) identify and manage CV risk factors preoperatively, or (2) exclude the highest-risk candidates from transplant by screening for absolute contraindications, namely significant obstructive CAD, severe HF, or severe PoPH. As outlined earlier, most CVD complications in the first year post-LT are noncoronary in origin and mostly consist of atrial fibrillation and HF. Prospective studies are required to determine whether aggressive risk factor management both before and after LT is beneficial in reducing the rates of post-LT CVD complications.

CLINICS CARE POINTS

- Intensive management of traditional cardiac risk factors including smoking, weight management, glucose, blood pressure and cholesterol is critical pre- and post-transplant in liver transplantation to reduce risk for cardiac events.
- Comprehensive echocardiogram should be performed in all liver transplant candidates and repeated at least every 6 months while awaiting transplant.
- Given the poor performance of noninvasive stress testing in the detection of CAD among patients with ESLD, coronary angiography, either invasive or noninvasive, is the gold standard for detecting CAD in LT transplant candidates.
- The Cardiovascular Risk in Orthotopic Liver Transplantation (CAR-OLT) score is a CVD risk prediction model that was derived in LT candidates and uses pre-transplant demographic, social, and clinical variables to estimate the risk of a major CVEs in the first year posttransplant. The score is available for clinical use at www.carolt.us.

DISCLOSURE

Dr. L.B. VanWagner receives investigator initiated grant support and consults for W.L. Gore & Associates, consults for Gerson Lehrman Group and consults for Noble Insights outside the submitted work.

REFERENCES

1. Kim WR, Lake JR, Smith JM, et al. OPTN/SRTR 2017 annual data report: liver. Am J Transplant 2019;19:184–283.
2. Roberts MS, Angus DC, Bryce CL, et al. Survival after liver transplantation in the United States: a disease-specific analysis of the UNOS database. Liver Transplant 2004;10(7):886–97.
3. Watt KDS, Pedersen RA, Kremers WK, et al. Evolution of causes and risk factors for mortality post-liver transplant: results of the NIDDK long-term follow-up study. Am J Transplant 2010;10(6):1420–7.
4. Izzy M, Vanwagner LB, Lee SS, et al. Understanding and managing cardiovascular outcomes in liver transplant recipients. Curr Opin Organ Transplant 2019; 24(2):148–55.
5. Serper M, Asrani SK. Liver transplantation and chronic disease management: moving beyond patient and graft survival. Am J Transplant 2020;20(3):629–30.
6. Vanwagner LB, Lapin B, Levitsky J, et al. High early cardiovascular mortality after liver transplantation. Liver Transplant 2014;20(11):1306–16.

7. Albeldawi M, Aggarwal A, Madhwal S, et al. Cumulative risk of cardiovascular events after orthotopic liver transplantation. Liver Transplant 2012;18(3):370–5.

8. VanWagner LB, Serper M, Kang R, et al. Factors associated with major adverse cardiovascular events after liver transplantation among a national sample. Am J Transplant 2016;16(9):2684–94.

9. VanWagner LB. A simple clinical calculator for assessing cardiac event risk in liver transplant candidates: the cardiovascular risk in orthotopic liver transplantation score. Clin Liver Dis 2018;11(6):145–8.

10. Madhwal S, Atreja A, Albeldawdi M, et al. Is liver transplantation a risk factor for cardiovascular disease? a meta-analysis of observational studies. Liver Transplant 2012;18(10):1140–6.

11. Coss E, Watt KDS, Pedersen R, et al. Predictors of cardiovascular events after liver transplantation: a role for pretransplant serum troponin levels. Liver Transplant 2011;17(1):23–31.

12. Raval Z, Harinstein ME, Skaro AI, et al. Cardiovascular risk assessment of the liver transplant candidate. J Am Coll Cardiol 2011;58(3):223–31.

13. Goldberg D, Ditah IC, Saeian K, et al. Changes in the prevalence of hepatitis C virus infection, nonalcoholic steatohepatitis, and alcoholic liver disease among patients with cirrhosis or liver failure on the waitlist for liver transplantation. Gastroenterology 2017;152(5). https://doi.org/10.1053/j.gastro.2017.01.003.

14. Wong RJ, Aguilar M, Cheung R, et al. Nonalcoholic steatohepatitis is the second leading etiology of liver disease among adults awaiting liver transplantation in the United States. Gastroenterology 2015;148(3):547–55.

15. Wedd JP, Harper AM, Biggins SW. MELD score, allocation, and distribution in the United States. Clin Liver Dis 2013;2(4):148–51.

16. Izzy M, Oh J, Watt KD. Cirrhotic cardiomyopathy after transplantation: neither the Transient nor innocent Bystander. Hepatology 2018;68(5):2008–15.

17. Claes K, Meier-Kriesche H-U, Schold JD, et al. Effect of different immunosuppressive regimens on the evolution of distinct metabolic parameters: evidence from the Symphony study. Nephrol Dial Transplant 2011;27(2):850–7.

18. Patel SS, Lin FP, Rodriguez VA, et al. The relationship between coronary artery disease and cardiovascular events early after liver transplantation. Liver Int 2019;39(7):1363–71.

19. Chatterjee A, Hage FG. Guidelines in review: 2014 ACC/AHA guideline on perioperative cardiovascular evaluation and management of patients undergoing noncardiac surgery: a report of the American College of Cardiology/American Heart Association Task Force on practice guidelines. J Nucl Cardiol 2014; 22(1):158–61.

20. Lee TH, Marcantonio ER, Mangione CM, et al. Derivation and prospective validation of a simple index for prediction of cardiac risk of major noncardiac surgery. Circulation 1999;100(10):1043–9.

21. Vanwagner LB, Harinstein ME, Runo JR, et al. Multidisciplinary approach to cardiac and pulmonary vascular disease risk assessment in liver transplantation: an evaluation of the evidence and consensus recommendations. Am J Transplant 2018;18(1):30–42.

22. Bargehr J, Trejo-Gutierrez JF, Patel T, et al. Preexisting atrial fibrillation and cardiac complications after liver transplantation. Liver Transplant 2015;21(3):314–20.

23. Dec GW, Kondo N, Farrell ML, et al. Cardiovascular complications following liver transplantation. Clin Transplant 1995;9(6):463–7.

24. Donovan CL, Marcovitz PA, Punch JD, et al. Two-dimensional and dobutamine stress echocardiography in the preoperative assessment of patients with end-stage liver disease prior to orthotopic liver transplantation. Transplantation 1996;61(8):1180–8.
25. ACC/AHA/ESC 2006 guidelines for management of patients with ventricular arrhythmias and the prevention of sudden cardiac death–executive summary: a report of the American College of Cardiology/American Heart Association Task Force and the European Society of Cardiology Committee for practice guidelines (Writing Committee to develop guidelines for management of patients with ventricular arrhythmias and the prevention of sudden cardiac death) developed in collaboration with the European Heart Rhythm Association and the Heart Rhythm Society. Eur Heart J 2006;27(17):2099–140.
26. Bernardi M, Calandra S, Colantoni A, et al. Q-T interval prolongation in cirrhosis: prevalence, relationship with severity, and etiology of the disease and possible pathogenetic factors. Hepatology 1998;27(1):28–34.
27. García González M, Hernandez-Madrid A, Lopez-Sanromán A, et al. Reversal of QT interval electrocardiographic alterations in cirrhotic patients undergoing liver transplantation. Transplant Proc 1999;31(6):2366–7.
28. Therapondos G, Flapan AD, Plevris JN, et al. Cardiac morbidity and mortality related to orthotopic liver transplantation. Liver Transplant 2004;10(12):1441–53.
29. Yancy CW, Jessup M, Bozkurt B, et al. ACC/AHA guideline for the management of heart failure: a report of the American College of Cardiology Foundation. American Heart Association Task Force on practice guidelines. J Am Coll Cardiol 2013;62:147–239.
30. Mittal C, Qureshi W, Singla S, et al. Pre-transplant left ventricular diastolic dysfunction is associated with post transplant acute graft rejection and graft failure. Dig Dis Sci 2013;59(3):674–80.
31. Dowsley TF, Bayne DB, Langnas AN, et al. Diastolic dysfunction in patients with end-stage liver disease is associated with development of heart failure early after liver transplantation. J Card Fail 2011;17(8). https://doi.org/10.1016/j.cardfail.2011.06.066.
32. Nagueh SF, Smiseth OA, Appleton CP, et al. Recommendations for the evaluation of left ventricular diastolic function by echocardiography: an update from the American Society of Echocardiography and the European Association of Cardiovascular Imaging. J Am Soc Echocardiogr 2016;29(4):277–314.
33. Katz AM, Rolett EL. Heart failure: when form fails to follow function. Eur Heart J 2015;37(5):449–54.
34. Lewis GA, Schelbert EB, Williams SB. Biological phenotypes of heart failure with preserved ejection fraction. J Am Coll Cardiol 2017;70:2186–200.
35. Maraj S, Jacobs LE, Maraj R, et al. Inducible left ventricular outflow tract gradient during dobutamine stress echocardiography: an association with intra-operative hypotension but not a contraindication to liver transplantation. Echocardiography 2004;21:681–5.
36. Wiese S, Hove J, Mo S, et al. Myocardial extracellular volume quantified by magnetic resonance is increased in cirrhosis and related to poor outcome. Liver Int 2018;38(9):1614–23.
37. Lossnitzer D, Steen H, Zahn A, et al. Myocardial late gadolinium enhancement cardiovascular magnetic resonance in patients with cirrhosis. J Cardiovasc Magn Reson 2010;12:47.
38. Izzy M, Vanwagner LB, Lin G, et al. Redefining cirrhotic cardiomyopathy for the modern era. Hepatology 2020;71(1):334–45.

39. Wray C. Liver transplantation in patients with cardiac disease. Semin Cardio-thorac Vasc Anesth 2018;22(2):111–21.
40. Carey EJ, Steidley DE, Aqel BA. Six-minute walk distance predicts mortality in liver transplant candidates. Liver Transplant 2010;16:1373–8.
41. Prentis JM, Manas DMD, Trenell MI, et al. Submaximal cardiopulmonary exer-cise testing predicts 90-day survival after liver transplantation. Liver Transplant 2012;18:152–9.
42. Tripathi D, Hayes PC. The role of carvedilol in the management of portal hyper-tension. Eur J Gastroenterol Hepatol 2010;22(8):905–11.
43. Wong F. Cirrhotic cardiomyopathy. Hepatol Int 2008;3(1):294–304.
44. Baik S, Fouad TR, Lee SS. Cirrhotic cardiomyopathy. Orphanet J Rare Dis 2007; 2(1):15.
45. Liu H, Jayakumar S, Traboulsi M, et al. Cirrhotic cardiomyopathy: implications for liver transplantation. Liver Transplant 2017;23(6):826–35.
46. Wiese S, Hove JD, Bendtsen F, et al. Cirrhotic cardiomyopathy: pathogenesis and clinical relevance. Nat Rev Gastroenterol Hepatol 2013;11(3):177–86.
47. Ferro JM, Viana P, Santos P. Management of neurologic manifestations in pa-tients with liver disease. Curr Treat Options Neurol 2016;18(8). https://doi.org/ 10.1007/s11940-016-0419-0.
48. Gaynor JJ, Moon JI, Kato T, et al. A cause-specific hazard rate analysis of prog-nostic factors among 877 adults who received primary orthotopic liver trans-plantation. Transplantation 2007;84(2):155–65.
49. Vanwagner LB, Holl JL, Montag S, et al. Blood pressure control according to clinical practice guidelines is associated with decreased mortality and cardio-vascular events among liver transplant recipients. Am J Transplant 2019; 20(3):797–807.
50. Ford ES, Ajani UA, Croft JB, et al. Explaining the decrease in U.S. Deaths from coronary disease, 1980–2000. Obstet Gynecol Surv 2007;62(10):664–5.
51. Carey WD, Dumot JA, Pimentel RR, et al. The prevalence of coronary artery dis-ease in liver transplant candidates over age 50. Transplantation 1995;59(6): 859–63.
52. Tiukinhoy-Laing SD, Rossi JS, Bayram M, et al. Cardiac hemodynamic and cor-onary angiographic characteristics of patients being evaluated for liver trans-plantation. Am J Cardiol 2006;98(2):178–81.
53. Skaro AI, Gallon LG, Lyuksemburg V, et al. The impact of coronary artery dis-ease on outcomes after liver transplantation. J Cardiovasc Med 2016;17(12): 875–85.
54. Snipelisky DF, Mcree C, Seeger K, et al. Coronary interventions before liver transplantation might not avert postoperative cardiovascular events. Tex Heart Inst J 2015;42(5):438–42.
55. Safadi A, Homsi M, Maskoun W, et al. Perioperative risk predictors of cardiac outcomes in patients undergoing liver transplantation surgery. Circulation 2009;120(13):1189–94.
56. Kadayifci A, Tan V, Ursell PC, et al. Clinical and pathologic risk factors for athero-sclerosis in cirrhosis: a comparison between NASH-related cirrhosis and cirrhosis due to other aetiologies. J Hepatol 2008;49(4):595–9.
57. Vanwagner LB, Bhave M, Te HS, et al. Patients transplanted for nonalcoholic steatohepatitis are at increased risk for postoperative cardiovascular events. Hepatology 2012;56(5):1741–50.

58. Targher G, Bertolini L, Padovani R, et al. Increased prevalence of cardiovascular disease in Type 2 diabetic patients with non-alcoholic fatty liver disease. Diabet Med 2006;23(4):403–9.
59. Targher G, Arcaro G. Non-alcoholic fatty liver disease and increased risk of cardiovascular disease. Atherosclerosis 2007;191(2):235–40.
60. Findlay J, Keegan M, Pellikka P, et al. Preoperative dobutamine stress echocardiography, intraoperative events, and intraoperative myocardial injury in liver transplantation. Transplant Proc 2005;37(5):2209–13.
61. Plevak DJ. Stress echocardiography identifies coronary artery disease in liver transplant candidates. Liver Transplant Surg 1998;4(4):337–9.
62. Plotkin JS, Benitez RM, Kuo PC, et al. Dobutamine stress echocardiography for preoperative cardiac risk stratification in patients undergoing orthotopic liver transplantation. Liver Transplant Surg 1998;4(4):253–7.
63. Williams K, Lewis JF, Davis G, et al. Dobutamine stress echocardiography in patients undergoing liver transplantation evaluation. Transplantation 2000;69(11): 2354–6.
64. Harinstein ME, Flaherty JD, Ansari AH, et al. Predictive value of dobutamine stress echocardiography for coronary artery disease detection in liver transplant candidates. Am J Transplant 2008;8(7):1523–8.
65. Davidson CJ, Gheorghiade M, Flaherty JD, et al. Predictive value of stress myocardial perfusion imaging in liver transplant candidates. Am J Cardiol 2002;89(3):359–60.
66. Soldera J, Camazzola F, Rodríguez S, et al. Cardiac stress testing and coronary artery disease in liver transplantation candidates: meta-analysis. World J Hepatol 2018;10(11):877–86.
67. Lester SJ, Hurst RT. Liver transplantation: do you have the heart for it? Liver Transplant 2006;12(4):520–2.
68. Hou ZH, Lu B, Gao Y, et al. Prognostic value of coronary CT angiography and calcium score for major adverse cardiac events in outpatients. JACC Cardiovasc Imaging 2012;5:990–9.
69. Mitchell JD, Fergestrom N, Gage BF, et al. Impact of statins on cardiovascular outcomes following coronary artery calcium scoring. J Am Coll Cardiol 2018; 72:3233–42.
70. Kemmer N, Case J, Chandna S, et al. The role of coronary calcium score in the risk assessment of liver transplant candidates. Transplant Proc 2014;46(1): 230–3.
71. Winther S, Svensson M, Jorgensen HS, et al. Diagnostic and myocardial perfusion imaging in kidney transplantatino candidates. JACC Cardiovasc Imaging 2015;8:553–62.
72. Campbell PT, Vanwagner LB. Mind the gap: statin underutilization and impact on mortality in liver transplant recipients. Liver Transplant 2019;25(10):1477–9.
73. Parekh J, Corley DA, Feng S. Diabetes, hypertension and hyperlipidemia: prevalence over time and impact on long-term survival after liver transplantation. Am J Transplant 2012;12(8):2181–7.
74. Laish I, Braun M, Mor E, et al. Metabolic syndrome in liver transplant recipients: prevalence, risk factors, and association with cardiovascular events. Liver Transplant 2011;17(1):15–22.
75. Patel SS, Rodriguez VA, Siddiqui MB, et al. The impact of coronary artery disease and statins on survival after liver transplantation. Liver Transplant 2019; 25(10):1514–23.

76. Fussner LA, Heimbach JK, Fan C, et al. Cardiovascular disease after liver transplantation: when, what, and who is at risk. Liver Transplant 2015;21(7):889–96.
77. Garg A, Armstrong WF. Echocardiography in liver transplant candidates. JACC Cardiovasc Imaging 2013;6(1):105–19.
78. Alper I, Ulukaya S, Demir F, et al. Effects of cardiac valve dysfunction on perioperative management of liver transplantation. Transplant Proc 2009;41(5): 1722–6.
79. Peeraphatdit TB, Nkomo VT, Naksuk N, et al. Long-term outcomes after transcatheter and surgical aortic valve replacement in patients with cirrhosis: a guide for the hepatologist. Hepatology 2020. https://doi.org/10.1002/hep.31193.
80. Kuo PC, Plotkin JS, Gaine S, et al. Portopulmonary hypertension and the liver transplant candidate. Transplantation 1999;67(8):1087–93.
81. Lentine KL, Costa SP, Weir MR, et al. Cardiac disease evaluation and management among kidney and liver transplantation candidates. Circulation 2012; 126(5):617–63.
82. Martínez-Palli G, Taurà P, Balust J, et al. Liver transplantation in high-risk patients: hepatopulmonary syndrome and portopulmonary hypertension. Transplant Proc 2005;37(9):3861–4.
83. Swanson KL, Wiesner RH, Nyberg SL, et al. Survival in portopulmonary hypertension: Mayo clinic experience categorized by treatment subgroups. Am J Transplant 2008;8(11):2445–53.
84. Hemnes AR, Robbins IM. Sildenafil monotherapy in portopulmonary hypertension can facilitate liver transplantation. Liver Transplant 2009;15(1):15–9.
85. Krowka M. Pulmonary hemodynamics and perioperative cardiopulmonary-related mortality in patients with portopulmonary hypertension undergoing liver transplantation. Liver Transplant 2000;6(4):443–50.
86. Ashfaq M, Chinnakotla S, Rogers L, et al. The impact of treatment of portopulmonary hypertension on survival following liver transplantation. Am J Transplant 2007;7(5):1258–64.
87. Sussman N, Kaza V, Barshes N, et al. Successful liver transplantation following medical management of portopulmonary hypertension: a single-center series. Am J Transplant 2006;6(9):2177–82.
88. Krowka MJ, Mandell MS, Ramsay MA, et al. Hepatopulmonary syndrome and portopulmonary hypertension: a report of the multicenter liver transplant database. Liver Transplant 2004;10(2):174–82.
89. Krowka MJ, Fallon MB, Kawut SM, et al. International liver transplant society practice guidelines. Transplantation 2016;100(7):1440–52.
90. Assmann G, Schulte H. The Prospective Cardiovascular Münster (PROCAM) study: prevalence of hyperlipidemia in persons with hypertension and/or diabetes mellitus and the relationship to coronary heart disease. Am Heart J 1988;116(6):1713–24.
91. Maira TD, Rubin A, Puchades L, et al. Framingham score, renal dysfunction, and cardiovascular risk in liver transplant patients. Liver Transplant 2015;21(6): 812–22.
92. Ridker PM, Buring JE, Rifai N, et al. Development and validation of improved algorithms for the assessment of global cardiovascular risk in women. JAMA 2007;297(6):611.
93. Goff DC Jr, Lloyd-Jones DM, Bennett G, et al. 2013 ACC/AHA guideline on the assessment of cardiovascular risk: a report of the American College of Cardiology/American Heart Association Task Force on practice guidelines [published

correction appears in J Am Coll Cardiol. 2014 Jul 1;63(25 Pt B):3026]. J Am Coll Cardiol 2014;63(25 Pt B):2935–59.

94. D'Agostino RB, Vasan RS, Pencina MJ, et al. General cardiovascular risk profile for use in primary care. Circulation 2008;117(6):743–53.

95. Huang S, Apinyachon W, Agopian VG, et al. Myocardial injury in patients with hemodynamic derangements during and/or after liver transplantation. Clin Transplant 2016;30(12):1552–7.

96. Keller T, Zeller T, Peetz D, et al. Sensitive troponin I assay in early diagnosis of acute myocardial infarction. N Engl J Med 2009;361(86):868–77.

97. Ford MK. Systematic review: prediction of perioperative cardiac complications and mortality by the revised cardiac risk index. Ann Intern Med 2010;152(1):26.

98. Gupta PK, Ramanan B, Lynch TG, et al. Development and validation of a risk calculator for prediction of mortality after infrainguinal bypass surgery. J Vasc Surg 2012;56(2):372–9.

99. Park Y-S, Moon Y-J, Jun I-G, et al. Application of the revised cardiac risk index to the model for end-stage liver disease score improves the prediction of cardiac events in patients undergoing liver transplantation. Transplant Proc 2018;50(4): 1108–13.

100. Bilimoria KY, Liu Y, Paruch JL, et al. Development and evaluation of the universal ACS NSQIP surgical risk calculator: a decision aid and informed consent tool for patients and Surgeons. J Am Coll Surg 2013;217(5). https://doi.org/10.1016/j. jamcollsurg.2013.07.385.

101. Vanwagner LB, Ning H, Whitsett M, et al. A point-based prediction model for cardiovascular risk in orthotopic liver transplantation: the CAR-OLT score. Hepatology 2017;66(6):1968–79.

102. Roccaro GA, Goldberg DS, Hwang W-T, et al. Sustained posttransplantation diabetes is associated with long-term major cardiovascular events following liver transplantation. Am J Transplant 2017;18(1):207–15.

103. Cífková R, Pitha J, Trunecuka P, et al. Blood pressure, endothelial function and circulating endothelin concentrations in liver transplant recipients. J Hypertens 2001;19(8):1359–67.

104. Patel SS, Nabi E, Guzman L, et al. Coronary artery disease in decompensated patients undergoing liver transplantation evaluation. Liver Transplant 2018; 24(3):333–42.

105. Pagadala M, Dasarathy S, Eghtesad B, et al. Posttransplant metabolic syndrome: an epidemic waiting to happen. Liver Transplant 2009;15(12):1662–70.

Beyond Ice and the Cooler
Machine Perfusion Strategies in Liver Transplantation

Check for updates

David D. Aufhauser Jr, MD[a], David P. Foley, MD[b],*

KEYWORDS

- Steatosis • Donation after cardiac death • Hypothermic machine perfusion
- Normothermic machine perfusion • Normothermic regional perfusion
- Organ rehabilitation

KEY POINTS

- Machine perfusion is a promising preservation technique to reduce the risks associated with transplant of marginal (steatotic, elderly, and donation after circulatory death) hepatic allografts.
- Multiple strategies for machine perfusion are under investigation, including in situ and ex situ approaches; hypothermic, subnormothermic, and normothermic temperatures; oxygenated and deoxygenated perfusate; and portal vein alone or combined portal vein and hepatic artery perfusion.
- Machine perfusion may facilitate assessment of organ viability and enable liver-directed therapy before transplant.
- Clinical trials suggest machine perfusion may improve the use of hepatic allografts, mitigate ischemia-reperfusion injury, and reduce the incidences of early allograft dysfunction, biliary complications, and ischemic cholangiopathy.

INTRODUCTION

Static cold storage (SCS) of hepatic allografts in preservation solution has long been the standard of care in liver transplant. The introduction of University of Wisconsin solution for SCS in the 1980s facilitated excellent posttransplant outcomes and led to the rapid growth in the field.[1] However, current challenges require new approaches to organ preservation. The demand for hepatic allografts in the United States greatly outpaces supply.[2] Efforts to alleviate the shortage require more aggressive use of marginal hepatic allografts, including those from older donors (those

[a] Department of Surgery, Division of Transplantation, University of Wisconsin, 600 Highland Avenue, MC 7375, Madison, WI 53792, USA; [b] Department of Surgery, Division of Transplantation, University of Wisconsin, CSC H5/701, 600 Highland Avenue, Madison, WI 52792, USA
* Corresponding author.
E-mail address: foley@surgery.wisc.edu

Clin Liver Dis 25 (2021) 179–194
https://doi.org/10.1016/j.cld.2020.08.013
1089-3261/21/© 2020 Elsevier Inc. All rights reserved.

aged >70 years), those with more steatosis, and those from donors after circulatory death (DCD). Marginal donor allografts are more vulnerable to ischemic injury and have higher rates of primary nonfunction (PNF), early allograft dysfunction (EAD), and biliary complications, including ischemic cholangiopathy (IC).[3,4] Techniques that reduce ischemia-reperfusion injury (IRI) in these higher-risk grafts could improve post-transplant outcomes and reduce reluctance to use higher-risk organs.[5] Changes in organ allocation policy over the last decade to facilitate wider geographic sharing may also contribute to longer periods of cold ischemia and reinforce the need for alternatives to SCS.[6] Novel strategies to preserve hepatic allografts between organ recovery and transplant may reduce the risks associated with more aggressive organ use and help alleviate organ shortages.

In renal transplantation, machine perfusion (MP) of ex situ organs reduces the risk of delayed graft function and improves early allograft function compared with SCS.[7,8] MP has achieved widespread adaptation in renal transplantation and has emerged as the next frontier of organ preservation in liver transplants in hopes that it will yield similar benefit. The technology promises to reduce ischemic injury, to open new routes for organ rehabilitation, to enable viability assessment of higher-risk organs, and to improve transplant logistics. Several groups have developed various different techniques of MP. This article reviews potential benefits of MP, summarizes current human clinical trials supporting particular strategies and devices, and discusses future direction as this field develops.

BENEFITS OF MACHINE PERFUSION
Ischemia Reperfusion Injury

Traditional SCS relies on depressed temperature and preservation solutions that mimic intracellular contents to reduce cellular metabolism. Although this strategy significantly reduces metabolic demand in the stored organ, some anaerobic activity continues and leads to a host of intracellular changes. Reperfusion with oxygenated blood exacerbates the injury and leads to cascading organ damage through multiple intracellular and extracellular pathways, including ATP depletion, mitochondrial damage, generation of reactive oxygen species (ROS), apoptosis and necrosis, microcirculatory failure, inflammatory cytokine release, innate immune activation, and platelet aggregation.[9–11] This pattern on injury is referred to as IRI. IRI manifests itself in transplanted hepatic allografts through PNF, EAD, biliary complications, and reduced graft survival. The risk posed by IRI limit logistic flexibility in liver transplantation; for example, rates of PNF start increasing significantly as cold ischemic time (CIT) passes 7.5 hours,[12] and graft and patient survival increases with CIT beyond 12 hours.[13]

IRI is particularly marked in DCD allografts. Donation after brain death (DBD) permits controlled flush of organs with preservation solutions and rapid cooling of the liver at the time of circulatory arrest. In contrast, DCD recoveries are preceded by a variable period of hypoxia and hypotension before circulatory arrest, verification and declaration of death, and finally organ flushing/cooling. This period is known as warm ischemic time (WIT) and can greatly increase IRI. The warm ischemia inherent to the DCD process can clinically manifest itself in the recipient through a significant intraoperative, postreperfusion syndrome, and through posttransplant complications including PNF and non-anastomotic biliary strictures, commonly referred to as IC. IC complicates 5% to 30% of DCD livers and frequently necessitates retransplant.[14] However, WIT is not the sole determinant of subsequent IC, and other factors, such as donor age, anastomotic type, and surgical procurement, may also influence the development of IC.

Machine Perfusion Strategies

MP is intended to reduce IRI and improve posttransplant outcomes and comes in 2 principal varieties: ex situ and in situ. Ex situ MP begins with standard surgical recovery of the liver, including cross clamp and a traditional flush with preservation solution. Following the donor hepatectomy, the organ is cannulated for ex situ MP. Ex situ MP can be applied to both DBD and DCD scenarios. There are numerous variations of ex situ MP. Cannulation can include just the portal vein (single) or both the portal vein and the hepatic artery (dual). MP can occur at a variety of temperatures, including hypothermic MP (HMP), subnormothermic machine perfusion (SNP), normothermic machine perfusion (NMP), and normothermic regional perfusion (NRP). It can use a variety of different perfusion solutions, ranging from modified University of Wisconsin solution to human blood products. The perfusate can be oxygenated or nonoxygenated by circuit. The theoretic advantages of these different approaches are outlined later.

HMP circulates either oxygenated or nonoxygenated preservation solution ex situ and typically aims for temperatures between 4°C and 12°C. HMP has shown significant benefit in renal transplantation and has achieved widespread adaptation in that field.[7,8] HMP may benefit organs in multiple ways. HMP may act to flush out proinflammatory cytokines, reduce upregulation of cell adhesion molecules, and attenuate other acute phase reactants that contribute to postreperfusion inflammation.[15–17] Animal models of hypothermic oxygenated perfusion (HOPE) suggest that the strategy can also mitigate ATP depletion, reduce mitochondrial stress, and mitigate cellular necrosis during organ storage.[18]

SNP is another ex situ technique. It occurs at temperatures between 20°C and 30°C and typically circulates an oxygenated preservation solution. The rationale for this approach rests on animal models showing that more gradual rewarming of preserved livers decreases oxidative stress and mitochondrial strain compared with SNP by allowing the progressive normalization of cellular metabolism.[19–21] Although there are extensive data supporting SNP in animal models, it has not yet been tested in human clinical trials.

NMP is an ex situ approach that aims to mimic physiologic conditions by perfusing the liver with oxygenated blood and nutrients at physiologic temperatures (35°C–38°C). The strategy aims to restore normal cellular metabolism during liver storage and to facilitate viability assessment in a near-physiologic state. In animal models of NMP, the approach leads to decreased transaminase levels, restoration of tissue ATP concentrations, and increased bile production during storage compared with SCS.[21] After reperfusion, NMP livers show increased oxygen extraction, decreased transaminase and bilirubin levels, decreased hepatocyte and bile duct necrosis, and increased hepatic artery perfusion.[22] These studies suggest that the NMP strategy significant mitigates IRI during liver transplant.

A hybrid technique known as controlled oxygenated rewarming (COR) attempts to realize the benefits of both HMP and NMP by sequentially applying a period of HMP, slow rewarming to normothermic temperatures, and an interval of NMP with viability testing. Preclinical models of COR show increased concentrations of hepatic ATP, decreased tissue oxidative injury, and increased bile production and lactate clearance during NMP compared with livers preserved with NMP.[23,24]

NRP differs from the previous strategies because MP occurs in situ in the donor rather than ex situ and because it is intended for use only in DCD scenarios. NRP involves the normal withdrawal and declaration phase of DCD donation followed by rapid arterial and venous cannulation and initiation of perfusion using a cardiopulmonary bypass or extracorporeal membrane oxygenation circuit. Target flows are typically between 1.7 and 4 L/min with goal temperatures between 35.5°C and 37.5°C. The circuit restores circulation to abdominal organs for an observation period of around 2 hours, during which time hepatic quality and function are assessed. After this period of observation, the organs are flushed with cold traditional preservation solution, removed from the body, and subjected to SCS for transport and preservation until transplant.[25,26]

Viability Assessment

The assessment of whether an organ is suitable for transplant has traditionally relied on pretransplant clinical history, pretransplant biochemical function, gross inspection of organ appearance, and histologic inspection of a biopsy specimen. MP offers the potential to improve on these metrics and allow more accurate assessment of the organ viability. By reducing the uncertainty associated with marginal liver allografts, MP may facilitate greater use of these organs. Proposed metrics for assessing organ viability are listed in **Box 1**. Ex situ devices allow hemodynamic assessment of portal vein and hepatic artery flows and resistance.[27] Serial biochemical assessment of

---

Box 1
Markers of organ viability

Hemodynamics

Portal vein flow

Portal vein resistance

Hepatic artery flow

Hepatic artery resistance

Hepatocellular injury

Aspartate transaminase

Alanine transaminase

Bilirubin

Alkaline phosphatase

Lactate dehydrogenase

Physiologic function

pH

Lactate

Albumin

Urea

Lactate

Glucose

Bile

Quantity

pH

Bicarbonate

Glucose

markers, including alanine transaminase (ALT), aspartate transaminase (AST), lactate dehydrogenase, bilirubin, alkaline phosphatase, pH, lactate, albumin, and urea, are possible with any MP approach.[28] Assessment of novel biomarkers during perfusion, such as mitochondrial flavin, may offer additional insights into graft viability.[29] Techniques that more closely restore normal hepatic metabolism (SMP, NMP, COR, and NRP) allow more direct assessment of a liver's physiologic function, such as quantification of bile production and measurement of biliary chemistries.[30–33] The kinetics of many of these metrics are likely as important as the absolute values; a trend toward normalization of values may be more predictive of allograft function than a static set of laboratory tests.[25]

Protocols to assess organ viability are in evolution and have varied both between MP techniques and between individual clinical trials. Early clinical trials adapted conservative parameters for viability assessment of MP organs. For example, an early NRP trial serially measured ALT and lactate from the perfusate every 30 minutes to facilitate assessment of organ function. The investigators describe initially using ALT less than 200 IU/L as a cutoff for using the organ before moving the threshold to less than 500 IU/L because of promising results with the lower threshold.[25] In another NMP trial, the only NMP liver to develop PNF had persistently increased lactate level throughout the period of MP.[34] As MP technology matures, protocols and scores for organ viability assessment are likely to become more precisely defined.

Organ Rehabilitation

MP introduces the possibility of administering pretransplant therapy to potential hepatic allografts, a practice known as organ rehabilitation. This strategy allows targeted therapy to the liver alone, facilitating use of agents that may be toxic to other organs or unethical to administer to DCD donors before circulatory arrest. Organ rehabilitation has not yet been substantially tested in human clinical transplantation, but several potential therapies have been investigated in preclinical models using discarded human livers and animal models. Reported approaches to organ rehabilitation using MP include administration of antiinflammatory medications (such as prostaglandin E1, N-acetylcysteine, and sevoflurane),[35,36] RNA interference (against Fas, enkephalin, or p53),[37,38] and immunomodulation with cell therapies or extracellular vesicles.[39,40] One particularly promising avenue for organ rehabilitation is the use of MP to reduce fat content in steatotic liver allografts, which account for a large fraction of discarded organs. Preclinical models have shown significant improvement in graft steatosis with NMP alone when perfused for a period as short as 3 hours and suggest that this effect may be augmented by the addition of defatting agents to the perfusate that promote lipid oxidation and export.[41–43] Organ rehabilitation has the potential to augment the advantages of MP with many promising avenues for investigation as it achieves more widespread application.

Improve Logistics

Traditional SCS limits storage time because of adverse outcomes observed with increasing CIT.[12,13] This limit creates significant logistic hurdles, including unpredictable operating room hours, team member fatigue, and high transportation costs. MP promises to reduce these hurdles by extending the limits of storage time and increasing the ability to start liver transplants at predictable times. For example, in the Consortium for Organ Preservation in Europe (COPE) trial, NMP livers showed decreased hepatocellular injury despite participating clinicians taking advantage of the logistic flexibility afforded by technology. NMP livers in that trial had median preservation times of more than 4 hours longer than SCS livers (discussed later).[34]

Successful liver transplant after 26 hours of NMP has been reported in humans and after storage times of 72 hours with NMP have been described in animal models.[44–46] These increases in temporal limits of storage significantly increase logistic flexibility in transplantation.

HUMAN CLINICAL TRIALS
Hypothermic Machine Perfusion

Human clinical trials of HMP are summarized in **Table 1**. The first human clinical trial of HMP was conducted in 2010 by Guarrera and colleagues[27] using a nonoxygenated system. The prospective study included 20 recipients of HMP-preserved DBD livers who were compared with 20 matched SCS comparators. The investigators reported nonsignificant trends toward decreased EAD (5% HMP vs 25% SCS) and biliary complications (10% vs 20%) as well as significant reductions in recipient serum AST, ALT, bilirubin, and creatinine levels.[27] It was the first study to show feasibility of the concept and had hints of the technology's promise.

A follow-up study from the same group in 2015 revealed similar benefit. Thirty-one HMP expanded criteria donor (ECD) livers that had been declined by all United Network for Organ Sharing (UNOS) centers in their region were compared with 31 matched SCS ECD livers. The investigators described similar incidences of EAD (19% HMP vs 30% SCS) and similar 1-year patient survivals (84% HMP vs 80% SCS) between the groups. However, HMP livers showed significantly reduced rates of biliary complications (13% vs 42%); lower serum AST, ALT, bilirubin, and creatinine levels; and significantly shorter hospital stays (14 days vs 20 days).[28] The results show the ability of HMP to salvage livers that would have otherwise been declined and decrease complications. In addition, the technology used in this study required livers to be recovered and subjected to SCS during transit to the transplant center where HMP was initiated. Close to 40% of the ischemic time in the HMP arm was SCS before perfusion. The back-to-base strategy used here has significant logistic advantages for a transplant team and avoids the need to transport perfusion equipment. However, prolonged SCS before HMP may compromise some of the benefits offered by MP.

HMP has also been evaluated in DCD liver transplantation with promising results. Most of these studies involve devices that include an oxygenator in the perfusion circuit, a modification known as HOPE. A group at the University Hospital in Zurich has described using HOPE in DCD donors whereby inflow perfusion occurs through the portal vein alone. Their 2014 pilot study compared 8 HOPE-preserved DCD livers with median WIT of 38 minutes with 8 matched DBD livers and reported similar rates of EAD (0% each group), biliary complications (25% each group), and early graft survival (100% each group) between the groups.[47] A 2015 follow-up study compared 25 HOPE-preserved DCD livers at 1 center with 50 SCS DCD livers at 2 separate centers. HOPE livers showed lower peak ALT level (1239 IU/L vs 2065 IU/L), EAD (20% vs 44%), IC (0% vs 22%), overall biliary complications (20% vs 46%), and 1-year graft survival (90% vs 69%). The HOPE DCD outcomes were also similar to a second control group of 50 matched DBD liver transplants.[48]

A group in the Netherlands has also explored application of HOPE to DCD livers through a system that perfuses the liver through both the portal vein and the hepatic artery. In a trial comparing 10 HOPE DCD livers with 20 SCS DCD controls, the investigators report 100% 1-year graft and patient survival in the HOPE group compared with 67% and 85% in the SCS group, respectively. They identified 1 case (10%) of IC in the HOPE group compared with 9 cases (45%) in the SCS group, but these differences were not statistically significant because the study was underpowered.

Table 1
Select clinical trials in hypothermic machine perfusion

Author, Year	Technology	Donor Type	Number of Patients	EAD (%)	Biliary Complications (%)	IC (%)	Primary Nonfunction (%)	1-y Graft Survival (%)	1-y Patient Survival (%)
Guarrera et al,[27] 2010	HMP	DBD	40 (20 HMP and 20 SCS)	5 HMP vs 25 SCS	10 HMP vs 20 SCS	0 HMP vs 0 SCS	0 HMP vs 0 SCS	90 HMP vs 90 SCS	90 HMP vs 90 SCS
Guarrera et al,[28] 2015	HMP	ECD DBD	61 (31 HMP and 30 SCS)	19 HMP vs 30 SCS	13 HMP vs 42 SCS[a,b]	0 HMP vs 0 SCS	3 HMP vs 7 SCS	80 HMP vs 80 SCS	84 HMP vs 80 SCS
Dutkowsk et al,[47] 2014	HOPE	DCD HOPE and DBD SCS	16 (8 DCD HOPE and 8 DBD SCS)	0 DCD HOPE vs 0 DBD SCS	25 DCD HOPE vs 25 DBD SCS	0 DCD HOPE vs 0 DBD SCS	0 DCD HOPE vs 0 DBD SCS	—	—
Dutkowsk et al,[48] 2015	HOPE	DCD	75 (25 HOPE and 50 SCS)	20 HOPE vs 44 SCS[a]	20 HOPE vs 46 SCS[a]	0 HOPE vs 22 SCS[a]	0 HOPE vs 6 SCS	90 HOPE vs 69 SCS	—
van Rijn et al,[49] 2017	HOPE	DCD	30 (10 HOPE and 20 SCS)	0 HOPE vs 10 SCS	—	10 in HOPE vs 45 SCS	0 HOPE vs 0 SCS	100 HOPE vs 67 SCS	100 HOPE vs 85 SCS

[a] $P<.05$.
[b] $P<.01$.
Data from Refs.[27,28,47–49]

Significant reductions in peak serum ALT level, postoperative day 7 serum bilirubin level, and postoperative day 30 ALT, GGT, AP, and bilirubin levels were seen in HOPE livers compared with SCS livers.[49]

HOPE technology is currently being evaluated in the Perfusion to Improve Liver Outcomes in Transplantation (PILOT) trial in the United States, a phase 3 randomized multicenter clinical trial (NCT03484455) comparing the LifePort Liver Transporter HOPE system (Organ Recovery Systems, Itasca, IL) with conventional SCS. The Liver Assist device (Organ Assist, Groningen, The Netherlands) also has multiple ongoing HOPE clinical trials, including randomized studies, comparing the effects of preservation with the HOPE versus SCS on posttransplant hepatocellular injury markers (NCT01317342), on rates of IC after DCD liver transplant (NCT02584283), and on hepatocellular injury markers and outcomes in extended-criteria DBD donors (NCT03124641).

Normothermic Machine Perfusion

Several studies have shown the feasibility and efficiency of NMP (**Table 2**). The first case report of successful transplant of a human liver after NMP came out of the University of Cambridge in 2015. This report described the transplant of a DCD liver after 5 hours of SCS followed by 132 minutes of NMP using the Liver Assist device to provide pulsatile arterial and nonpulsatile portal perfusion.[50] A larger pilot study from the University of Birmingham in 2016 reported on an experience using NMP through either the Liver Assist device or the OrganOx *metra* device (OrganOx, Oxford, United Kingdom) on 6 hepatic allografts that previously had been declined for transplant. Organs were assessed for viability after 3 hours of perfusion, defined by lactate level of less than 2.5 mmol/L, bile production, stable pH greater than 7.3, arterial flow greater than 150 mL/min and portal flow greater than 500 mL/min, and homogeneous perfusion of the liver. Five of the 6 organs passed this viability assessment and were transplanted. The 5 recipients had no EAD, PNF, biliary complication, or 30-day graft loss.[51] This study suggests NMP's potential to expand the donor pool by facilitating salvage of declined allografts.

Larger studies in NMP have primarily used the OrganOx *metra* device. A trial of NMP at the University of Oxford in 2016 included 20 NMP livers compared with 40 matched SCS controls. The investigators reported similar rates of EAD (15% NMP vs 23% SCS), PNF (0% in each group), and 30-day graft survival (100% NMP vs 97.5% SCS). NMP livers had significantly reduced serum peak AST levels compared with SCS livers (417 vs 902).[52] A similar Canadian safety and feasibility trial with the same NMP device had similar results with no significant differences in EAD (56% NMP vs 30% SCS), PNF (0% each group), and 30-day graft survival (90% NMP vs 100% SCS).[53]

The largest of these studies is the COPE trial, a multicenter randomized controlled trial in Europe that included 220 liver transplants randomized to either NMP or SCS.[34] The study had several remarkable findings. First, discard rates were significantly higher in livers preserved with SCS (24%) than NMP (12%). Second, DCD livers preserved with NMP had significantly longer median periods of warm ischemia (21 minutes) than those preserved with SCS (16 minutes). Third, NMP-preserved livers had longer median preservations times (11 hours 54 minutes) than SCS livers (7 hours 45 minutes). Compared with SCS liver, NMP livers had a 49% reduction in peak AST level and a 74% reduction in EAD. There was no difference in IC rates, although only 1 patient in each developed the complication. There was a single case of PNF in the NMP arm. There was no difference in graft or patient survival. The reductions in AST level and EAD and equivalent graft and patient survival are particularly remarkable

Table 2
Select clinical trials in normothermic machine perfusion

Author, Year	Technology	Donor Type	Number of Patients	EAD (%)	Biliary Complications (%)	IC (%)	Primary Nonfunction (%)	1-y Graft Survival (%)	1-y Patient Survival (%)
Mergental et al,[51] 2016	NMP	DBD and DCD	5 NMP	0	0	0	0	—	—
Ravikumar et al,[52] 2016	NMP	DBD and DCD	60 (20 NMP and 40 SCS)	15 NMP vs 23 SCS	—	—	0 NMP vs 0 SCS	—	—
Bral et al,[53] 2017	NMP	DBD and DCD	40 (10 NMP and 30 SCS)	56 NMP vs 30 SCS	0 NMP vs 15 SCS	—	0 NMP vs 0 SCS	—	—
Nasralla et al,[34] 2018	NMP	DBD and DCD	222 (121 NMP and 101 SCS)	10 NMP s 30 SCS[a]	41 NMP vs 42 SCS	1 NMP vs 1 SCS	1 NMP vs 0 SCS	95 NMP vs 96 SCS	96 NMP vs 97 SCS
van Leeuwen etal,[54] 2019	COR	DCD	35 (11 COR and 24 SCS)	—	27 COR vs18 SCS	9 COR vs 18 SCS	0 COR vs 8 SCS	100 COR vs 80 SCS	—
Ceresa et al,[59] 2019	NMP	DBD AND DCD	31 SCS-NMP	13	6	0	0	84	—
Bral el al,[60] 2019	NMP	DBD AND DCD	43 (26 SCS-NMP and 17 NMP)	19 SCS-NMP vs 35 NMP	5 SCS-NMP vs 24 NMP	0 SCS-NMP vs 0 NMP	0 SCS-NMP vs 0 NMP	—	—

[a] $P<.01$.
Data from Refs.[34,51–54,59,60]

given that the NMP group had lower discard rates, longer preservation times, and longer WIT in the DCD subset, all factors that portend poor outcomes with traditional preservation approaches.[34] Outside of study design, these factors suggest that NMP has the ability to alter practice patterns by reducing discards and increasing acceptable preservation times.

Additional clinical trials using the OrganOx system are ongoing, including a multi-center study in the United States examining the impact of the device on the rate of EAD (NCT02775162) and a single-center study at the University of Toronto examining the device's impact on rates of PNF, retransplant, and patient survival (NCT02478151). Investigators are studying a separate NMP device, the Organ Care System (Transmedics, Andover, MA) in a multi-institution randomized trial designed to determine its impact on EAD (NCT02522871).

Controlled Oxygenated Rewarming

A pilot study of COR in human liver transplants has established the feasibility of this technique. A group from the University of Groningen assessed the ability to rescue so-called orphan livers that were previously refused for transplant by resuscitating the allografts with 2 hours of HMP followed by COR at 1°C every 2 minutes until reaching 37°C and finally a 2.5-hour period of NMP for viability testing and continued NMP until transplant using the Liver Assist device. This strategy enabled the investigators to salvage 11 of 16 previously declined livers (69%), all of which were DCD. They describe excellent posttransplant outcomes in these livers, including no PNF, no HAT, a single case of IC (9%), 3 anastomotic biliary strictures (27%), and 100% graft and patient survival through 1 year. These outcomes compared favorably with matched DCD transplants, although the study was underpowered to detect statistical differences.[54] These pilot results are encouraging, although future investigation is needed to directly compare the outcomes following HMP, COR, and NMP.

Normothermic Regional Reperfusion

NRP is a variation on MP that has shown significant promise to improve outcomes in DCD liver transplantation, primarily through protection from IC. Human trials of NRP are summarized in **Table 3**. In Spain, NRP has become common and has been used in 25% of controlled DCD cases since 2012. In a retrospective cohort study from national Spanish data collected between 2012 and 2016, Hessheimer and colleagues[55] describe 370 potential DCD liver donors, of whom 152 were recovered using NRP and 218 using standard super-rapid recovery (SRR) techniques. The 2 approaches had similar rates of organ use (64% NRP vs 57% SRR), incidence of EAD (22% NRP vs 29% SRR), incidence of PNF (2% NRP vs 4% SRR), and 1-year graft survival (87% NRP vs 78% SRR). However, NRP allograft had significantly lower rates of IC (2% NRP vs 12% SRR) and overall biliary complications (9% NRP vs 29% SRR).[55]

Protection from IC and biliary complications with NRP has been observed in other studies as well. A large nonrandomized experience at 2 UK transplant centers retrospectively compared 43 NRP and 187 SCS DCD liver transplants. The NRP livers showed significant reductions in EAD (12% with NRP vs 32% with SCS), 30-day graft loss (2% with NRP vs 12%), IC (0% with NRP vs 27% with SCS), and anastomotic stricture (7% with NRP vs 27% with SCS).[25] The study was not randomized and NRP donors tended to be younger with lower US donor risk index, but the reduction in IC and biliary stricture incidence is notable despite the modestly higher donor quality in the NRP arm. Other, smaller studies have described similarly low rates of IC with NRP.[56–58]

Table 3
Select clinical trials in normothermic regional perfusion

Author, Year	Donor Type	Number of Patients	Use (%)	EAD (%)	Biliary Complications (%)	IC (%)	Primary Nonfunction (%)	1-y Graft Survival (%)	1-y Patient Survival (%)
Jimenez-Galanes et al,[56] 2009	DCD and DBD	60 (20 uncontrolled DCD NRP vs 40 DBD SCS)	—	—	—	5 DCD NRP vs 0 DBD SCS	10 DCD NRP vs 3 DBD SCS	80 DCD NRP vs 88 DBD SCS	86 DCD NRP vs 88 DBD SCS
Minambres et al,[58] 2017	DCD	11 NRP	41	—	—	0	9	90	90
Hessheimer et al,[55] 2018	DCD	370 (152 NRP and 218 SCS)	64 NRP vs 57 SCS	22 NRP vs 29 SCS	9 NRP vs 24 SCS[b]	2 NRP vs 12 SCS[a]	2 NRP vs 4 SCS	87 NRP vs 78 SCS	—
Watson et al,[25] 2018	DCD	230 (43 NRP vs 187 SCS)	—	12 NRP vs 32[b]	—	0 NRP vs 27 SCS[b]	—	0 NRP vs 7 SCS	—

[a] $P<.05$.
[b] $P<.01$.

Data from Refs.[22,55,56,58]

BACK TO BASE

Transportation of MP devices between donor and recipient hospitals poses significant logistic challenges. As a result, many of the trials discussed in this article, including all of the HMP and COR studies, used a strategy of sequential SCS for transport followed by MP at the recipient center.[27,28,47–49,51,54] This approach is referred to as back to base. By contrast, the NMP trials that have been reported tended to begin MP at the donor hospital and continue it for the duration of preservation.[34,52,53]

Much remains unresolved about the relative merits of an immediate MP approach versus a back-to-base approach and about whether the advantages of each strategy differ based on the temperature of perfusion. In NMP, the back-to-base approach has been explored in 2 pilot studies, both using the OrganOx *metra* device. In the United Kingdom, a prospective multicenter study of 31 patients explored outcomes following liver transplant with sequential preservation with SCS followed by NMP. With a median duration of SCS of 6 hours and of NMP of 8 hours, the investigators reported a 13% rate of EAD, a 6% rate of biliary complications, and no IC. Graft survival at 30 days (94%) and patient survival at 1 year (84%) were acceptable.[59] In Canada, a single-center study compared 26 back-to-base NMP-preserved liver transplants with mean SCS time of 6 hours with 19 immediate NMP-preserved transplants. Both groups had 100% 30-day graft and patient survival, and there were no significant differences in rates of PNF, EAD, or biliary complications.[60] These studies suggest that back-to-base application of NMP is safe and feasible, but larger efforts are needed to ensure that this approach realizes the full potential of this technology.

COST-EFFECTIVENESS

There are few data on the cost-effectiveness of liver MP. One early single-center study reported a 15% increase in total orthotopic liver transplant costs with NMP, primarily caused by the cost of the devices and disposables. However, apart from device costs, the technology decreased other costs by 36% through decreased transfusions requirement, decreased intensive care unit stay, and decreased length of hospitalization.[61] MP is more established and more heavily used in renal transplants, where the technology has been established to be cost-effective.[62] As liver MP technology matures and costs decrease, it may show similar benefit.

SUMMARY

The early experience with liver MP shows the immense promise of this approach to improve outcomes from transplanting higher-risk hepatic allografts, to enhance transplant logistics, and to facilitate novel treatments of IRI during preservation. In clinical studies, NMP-preserved livers consistently have decreased markers of liver injury despite longer preservation time compared with SCS-preserved organs. Large studies in both HOPE and NRP have shown reductions in IC in DCD liver transplantation. NMP and HMP platforms have both shown promise in salvaging organs that were declined with traditional SCS-preservation.

However, many questions about to how to optimally apply this technique remain. Which MP strategy and temperature delivers the best outcomes? Should this technology be applied universally to all allografts or only to select marginal organs? What is the optimal and maximum duration of perfusion? What metrics are most accurate in predicting viability of perfused organs? What therapies should be administered to perfused organs? As the technology moves out of clinical trials and sees more widespread application, transplant surgeons and hepatologists must answer these questions to make sure the field realizes the full potential of this technology.

CLINICS CARE POINTS

- Machine perfusion may improve outcomes after liver transplantation from higher risk donors.
- Advantages of machine perfusion may include reduced ischemia-reperfusion injury, ischemic cholangiopathy, and early allograft dysfunction; improved organ viability assessment; and expansion of acceptable preservation times.
- Optimal machine perfusion approaches are still being established.

DISCLOSURE

The authors have nothing to disclose.

REFERENCES

1. Kalayoglu M, Sollinger HW, Stratta RJ, et al. Extended preservation of the liver for clinical transplantation. Lancet 1988;1(8586):617–9.
2. Kwong A, Kim WR, Lake JR, et al. OPTN/SRTR 2018 annual data report: liver. Am J Transplant 2020;20(Suppl s1):193–299.
3. Feng S, Goodrich NP, Bragg-Gresham JL, et al. Characteristics associated with liver graft failure: the concept of a donor risk index. Am J Transplant 2006;6(4): 783–90.
4. Jay CL, Lyuksemburg V, Ladner DP, et al. Ischemic cholangiopathy after controlled donation after cardiac death liver transplantation: a meta-analysis. Ann Surg 2011;253(2):259–64.
5. Dutkowski P, de Rougemont O, Clavien PA. Machine perfusion for 'marginal' liver grafts. Am J Transplant 2008;8(5):917–24.
6. Gentry SE, Chow EK, Wickliffe CE, et al. Impact of broader sharing on the transport time for deceased donor livers. Liver Transpl 2014;20(10):1237–43.
7. Jochmans I, Moers C, Smits JM, et al. Machine perfusion versus cold storage for the preservation of kidneys donated after cardiac death: a multicenter, randomized, controlled trial. Ann Surg 2010;252(5):756–64.
8. Moers C, Smits JM, Maathuis MH, et al. Machine perfusion or cold storage in deceased-donor kidney transplantation. N Engl J Med 2009;360(1):7–19.
9. Chouchani ET, Pell VR, Gaude E, et al. Ischaemic accumulation of succinate controls reperfusion injury through mitochondrial ROS. Nature 2014;515(7527): 431–5.
10. Clavien PA, Harvey PR, Strasberg SM. Preservation and reperfusion injuries in liver allografts. An overview and synthesis of current studies. Transplantation 1992;53(5):957–78.
11. de Rougemont O, Lehmann K, Clavien PA. Preconditioning, organ preservation, and postconditioning to prevent ischemia-reperfusion injury to the liver. Liver Transpl 2009;15(10):1172–82.
12. Stahl JE, Kreke JE, Malek FA, et al. Consequences of cold-ischemia time on primary nonfunction and patient and graft survival in liver transplantation: a meta-analysis. PLoS One 2008;3(6):e2468.

13. Adam R, Bismuth H, Diamond T, et al. Effect of extended cold ischaemia with UW solution on graft function after liver transplantation. Lancet 1992;340(8832): 1373–6.

14. Hessheimer AJ, Cardenas A, Garcia-Valdecasas JC, et al. Can we prevent ischemic-type biliary lesions in donation after circulatory determination of death liver transplantation? Liver Transpl 2016;22(7):1025–33.

15. Guarrera JV, Henry SD, Chen SW, et al. Hypothermic machine preservation attenuates ischemia/reperfusion markers after liver transplantation: preliminary results. J Surg Res 2011;167(2):e365–73.

16. Henry SD, Nachber E, Tulipan J, et al. Hypothermic machine preservation reduces molecular markers of ischemia/reperfusion injury in human liver transplantation. Am J Transplant 2012;12(9):2477–86.

17. Tulipan JE, Stone J, Samstein B, et al. Molecular expression of acute phase mediators is attenuated by machine preservation in human liver transplantation: preliminary analysis of effluent, serum, and liver biopsies. Surgery 2011;150(2): 352–60.

18. Dutkowski P, Furrer K, Tian Y, et al. Novel short-term hypothermic oxygenated perfusion (HOPE) system prevents injury in rat liver graft from non-heart beating donor. Ann Surg 2006;244(6):968–76 [discussion: 976–7].

19. Bruinsma BG, Yeh H, Ozer S, et al. Subnormothermic machine perfusion for ex vivo preservation and recovery of the human liver for transplantation. Am J Transplant 2014;14(6):1400–9.

20. Minor T, Efferz P, Fox M, et al. Controlled oxygenated rewarming of cold stored liver grafts by thermally graduated machine perfusion prior to reperfusion. Am J Transplant 2013;13(6):1450–60.

21. Shigeta T, Matsuno N, Obara H, et al. Impact of rewarming preservation by continuous machine perfusion: improved post-transplant recovery in pigs. Transplant Proc 2013;45(5):1684–9.

22. Boehnert MU, Yeung JC, Bazerbachi F, et al. Normothermic acellular ex vivo liver perfusion reduces liver and bile duct injury of pig livers retrieved after cardiac death. Am J Transplant 2013;13(6):1441–9.

23. Boteon YL, Laing RW, Schlegel A, et al. Combined hypothermic and normothermic machine perfusion improves functional recovery of extended criteria donor livers. Liver Transpl 2018;24(12):1699–715.

24. Westerkamp AC, Karimian N, Matton AP, et al. Oxygenated hypothermic machine perfusion after static cold storage improves hepatobiliary function of extended criteria donor livers. Transplantation 2016;100(4):825–35.

25. Watson CJE, Hunt F, Messer S, et al. In situ normothermic perfusion of livers in controlled circulatory death donation may prevent ischemic cholangiopathy and improve graft survival. Am J Transplant 2019;19(6):1745–58.

26. Oniscu GC, Randle LV, Muiesan P, et al. In situ normothermic regional perfusion for controlled donation after circulatory death–the United Kingdom experience. Am J Transplant 2014;14(12):2846–54.

27. Guarrera JV, Henry SD, Samstein B, et al. Hypothermic machine preservation in human liver transplantation: the first clinical series. Am J Transplant 2010;10(2): 372–81.

28. Guarrera JV, Henry SD, Samstein B, et al. Hypothermic machine preservation facilitates successful transplantation of "orphan" extended criteria donor livers. Am J Transplant 2015;15(1):161–9.

29. Muller X, Schlegel A, Kron P, et al. Novel real-time prediction of liver graft function during hypothermic oxygenated machine perfusion before liver transplantation. Ann Surg 2019;270(5):783–90.

30. Linares-Cervantes I, Echeverri J, Cleland S, et al. Predictor parameters of liver viability during porcine normothermic ex situ liver perfusion in a model of liver transplantation with marginal grafts. Am J Transplant 2019;19(11):2991–3005.

31. op den Dries S, Karimian N, Sutton ME, et al. Ex vivo normothermic machine perfusion and viability testing of discarded human donor livers. Am J Transplant 2013;13(5):1327–35.

32. Watson CJE, Kosmoliaptsis V, Pley C, et al. Observations on the ex situ perfusion of livers for transplantation. Am J Transplant 2018;18(8):2005–20.

33. Matton APM, de Vries Y, Burlage LC, et al. Biliary bicarbonate, pH, and glucose are suitable biomarkers of biliary viability during ex situ normothermic machine perfusion of human donor livers. Transplantation 2019;103(7):1405–13.

34. Nasralla D, Coussios CC, Mergental H, et al. A randomized trial of normothermic preservation in liver transplantation. Nature 2018;557(7703):50–6.

35. Goldaracena N, Echeverri J, Spetzler VN, et al. Anti-inflammatory signaling during ex vivo liver perfusion improves the preservation of pig liver grafts before transplantation. Liver Transpl 2016;22(11):1573–83.

36. Hara Y, Akamatsu Y, Maida K, et al. A new liver graft preparation method for uncontrolled non-heart-beating donors, combining short oxygenated warm perfusion and prostaglandin E1. J Surg Res 2013;184(2):1134–42.

37. Gillooly AR, Perry J, Martins PN. First report of siRNA uptake (for RNA Interference) during ex vivo hypothermic and normothermic liver machine perfusion. Transplantation 2019;103(3):e56–7.

38. Beal EW, Kim JL, Reader BF, et al. [D-Ala(2), D-Leu(5)] enkephalin improves liver preservation during normothermic ex vivo perfusion. J Surg Res 2019;241: 323–35.

39. Dengu F, Abbas SH, Ebeling G, et al. Normothermic machine perfusion (NMP) of the liver as a platform for therapeutic interventions during ex-vivo liver preservation: a review. J Clin Med 2020;9(4):1046.

40. Chin LY, Carroll C, Raigani S, et al. Ex vivo perfusion-based engraftment of genetically engineered cell sensors into transplantable organs. PLoS One 2019;14(12): e0225222.

41. Jamieson RW, Zilvetti M, Roy D, et al. Hepatic steatosis and normothermic perfusion-preliminary experiments in a porcine model. Transplantation 2011; 92(3):289–95.

42. Nagrath D, Xu H, Tanimura Y, et al. Metabolic preconditioning of donor organs: defatting fatty livers by normothermic perfusion ex vivo. Metab Eng 2009; 11(4–5):274–83.

43. Boteon YL, Attard J, Boteon A, et al. Manipulation of lipid metabolism during normothermic machine perfusion: effect of defatting therapies on donor liver functional recovery. Liver Transpl 2019;25(7):1007–22.

44. Watson CJ, Randle LV, Kosmoliaptsis V, et al. 26-hour storage of a declined liver before successful transplantation using ex vivo normothermic perfusion. Ann Surg 2017;265(1):e1–2.

45. Pienaar BH, Lindell SL, Van Gulik T, et al. Seventy-two-hour preservation of the canine liver by machine perfusion. Transplantation 1990;49(2):258–60.

46. Butler AJ, Rees MA, Wight DG, et al. Successful extracorporeal porcine liver perfusion for 72 hr. Transplantation 2002;73(8):1212–8.

47. Dutkowski P, Schlegel A, de Oliveira M, et al. HOPE for human liver grafts obtained from donors after cardiac death. J Hepatol 2014;60(4):765–72.
48. Dutkowski P, Polak WG, Muiesan P, et al. First comparison of hypothermic oxygenated perfusion versus static cold storage of human donation after cardiac death liver transplants: an international-matched case analysis. Ann Surg 2015; 262(5):764–70 [discussion: 770–1].
49. van Rijn R, Karimian N, Matton APM, et al. Dual hypothermic oxygenated machine perfusion in liver transplants donated after circulatory death. Br J Surg 2017;104(7):907–17.
50. Watson CJ, Kosmoliaptsis V, Randle LV, et al. Preimplant normothermic liver perfusion of a suboptimal liver donated after circulatory death. Am J Transplant 2016;16(1):353–7.
51. Mergental H, Perera MT, Laing RW, et al. Transplantation of declined liver allografts following normothermic ex-situ evaluation. Am J Transplant 2016;16(11): 3235–45.
52. Ravikumar R, Jassem W, Mergental H, et al. Liver transplantation after ex vivo normothermic machine preservation: a phase 1 (First-in-Man) clinical trial. Am J Transplant 2016;16(6):1779–87.
53. Bral M, Gala-Lopez B, Bigam D, et al. Preliminary single-center canadian experience of human normothermic ex vivo liver perfusion: results of a clinical trial. Am J Transplant 2017;17(4):1071–80.
54. van Leeuwen OB, de Vries Y, Fujiyoshi M, et al. Transplantation of high-risk donor livers after ex situ resuscitation and assessment using combined hypo- and normothermic machine perfusion: a prospective clinical trial. Ann Surg 2019; 270(5):906–14.
55. Hessheimer A, Coll E, Valdivieso A, et al. Superior outcomes using normothermic regional perfusion in CDCD liver transplantation. Transplantation 2018;102:S380.
56. Jimenez-Galanes S, Meneu-Diaz MJ, Elola-Olaso AM, et al. Liver transplantation using uncontrolled non-heart-beating donors under normothermic extracorporeal membrane oxygenation. Liver Transpl 2009;15(9):1110–8.
57. De Carlis R, Di Sandro S, Lauterio A, et al. Successful donation after cardiac death liver transplants with prolonged warm ischemia time using normothermic regional perfusion. Liver Transpl 2017;23(2):166–73.
58. Minambres E, Suberviola B, Dominguez-Gil B, et al. Improving the outcomes of organs obtained from controlled donation after circulatory death donors using abdominal normothermic regional perfusion. Am J Transplant 2017;17(8): 2165–72.
59. Ceresa CDL, Nasralla D, Watson CJE, et al. Transient cold storage prior to normothermic liver perfusion may facilitate adoption of a novel technology. Liver Transpl 2019;25(10):1503–13.
60. Bral M, Dajani K, Leon Izquierdo D, et al. A back-to-base experience of human normothermic ex situ liver perfusion: does the chill kill? Liver Transpl 2019; 25(6):848–58.
61. Pezzati D, Liu Q, Hassan H, et al. A cost analysis on normothermic machine perfusion at a single center. Am J Transplant 2017;17 (suppl 3).
62. Groen H, Moers C, Smits JM, et al. Cost-effectiveness of hypothermic machine preservation versus static cold storage in renal transplantation. Am J Transplant 2012;12(7):1824–30.

Paradigm Shift in Utilization of Livers from Hepatitis C–Viremic Donors into Hepatitis C Virus–Negative Patients

Eric F. Martin, MD

KEYWORDS

- Hepatitis C virus • Liver transplantation • HCV-positive donor • HCV-viremic donor

KEY POINTS

- Patients with hepatitis C virus (HCV) infection are now being cured at consistently high rates regardless of genotype, treatment experience, renal function, or severity of liver disease in both the pretransplant and the posttransplant settings.
- There is no difference in patient or graft survival of HCV-infected recipients using organs from HCV-viremic donors compared with HCV-negative donors.
- The opioid epidemic has resulted in a dramatic increase in the number of new HCV infections, including HCV-positive donors.
- The post–direct-acting antiviral era has resulted in an increased utilization of HCV-viremic organs, including HCV-viremic livers transplanted into HCV-negative recipients.
- Early graft outcomes are similar for HCV-viremic and HCV-negative recipients regardless of donor HCV viremia.

INTRODUCTION

There are approximately 2.4 million people infected with chronic hepatitis C virus (HCV) in the United States.[1] It is estimated that 20% to 30% of those with chronic HCV will progress to cirrhosis after 20 to 30 years with an additional 2% to 5% annual risk of developing end-stage liver disease (ESLD).[2,3] Liver transplantation (LT) remains the most durable and curative treatment for patients with ESLD. Despite record-breaking numbers of LTs performed in the United States in each of the last 7 years, the demand for LT continues to exceed the supply of available donors.[4,5] The emergence of highly effective and well-tolerated direct-acting antiviral (DAA) therapy has transformed the clinical course and management of HCV. Although the widespread availability of DAA therapy has resulted in a decrease in the number of LTs performed each year for patients with ESLD because of chronic HCV, the incidence of HCV has

Division of Digestive Health and Liver Disease, University of Miami Miller School of Medicine, 1120 Northwest 14th Street, Suite 1112, Miami, FL 33136, USA
E-mail address: efm10@miami.edu

Clin Liver Dis 25 (2021) 195–207
https://doi.org/10.1016/j.cld.2020.08.009
1089-3261/21/© 2020 Elsevier Inc. All rights reserved.
liver.theclinics.com

increased in the last decade owing in large part to the opioid epidemic. Given the high wait-list mortality for patients with ESLD, the insufficient supply of donor livers, the opioid epidemic, and the accessibility of highly effective DAA therapy, there is an increasing interest in transplanting HCV-positive organs. This review lays out the historic framework that has led to the current fundamental changes in the author's approach to the management of patients with HCV in both the pretransplant and the posttransplant settings that now include the transplantation of HCV-viremic livers into HCV-negative recipients.

HISTORY OF HEPATITIS C VIRUS AND LIVER TRANSPLANT

Since the first successful LT in 1967,[6] significant advancements have been made in surgical techniques, postoperative care, and immunosuppressive therapy. Such developments have resulted in a dramatic increase in the annual rates of LT in the United States and abroad. Specifically, the annual rates of LT have more than quadrupled in the United States during the last 30 years, with 1713 LTs performed in 1988 compared with more than 8000 LTs in each of the last 3 years, including a record-setting 8896 LTs in 2019.[5] The emergence of DAA therapy has resulted in a dramatic decrease in both wait-list registrations and LTs for HCV-related indications, with a decrease in the rate of LT wait-listing for HCV complicated by decompensated cirrhosis by more than 30% in the post-DAA era.[7] Further reductions are expected with improved testing, linkage to care, and access to DAA therapy.[7] Despite the decline in HCV-related LT wait-list additions and LTs, the total number of LTs performed each year in the United States continues to increase with 11,844 patients added in 2018 compared with 11,340 in 2016.[8] This increase is in large part due to the increasing disease burden related to alcoholic liver disease (ALD) and nonalcoholic steatohepatitis (NASH).[9] In fact, HCV, which was the most common indication for LT during the last 2 decades, was surpassed in 2016 by both ALD and NASH as the 2 most common indications for LT.[10]

Despite the tremendous numbers of LTs performed each year, currently 13,000 people remain on the wait list for LT,[5] which is further confounded by an annual overall wait-list mortality of nearly 13 deaths per 100 wait list-years.[8] The unrelenting disparity between the need for LT and the shortage of donor organs continues to challenge the transplant community. Efforts to expand the liver donor pool while implementing the most equitable and efficacious organ allocation policies remain under constant scrutiny. Such efforts have included improvements in education and awareness of organ donation, medical and surgical advances in living donor and split donor transplantation, as well as the use of grafts from extended criteria donors (ECDs) or the so-called marginal grafts.[11] Although ECD is more clearly defined in kidney transplantation, there is no clear definition for what constitutes an ECD liver, but generally includes categories such as hepatic steatosis, advanced donor age, donation after cardiac death, increased ischemic time, and donors with increased risk of infectious disease transmission, such hepatitis B core antibody and HCV-positive donors.[12] ECDs understandably create concerns regarding inferior graft and patient survival; however, these grafts can be used safely through careful selection of donor and recipient risk with acceptable outcomes.

DEFINITION AND INTERPRETATION OF HEPATITIS C VIRUS–POSITIVE DONOR

HCV is a positive-strand RNA virus and is identified by nucleic acid testing (NAT), which directly measures viral RNA using polymerase chain reaction (PCR) that is detectable within 3 to 5 days after exposure (**Fig. 1**). Serologic conversion then results in the formation of anti-HCV immunoglobulin G antibodies that are detectable by

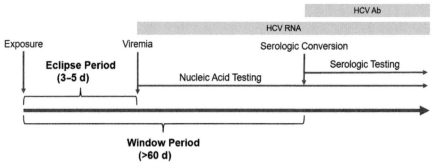

Fig. 1. HCV testing from time of initial exposure. Ab, antibody.

serologic tests, such as enzyme immunoassays, within 2 to 6 months after exposure (see **Fig. 1**). Historically, HCV-positive donors were identified based only on serologic testing and often labeled as "seropositive donors."[13] In fact, the Organ Procurement and Transplantation Network (OPTN) did not mandate documentation of donor HCV NAT until March 31, 2015. Therefore, the implementation of NAT, which more accurately assesses the risk of infectious transmission, requires redefining the term HCV-positive donor.[13] This distinction is important because donors with positive HCV antibody but without viremia do not transmit HCV unless they have been identified as Public Health Service (PHS) increased risk at which point the risk of transmission is still extremely low.[14] As such, historical outcomes data involving HCV-positive donors are limited and should be interpreted with caution because they do not adequately differentiate the presence or absence of viremia. A recent American Society of Transplantation (AST) consensus conference endorsed the replacement of the term HCV-"positive" donor with HCV-"viremic" donor because it more accurately differentiates between the presence and absence of viremia, and, therefore, more directly conveys the risk of infectious transmission.[13] For consistency with the recommendations of the AST consensus conference, HCV-"positive" donors will be used in the rest of this review to refer to any clinical data in which seropositivity is known but NAT status is lacking.[13]

HEPATITIS C VIRUS AND THE OPIOID CRISIS

Much has been published about the escalating opioid crisis and its social and economic impact on public health. After an impressive decrease in new cases of HCV infection over the preceding decade, the consequential spread of HCV owing to the opioid epidemic has resulted in a dramatic 250% increase in new HCV infections in the United States between 2010 and 2016.[15] The impact of the opioid epidemic on organ donation is even more dramatic because there was nearly a 720% increase in drug overdose as the mechanism among adult organ donors in the United States between 2005 and 2018.[5] In an analysis of OPTN data between 2003 and 2014 by Goldberg and colleagues,[16] deceased donors who died of a drug overdose were younger (median age 31) than donors who died of cardiovascular disease (median age 47) and stroke (median age 52). In addition, the liver quality of the donor livers attributable to a drug overdose was significantly better and associated with longer graft survival than those of donors who died of cardiovascular disease.[16]

UTILIZATION AND DISCARD RATES OF HEPATITIS C VIRUS–VIREMIC LIVERS

Although donors who died of a drug overdose had the highest overall donation rates, the mean number of organs transplanted per donor was significantly lower for donors who died of a drug overdose compared with donors who died of a gunshot wound, blunt injury, and asphyxiation.[16] Data suggest the primary reason for the underutilization of organs from donors who died of a drug overdose is the concern of disease transmission of hepatitis B virus (HBV), HCV, and human immunodeficiency virus (HIV).[17] Historically, transplant providers were reluctant to transplant organs from PHS increased-risk donors because of the concern for potential transmission of HBV, HCV, and HIV. These concerns were often echoed by patient apprehension at time of organ offer, and, thus, the discard rate of these otherwise good-quality organs was historically high. Approximately 28% of HCV-"positive" livers were discarded each year between 2005 and 2010, which declined to 22% in 2011 and 11% in 2015.[18] Fortunately, this gap appears to have closed based on analysis of Scientific Registry of Transplant Recipients (SRTR) data from 2018 that revealed HCV antibody–positive donor livers were no more likely to be discarded than HCV antibody–negative livers (7.6% vs 8.5%).[8] In addition, despite fewer wait-list registrants with HCV infection, the proportion of adults willing to accept HCV-positive donors nearly doubled from 19.8% in 2016 to 34.6% in 2018.[8] This impressive turnaround likely reflects the willingness of HCV-negative transplant candidates to accept HCV-positive donors in the DAA era coupled by the reevaluation of what was previously considered a strong risk factor for organ discard. Therefore, preventing underutilization of such organs remains critically important to continue to offset the organ shortage.

NATURAL HISTORY OF RECURRENT HEPATITIS C VIRUS AFTER LIVER TRANSPLANTATION

Patients with active HCV infection at time of LT experience universal recurrence of HCV infection. Furthermore, the natural history of chronic HCV is accelerated after LT with 20% to 54% progressing to cirrhosis within 5 years.[19–23] Graft failure because of fibrosing cholestatic hepatitis (FCH), which is one of the most feared complications of HCV after LT, is a severe form of recurrent viral hepatitis that may develop as early as 2 to 3 months and is marked by cholestatic hepatic dysfunction with high levels of HCV viremia. Estimated to occur in 2% to 5% of HCV-viremic recipients, the incidence of FCH in the case of HCV-naïve recipients with HCV-viremic organs remains unclear. Historically, despite anecdotal reports of rescue therapy with antivirals and reduction of immunosuppression, most cases of FCH rapidly progressed to graft failure and death often within the first year after LT.[21] More recently, successful treatment with DAAs has been reported with sustained virological response (SVR) of 96% in 1 case series following treatment of 23 patients who developed FCH.[24]

TREATMENT OF HEPATITIS C VIRUS AFTER LIVER TRANSPLANT

Before the introduction of DAA therapy, treatment of HCV consisted primarily of pegylated interferon (PEG-IFN) and ribavirin-based regimens. Unfortunately, the poor efficacy and tolerability of PEG-IFN and ribavirin-based regimens in the pre-DAA era resulted in an overall 10% reduction in patient and graft survival at 10 years when compared with transplants for other indications.[25] The second- and third-generation DAAs have proven to be highly effective interferon-free regimens with consistently high SVR rates regardless of genotype, treatment experience, renal function, or severity of liver disease.

The safety and efficacy of DAAs are also well studied in post-LT patients with cure rates that exceed 95% regardless of genotype, treatment experience, or allograft cirrhosis.[26–31] DAAs are well-tolerated post-LT with minimal interactions with the commonly prescribed post-LT medications.

TRANSPLANTATION OF HEPATITIS C VIRUS–POSITIVE DONORS INTO HEPATITIS C VIRUS–POSITIVE RECIPIENTS

The initial interest for transplanting HCV-positive donors into HCV-positive LT recipients was tempered by the concerns of poor graft function because of accelerated progression of HCV infection. However, studies have consistently reported that HCV-"positive" recipients receiving HCV-"positive" livers have comparable survival to those receiving HCV-negative livers.[32–38] There was a dramatic increase in the use of HCV-"positive" livers into HCV-"positive" recipients from 6.9% in 2010 to 16.9% in 2015, which coincided with the introduction of DAA.[18] The interpretations of these earlier studies, however, are limited because most of the outcomes data included HCV-"positive" donors and did not specify HCV NAT status.

HEPATITIS C VIRUS TRANSMISSION FROM SEROPOSITIVE, NONVIREMIC DONORS INTO HEPATITIS C VIRUS–NEGATIVE RECIPIENTS

It is well established that donors with positive HCV antibody and without HCV viremia do not transmit HCV unless the donor is designated as increased risk because of undetected HCV at the time of donor testing. Increased risk donors (as defined by the US PHS guidelines) are at risk of recent HIV, HBV, and HCV infection and whose transplanted organs could be capable of inadvertently transmitting the virus to recipients despite negative routine serologic testing.[14] Most importantly, because most of these increased risk donors are actually negative for HIV, HBV, and HCV, the designation does in no way reflect the quality of the donated organs. However, not all PHS increased risk donors carry the same risk of infection. A well-cited metaanalysis reported pooled transmission risk of HCV as high as 32.4/10,000 (0.3%) if the risk factor was injection drug use compared with as low as 0.8/10,000 if the donor had a history of recent incarceration.[39] This finding is emphasized in a recent prospective study of 26 consecutive HCV antibody–negative and/or HCV NAT–negative transplant recipients who received a liver graft from donors who were HCV antibody-positive and HCV NAT–negative. HCV transmission, which was defined as positive HCV PCR by 3 months after LT, occurred in 4 (16%), at a median follow-up of 11 months. Importantly, HCV transmission occurred only in patients who received HCV antibody-positive livers from donors who died of a drug overdose.[40] With that said, the disease transmission from PHS increased risk donors overall is extremely rare.[41,42] In fact, the risk of dying on the wait list far exceeds the risk of disease transmission from a donor identified as PHS increased risk.

TRANSPLANTATION OF HEPATITIS C VIRUS–VIREMIC DONORS INTO HEPATITIS C VIRUS–NEGATIVE RECIPIENTS

The apprehension concerning transplantation of HCV-viremic grafts into HCV-negative recipients arises in part from the ethical concerns of introduction of an active virus known to cause progressive liver disease into an immunocompromised host. However, the rationale in support of this approach is based on the potential advantages of a decrease in the waiting time (and with it a decrease in wait-list mortality) coupled with the ability to be transplanted at a lower model for end-stage liver disease (MELD) score using organs that previously were more likely to be discarded than transplanted with access to highly effective, safe, and tolerable DAA therapy.

Outcomes

The number of LTs using HCV-positive donors into HCV-negative recipients dramatically increased from 6 in 2014 (first complete year of DAA era) to 548 in 2019[5] (**Fig. 2**). Meanwhile, during the same time period, the number of LTs including HCV-positive donors into HCV-positive recipients decreased by nearly 50% from 2166 in 2014 to 1138 in 2019 (see **Fig. 1**). These data are limited because OPTN data collection for donor HCV NAT began March 31, 2015 compared with recipient HCV NAT, which began February 28, 2018. LT from HCV-viremic donors into HCV NAT–negative recipients represented 1.3% and 2.2% of all LTs in 2018 and 2019, respectively.

Although early results are encouraging, there is a paucity of data with a small number of published cases and variable treatment approaches using HCV-viremic livers into HCV-negative recipients (**Table 1**).[43–45] Interestingly, in 1 prospective observational study that reported an SVR12 of 100%, 7 recipients had a history of HCV that was successfully treated before LT and were nonviremic at time of LT.[46] Another noteworthy finding was the relatively high rate of acute rejection (30%), which included 2 cases of acute rejection cellular rejection and 1 case of antibody-mediated rejection.[46] Although the sample size was small, the rate of biopsy-proven acute rejection observed in the study by Kwong and colleagues[46] exceeds the range of what is reported in the general post-LT population (15.6%–26.9%).[47] It is well established that LT recipients with HCV infection are at increased risk of acute rejection. Specifically, HCV treatment in the post-LT period is associated with rejection and immune

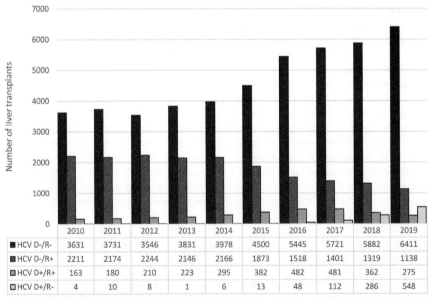

	2010	2011	2012	2013	2014	2015	2016	2017	2018	2019
■ HCV D-/R-	3631	3731	3546	3831	3978	4500	5445	5721	5882	6411
■ HCV D-/R+	2211	2174	2244	2146	2166	1873	1518	1401	1319	1138
▨ HCV D+/R+	163	180	210	223	295	382	482	481	362	275
□ HCV D+/R-	4	10	8	1	6	13	48	112	286	548

Fig. 2. Annual number of LTs in the United States based on donor and recipient HCV status between 2010 and 2019.[5] HCV D+/R+, HCV-positive recipients whose donor was HCV-negative; HCV D–/R+, HCV-positive recipients whose donor was HCV-negative; HCV-negative recipients whose donor was HCV-positive. OPTN data collection for donor HCV NAT began March 31, 2015. OPTN data collection for recipient HCV NAT began February 28, 2018. (*Data from* U.S. Department of Health and Human Services. Available at: https://optn.transplant.hrsa.gov/data/view-data-reports/. Accessed June 1, 2020.)

Table 1
Transplantation of hepatitis C virus–viremic livers into hepatitis C virus–negative recipients

References	Study Type	Number of Patients	HCV Genotype	DAA Therapy × Weeks	Median Allocation MELD at LT	Median Time from Listing to LT (d)	Median Time from Consent to LT (d)	Median Time to Treatment (d)	SVR12, %
Anwar et al,[53] 2020	Matched cohort	30	1a (16), 1a/1b (1), 2b (2), 3 (12)	GLE/PIB (27), SOF/VEL (3)	21 vs 21 (P = .41)	63 vs 50 (P = .15)	72 vs 50 (P = .27)	47	63[a]
Crismale et al,[54] 2020	Prospective observational study	13 (8 LT, 5 SLK)	1a (10), 1b (1), 3 (2)	SOF-based regimen[b](7), GLE/PIB (6)	30	329	96	42	93
Kwong et al,[46] 2019	Prospective observational study	10	1a (2), 1b (1), 2 (1), 2b (2), 3 (4)	SOF/VEL × 12 (6), LED/SOF × 12–24 (3), SOF/DCV/RBV × 24 (1)	33	Not reported	Not reported	43	100
Bethea et al,[55] 2020	Open-labeled, unblinded single-center trial	10[c]	1a (8), 3 (2)	GLE/PIB (10)	32	260	69.5	1.5	100

Abbreviations: GLE/PIB, glecaprevir/pibrentasvir; LED/SOF, ledipasvir/sofosbuvir; SLK, simultaneous liver/kidney; SOF/DCV/RBV, sofosbuvir/daclatasvir/ribavirin; SOF/VEL, sofosbuvir/velpatasvir.

[a] Only 19/32 (63%) achieved SVR12; 6/30 (20%) completed EOT pending SVR12, and 5/30 (17%) were still on HCV treatment.
[b] Did not specify which SOF-based regimen.
[c] Four underwent SLK.

Data from Refs.[46,53–55]

graft dysfunction that is thought to result from declining immunosuppression levels and/or alterations in the immune profile after eradication of HCV.[48,49]

In a recent analysis of SRTR data by Cotter and colleagues,[43] the 1- and 2-year graft survivals of 87 HCV-negative transplant recipients who received an allograft from HCV-viremic donors were similar to HCV-negative transplant recipients who received an allograft from donors who were HCV NAT negative (1-year 93% vs 93%, 2-year 86% vs 88%).

Patient Selection

In the case of an HCV-infected patient who is wait listed for LT, modeling data suggest that it is cost-effective to delay treatment of HCV until after LT when the allocation MELD exceeds 23 to 27.[44] On the other hand, another Markov-based model suggests that HCV-negative LT candidates with an MELD score greater than 20 may benefit from a shortened waiting time after accepting an HCV-infected liver.[45] Last, a more recent Markov-based model found that accepting any liver regardless of HCV status showed a survival benefit when the recipient's MELD was ≥20.[50] Importantly, the relative benefit of accepting a liver from an HCV-viremic donor differs across UNOS regions and has changed rapidly over the last several years.[51]

Donor Selection

Although there are no current consensus guidelines on the threshold of underlying fibrosis in procured HCV-positive grafts compared with HCV-negative grafts in the DAA era, the general acceptable threshold is less than stage 3 fibrosis (F3).[33] Other risks for progression of preexisting fibrosis include donor age, degree of steatosis, and severity of necroinflammation.[33] Although mitigated by early DAA therapy, additional studies are warranted to clarify these concerns.

Treatment Concerns

One of the main concerns with this approach that may prevent the expanded use of HCV-viremic organs outside of a clinical study is the timely acquisition of HCV treatment. DAAs are typically approved for chronic HCV with further restrictions based on the presence of advanced hepatic fibrosis. On the other hand, transplantation of HCV-viremic livers into HCV-negative recipients involves treatment of acute donor-derived HCV before the development of infection-related comorbidities, which may result in treatment denial. The counterargument to this point is that although the cost of caring for wait-listed patients is high, the potential savings from an earlier transplant would financially justify the use of DAA therapy with this approach. Therefore, well-designed clinical trials with compelling findings are needed to support inclusive payer coverage of DAA therapy.

The selection of DAA therapy for HCV-uninfected recipients of livers from HCV-viremic donors should follow the same principles as for those who develop recurrent HCV infection after LT (**Table 2**).[52] Unlike with nonhepatic transplants, a shorter duration of HCV therapy using a preemptive treatment approach is not currently recommended outside of a clinic trial setting for HCV-viremic livers into HCV-negative recipients because of the large reservoir of HCV in the transplanted liver allograft compared with non-liver HCV-viremic grafts.

The optimal timing of treatment of recurrent HCV after LT has not been well studied and requires addition clinical trials to better answer this question. The primary goal is to provide DAA therapy as early as clinically possible to avoid the development of severe acute hepatitis and other complications of HCV infection. Treatment options, whether preemptive (initiation of DAA treatment without confirmation of viremia of

Table 2
Recommended treatment of hepatitis C virus–uninfected recipients of livers from hepatitis C virus–viremic donors

Treatment-naïve and -experienced patients with genotype 1–6 infection in the allograft without cirrhosis	
Recommended	Duration, wk
Daily fixed-dose combination of glecaprevir/pibrentasvir (Mavyret)	12
Daily fixed-dose combination of sofosbuvir/velpatasvir (Epclusa)	12
Genotype 1 and 4 only: Daily fixed-dosed combination of elbasvir/ grazoprevir (Zepatier) for patients without baseline NS5A RASs for elbasvir	12
Genotype 1, 4, 5, or 6 only: Daily fixed-dose combination of ledipasvir/ sofosbuvir (Harvoni)	12

Data from Ghany, M.G., T.R. Morgan, and A.-I.H.C.G. Panel, Hepatitis C Guidance 2019 Update: American Association for the Study of Liver Diseases-Infectious Diseases Society of America Recommendations for Testing, Managing, and Treating Hepatitis C Virus Infection. Hepatology, 2020. 71(2): p. 686-721.

the recipient) or reactive (initiation of DAA treatment after confirmation of recipient viremia), are limited by the recipient's insurance coverage. There are emerging data that suggest preemptive treatment may reduce the risk of complications, such as FCH.

Organ Procurement and Transplantation Network Policy and Consensus Recommendations

OPTN policy mandates the screening of all donors and recipients for HCV using both serology and NAT; however, there is no OPTN policy that restricts transplantation of organs from HCV-viremic donors into any recipient, regardless of HCV status. With that said, according to guidelines provided by American Association for the Study of Liver Diseases and Infectious Diseases Society of America, the proper informed consent when considering use of HCV-viremic donor organs in HCV-negative recipients should include address the following concepts: (1) risk of transmission from an HCV-viremic donor; (2) risk of liver disease if HCV treatment is not available, significantly delayed, or unsuccessful; (3) benefits, namely reduced waiting time and possibly lower wait-list mortality; (4) unknown long-term consequences of HCV exposure; (5) risk of graft failure; and (6) risk of HCV transmission to the recipient's partner.[52] Likewise, transplant programs are recommended to develop strategies to document the aforementioned consent, assure timely access to HCV treatment, and ensure long-term follow-up of recipients (beyond SVR12).[52] Although early results are encouraging, longer-term data are needed using well-vetted clinical studies preferably with monitored institutional review board–approved protocols as per the AST consensus conference.[13] Such data are implicit if transplantation of HCV-viremic organs into HCV-negative recipients is to become standard of care.

SUMMARY

The emergence of highly effective and well-tolerated DAA therapy has transformed the clinical course and management of HCV in both the pretransplant and the posttransplant settings. The subsequent paradigm shift has led to a noticeable increase in the utilization of HCV-viremic organs, especially the utilization of HCV-viremic livers into HCV-negative recipients. Based on evolving data, the use of HCV-viremic livers can safely expand the donor pool with excellent posttransplant outcomes that are similar to other LT recipients regardless of donor HCV viremia status. Although the early outcomes data are encouraging, longer-term data are required to further validate the long-term benefit as well as justify consistent payer coverage of DAA medications before the utilization of HCV-viremic donors becomes standard of care.

CLINICS CARE POINTS

- Interpretation of donor HCV serologies is critical in understanding the potential risk of HCV transmission to the recipient. Clearful screening of all donor allografts for advanced hepatitis fibrosis is critical at time of donor selection when considering HCV-viremic organs.
- Although the optimal timing of treatment of recurrent HCV after LT is unknown, the primary goal is to provide DAA therapy as early as clinically possible to minimize the risk of severe acute hepatitis and other potential complications of HCV infection.
- The selection of DAA therapy for HCV-uninfected recipients of livers from HCV-viremic donors should follow the same principles as for those who develop recurrent HCV infection after LT.
- Shorter duration of HCV therapy using a preemptive approach is not currently recommended outside of a clinical trial for transplantation of HCV-viremic livers into HCV-negative recipients.
- Early results are encouraging; however, longer-term data are needed using well-vetted clinicals studies preferably with monitored institutional review board-approved protocols.

DISCLOSURE

The author has nothing to disclose.

REFERENCES

1. V.H.-S.S.A.M.C.f.D.C.a.P. Available at: https://www.cdc.gov/hepatitis/hcv/index.htm. Accessed June 1, 2020.
2. Fattovich G, Giustina G, Degos F, et al. Morbidity and mortality in compensated cirrhosis type C: a retrospective follow-up study of 384 patients. Gastroenterology 1997;112(2):463–72.
3. Lingala S, Ghany MG. Natural history of hepatitis C. Gastroenterol Clin North Am 2015;44(4):717–34.
4. Kim WR, Lake JR, Smith JM, et al. OPTN/SRTR 2015 annual data report: liver. Am J Transplant 2018;17(Suppl 1):174–253.
5. U.S. Department of Health and Human Services. Available at: https://optn.transplant.hrsa.gov/data/view-data-reports/. Accessed June 1, 2020.
6. Starzl TE, Groth CG, Brettschneider L, et al. Orthotopic homotransplantation of the human liver. Ann Surg 1968;168(3):392–415.
7. Flemming JA, Kim WR, Brosgart CL, et al. Reduction in liver transplant wait-listing in the era of direct-acting antiviral therapy. Hepatology 2017;65(3):804–12.
8. Kwong A, Kim WR, Lake JR, et al. OPTN/SRTR 2018 annual data report: liver. Am J Transplant 2020;20(Suppl s1):193–299.
9. Goldberg D, Ditah IC, Saeian K, et al. Changes in the prevalence of hepatitis C virus infection, nonalcoholic steatohepatitis, and alcoholic liver disease among

patients with cirrhosis or liver failure on the waitlist for liver transplantation. Gastroenterology 2017;152(5):1090–9.e1.

10. Cholankeril G, Ahmed A. Alcoholic liver disease replaces hepatitis C virus infection as the leading indication for liver transplantation in the United States. Clin Gastroenterol Hepatol 2018;16(8):1356–8.

11. Shetty A, Buch A, Saab S. Use of hepatitis C-positive liver grafts in hepatitis C-negative recipients. Dig Dis Sci 2019;64(5):1110–8.

12. Vodkin I, Kuo A. Extended criteria donors in liver transplantation. Clin Liver Dis 2017;21(2):289–301.

13. Levitsky J, Formica RN, Bloom RD, et al. The American Society of Transplantation consensus conference on the use of hepatitis C viremic donors in solid organ transplantation. Am J Transplant 2017;17(11):2790–802.

14. Seem DL, Lee I, Umscheid CA, et al. PHS guideline for reducing human immunodeficiency virus, hepatitis B virus, and hepatitis C virus transmission through organ transplantation. Public Health Rep 2013;128(4):247–343.

15. Liang TJ, Ward JW. Hepatitis C in injection-drug users - a hidden danger of the opioid epidemic. N Engl J Med 2018;378(13):1169–71.

16. Goldberg DS, Blumberg E, McCauley M, et al. Improving organ utilization to help overcome the tragedies of the opioid epidemic. Am J Transplant 2016;16(10): 2836–41.

17. Sibulesky L, Javed I, Reyes JD, et al. Changing the paradigm of organ utilization from PHS increased-risk donors: an opportunity whose time has come? Clin Transplant 2015;29(9):724–7.

18. Bowring MG, Kucirka LM, Massie AB, et al. Changes in utilization and discard of hepatitis C-infected donor livers in the recent era. Am J Transplant 2017;17(2): 519–27.

19. Berenguer M, Prieto M, San Juan F, et al. Contribution of donor age to the recent decrease in patient survival among HCV-infected liver transplant recipients. Hepatology 2002;36(1):202–10.

20. Berenguer M, Schuppan D. Progression of liver fibrosis in post-transplant hepatitis C: mechanisms, assessment and treatment. J Hepatol 2013;58(5):1028–41.

21. Gane EJ. The natural history of recurrent hepatitis C and what influences this. Liver Transpl 2008;14(Suppl 2):S36–44.

22. Gane EJ, Portmann BC, Naoumov NV, et al. Long-term outcome of hepatitis C infection after liver transplantation. N Engl J Med 1996;334(13):815–20.

23. Lai JC, Verna EC, Brown RS, et al. Hepatitis C virus-infected women have a higher risk of advanced fibrosis and graft loss after liver transplantation than men. Hepatology 2011;54(2):418–24.

24. Leroy V, Dumortier J, Coilly A, et al. Efficacy of sofosbuvir and daclatasvir in patients with fibrosing cholestatic hepatitis C after liver transplantation. Clin Gastroenterol Hepatol 2015;13(11):1993–2001.e1-2.

25. Cotter TG, Paul S, Sandıkçı B, et al. Improved graft survival after liver transplantation for recipients with hepatitis C virus in the direct-acting antiviral era. Liver Transpl 2019;25(4):598–609.

26. Agarwal K, Castells L, Müllhaupt B, et al. Sofosbuvir/velpatasvir for 12 weeks in genotype 1-4 HCV-infected liver transplant recipients. J Hepatol 2018;69(3): 603–7.

27. Altraif IH. Sofosbuvir plus ledipasvir for recurrent hepatitis C in liver transplant recipients. Liver Transpl 2017;23(4):554–6.

28. Charlton M, Gane E, Manns MP, et al. Sofosbuvir and ribavirin for treatment of compensated recurrent hepatitis C virus infection after liver transplantation. Gastroenterology 2015;148(1):108–17.

29. Kwo PY, Mantry PS, Coakley E, et al. An interferon-free antiviral regimen for HCV after liver transplantation. N Engl J Med 2014;371(25):2375–82.

30. Pillai AA, Maheshwari R, Vora R, et al. Treatment of HCV infection in liver transplant recipients with ledipasvir and sofosbuvir without ribavirin. Aliment Pharmacol Ther 2017;45(11):1427–32.

31. Reau N, Kwo PY, Rhee S, et al. Glecaprevir/pibrentasvir treatment in liver or kidney transplant patients with hepatitis C virus infection. Hepatology 2018;68(4): 1298–307.

32. Ballarin R, Cucchetti A, Spaggiari M, et al. Long-term follow-up and outcome of liver transplantation from anti-hepatitis C virus-positive donors: a European multicentric case-control study. Transplantation 2011;91(11):1265–72.

33. Lai JC, O'Leary JG, Trotter JF, et al. Risk of advanced fibrosis with grafts from hepatitis C antibody-positive donors: a multicenter cohort study. Liver Transpl 2012;18(5):532–8.

34. Marroquin CE, Marino G, Kuo PC, et al. Transplantation of hepatitis C-positive livers in hepatitis C-positive patients is equivalent to transplanting hepatitis C-negative livers. Liver Transpl 2001;7(9):762–8.

35. Northup PG, Argo CK, Nguyen DT, et al. Liver allografts from hepatitis C positive donors can offer good outcomes in hepatitis C positive recipients: a US National Transplant Registry analysis. Transpl Int 2010;23(10):1038–44.

36. O'Leary JG, Neri MA, Trotter JF, et al. Utilization of hepatitis C antibody-positive livers: genotype dominance is virally determined. Transpl Int 2012;25(8):825–9.

37. Saab S, Ghobrial RM, Ibrahim AB, et al. Hepatitis C positive grafts may be used in orthotopic liver transplantation: a matched analysis. Am J Transplant 2003;3(9): 1167–72.

38. Stepanova M, Locklear T, Rafiq N, et al. Long-term outcomes of heart transplant recipients with hepatitis C positivity: the data from the U.S. transplant registry. Clin Transplant 2016;30(12):1570–7.

39. Kucirka LM, Sarathy H, Govindan P, et al. Risk of window period hepatitis-C infection in high infectious risk donors: systematic review and meta-analysis. Am J Transplant 2011;11(6):1188–200.

40. Bari K, Luckett K, Kaiser T, et al. Hepatitis C transmission from seropositive, non-viremic donors to non-hepatitis C liver transplant recipients. Hepatology 2018; 67(5):1673–82.

41. Ellingson K, Seem D, Nowicki M, et al. Estimated risk of human immunodeficiency virus and hepatitis C virus infection among potential organ donors from 17 organ procurement organizations in the United States. Am J Transplant 2011;11(6): 1201–8.

42. Green M, Covington S, Taranto S, et al. Donor-derived transmission events in 2013: a report of the organ procurement transplant Network Ad Hoc Disease Transmission Advisory Committee. Transplantation 2015;99(2):282–7.

43. Cotter TG, Paul S, Sandıkçı B, et al. Increasing utilization and excellent initial outcomes following liver transplant of hepatitis C virus (HCV)-viremic donors into HCV-negative recipients: outcomes following liver transplant of HCV-viremic donors. Hepatology 2019;69(6):2381–95.

44. Chhatwal J, Samur S, Kues B, et al. Optimal timing of hepatitis C treatment for patients on the liver transplant waiting list. Hepatology 2017;65(3):777–88.

45. Bethea ED, Samur S, Kanwal F, et al. Cost effectiveness of transplanting HCV-infected livers into uninfected recipients with preemptive antiviral therapy. Clin Gastroenterol Hepatol 2019;17(4):739–747 e8.

46. Kwong AJ, Wall A, Melcher M, et al. Liver transplantation for hepatitis C virus (HCV) non-viremic recipients with HCV viremic donors. Am J Transplant 2019; 19(5):1380–7.

47. Levitsky J, Goldberg D, Smith AR, et al. Acute rejection increases risk of graft failure and death in recent liver transplant recipients. Clin Gastroenterol Hepatol 2017;15(4):584–593 e2.

48. Chan C, Schiano T, Agudelo E, et al. Immune-mediated graft dysfunction in liver transplant recipients with hepatitis C virus treated with direct-acting antiviral therapy. Am J Transplant 2018;18(10):2506–12.

49. Terrault NA, Berenguer M, Strasser SI, et al. International Liver Transplantation Society consensus statement on hepatitis C management in liver transplant recipients. Transplantation 2017;101(5):956–67.

50. Chhatwal J, Samur S, Bethea ED, et al. Transplanting hepatitis C virus-positive livers into hepatitis C virus-negative patients with preemptive antiviral treatment: a modeling study. Hepatology 2018;67(6):2085–95.

51. Mazur RD, Goldberg DS. Temporal changes and regional variation in acceptance of hepatitis C virus-viremic livers. Liver Transpl 2019;25(12):1800–10.

52. Ghany MG, Morgan TR. Hepatitis C guidance 2019 update: American Association for the Study of Liver Diseases-Infectious Diseases Society of America Recommendations for Testing, Managing, and Treating Hepatitis C Virus Infection. Hepatology 2020;71(2):686–721. https://pubmed.ncbi.nlm.nih.gov/?term=AASLD-IDSA+Hepatitis+C+Guidance+Panel%5BCorporate+Author%5D.

53. Anwar N, Kaiser TE, Bari K, et al. Use of hepatitis C nucleic acid test-positive liver allografts in hepatitis C virus seronegative recipients. Liver Transpl 2020;26(5): 673–80.

54. Crismale JF, Khalid M, Bhansali A, et al. Liver, simultaneous liver-kidney, and kidney transplantation from hepatitis C-positive donors in hepatitis C-negative recipients: a single-center study. Clin Transplant 2020;34(1):e13761.

55. Bethea E, Arvind A, Gustafson J, et al. Immediate administration of antiviral therapy after transplantation of hepatitis C-infected livers into uninfected recipients: implications for therapeutic planning. Am J Transplant 2020;20(6):1619–28.

Transplant of Elderly Patients

Is There an Upper Age Cutoff?

Claudia Cottone, MD[a],*, Nathalie A. Pena Polanco, MD[b],
Kalyan Ram Bhamidimarri, MD, MPH[c]

KEYWORDS

• Liver transplant • Elderly recipients • Old donors • Age limit

KEY POINTS

• Chronologic age is not a contraindication for liver transplant (LT); physiologic age is a more accurate indicator of functional status.

• The volume of wait-listed LT patients older than 65 years increased from 8.1% to 24.1% from 2002 to 2018.

• The volume of transplanted patients more than 65 years of age has increased from 6.8% in 2002 to 21.5% in 2019.

• Elderly LT recipients (older than 60 years) with body mass index greater than 30, hypertension, and diabetes mellitus type 2 have a 50% increased risk of postoperative cardiovascular mortality at 12 months and therefore need additional scrutiny during selection.

• Patient and graft survival rates after liver transplant in elderly recipients are lower compared with young recipients, but the survival benefit gained from LT is significant.

INTRODUCTION

Recent decades have witnessed an overall increase in life expectancy, particularly in developed countries, which in combination with decreased fertility rates has led to an increased prevalence of rapidly aging populations on a global landscape.[1] According to the 2019 United Nations (UN) data, 1 in 4 persons in Europe and North America will be more than 65 years old and those older than 80 years of age are expected to triple in number by 2050.[2] The increased life expectancy in the general population is also

[a] Department of Internal Medicine at Northwestern Medicine McHenry Hospital, Rosalind Franklin University of Medicine and Science, 4309 West Medical Center Drive, McHenry, IL 60050, USA; [b] Division of Digestive Health and Liver Diseases, University of Miami Miller School of Medicine, 1120 Northwest 14th Street, Suite 1105, Miami, FL 33136, USA; [c] Division of Digestive Health and Liver Diseases, University of Miami Miller School of Medicine, 1120 Northwest 14th Street, Suite 1144, Miami, FL 33136, USA
* Corresponding author.
E-mail address: Claudia.cottone13@gmail.com

Clin Liver Dis 25 (2021) 209–227
https://doi.org/10.1016/j.cld.2020.09.001
1089-3261/21/© 2020 Elsevier Inc. All rights reserved.

associated with an increased number of elderly patients who have end-stage liver disease (ESLD) and are in need of a liver transplant (LT). Based on a report from the World Health Organization, cirrhosis is the seventh most common cause of mortality in people older than 60 years.[1] Based on the Organ Procurement and Transplantation Network (OPTN) 2018 annual data report, the volume of wait-listed LT patients older than 65 years has steadily increased over time, representing 24.1% in 2018.[3] Not only the wait-listing trend but also the volume of LT in the same age group from 2002 to 2019 increased from 8% to 23% according to OPTN database[3] (**Fig. 1**). There are other noticeable trends with regard to the cause of ESLD and the indications for LT in the aging population. On one hand, chronic hepatitis C virus (HCV) in the elderly is decreasing but, in contrast, nonalcoholic steatohepatitis (NASH), alcoholic liver disease, and hepatocellular carcinoma (HCC) are increasing indications for LT.[4] As per current American Association for the Study of Liver Diseases (AASLD) guidelines, chronologic age in itself is not an absolute contraindication for LT.[5] Biological or physiologic age is the current strategy for patient selection for LT, accounting for factors other than just the chronologic age, such as nutritional status, functional status, lifestyle, and comorbid conditions. The stringent and individualized pretransplant selection of elderly patients has led to favorable posttransplant outcomes in several studies.[4,6–11] Although the feasibility of LT in elderly population does not seem to be problematic in terms of surgical technique and outcomes, the controversial issues are with regard to the ethical principles of utility and equity. This article reviews and summarizes the transplant outcomes in elderly patients, with a specific focus on patients older than 70 years of age, unless specified otherwise.

DISCUSSION
Pretransplant Evaluation Strategies

Cardiovascular
A rigorous cardiovascular pretransplant evaluation is paramount for every patient but more so in elderly NASH candidates because of increased prevalence of cardiovascular disease (CVD).[12] However, the ability to identify suitable candidates a priori who would

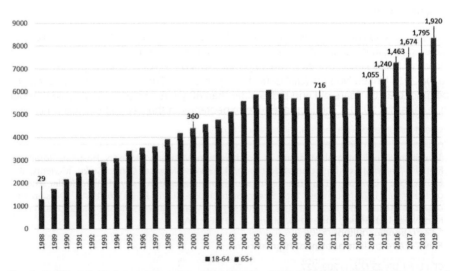

Fig. 1. Total adult LTs by recipients age from 1988 to 2019 (based on OPTN database as of June 18, 2020).

benefit from LT is difficult and is not well established. Patients with NASH have higher prevalence of coronary artery disease (CAD) and cardiovascular mortality at 1 year post-LT compared with other causes of liver diseases.[12] Age more than 60 years, a body mass index (BMI) greater than 30, hypertension, and diabetes mellitus (DM) type 2 are associated with an increased risk, as high as 50%, for early post-LT mortality.[13] Moderate to severe CAD is prevalent in up to 27% in LT candidates more than 50 years of age.[14] Cirrhotic cardiomyopathy, characterized by a blunted stress response, diastolic dysfunction, and QT prolongation is also a frequent finding during pre-LT screening (up to 50%) and its presence is associated with increased risk of overt heart failure in the early post-LT period.[15] Presence of atrial fibrillation pre-LT has been associated with increase intraoperative cardiac events, ventricular arrhythmias, cardiogenic shock, cardiac arrest, and deaths.[16] Portopulmonary hypertension (PPHTN) is prevalent in 4% to 8% of LT candidates, characterized by mean pulmonary artery pressure greater than 25 mm Hg in the setting of portal hypertension and is associated with higher perioperative mortality. However, data from large population studies do not show any significant difference in the rates of atrial fibrillation or PPHTN in the elderly.[16–18]

AASLD guidelines suggest electrocardiogram (ECG), transthoracic echocardiography (TTE), and pharmacologic stress test for all LT candidates. Cardiac computed tomography angiography, a noninvasive screening tool, has high sensitivity and specificity to detect coronary plaques and has a negative predictive value of 83% to 99% to screen for hemodynamically significant CAD.[19] Coronary artery calcium score (CACS) greater than 400 correlates well with high-risk CAD,[20] early cardiovascular events, and cardiac death after LT.[21] Older age and DM have also been associated with CACS greater than 400 in LT recipients.[21]

Coronary angiogram remains the gold standard for diagnosis and treatment of symptomatic CAD. Coronary angiography is endorsed in high-risk LT candidates with 3 or more risk factors: age older than 60 years, tobacco use, hypertension, DM, or dyslipidemia,[22] or in those with abnormal noninvasive cardiac testing. Revascularization before LT is recommended in those with coronary stenosis greater than 70% regardless of symptoms.[5] However, the role of angiogram in patients with asymptomatic ESLD is controversial because of the high incidence of postprocedure complications, bleeding, and contrast nephropathy, and the unclear survival benefit of revascularization in the absence of symptoms.[23] Uniform CVD screening protocols for the elderly transplant candidates are not well established; nonetheless, a thorough cardiovascular evaluation is imperative, especially in elderly and high risk patients.

Malignancies

Elderly patients with ESLD are at high risk of developing extrahepatic cancers (EHCs), with different incidence rates that vary with the cause of underlying liver disease. A recent population-based analysis reported increased rates of extrahepatic and liver malignancies among patients with chronic liver diseases.[24] Non-Hodgkin lymphomas, especially B-cell lymphomas and leukemias, are frequently observed in viral liver diseases (hepatitis B virus [HBV] and HCV), whereas gastrointestinal malignancies involving the colon, esophagus, and oropharynx are common in NASH and alcoholic liver disease.[24,25] Incidence of EHCs, both lymphoid and solid organ cancers, peaks in men after 65 years of age and in women after 75 years of age.[26] In LT recipients older than 70 years, malignancies are responsible for 20% of all-cause mortality after transplant.[4] Ear-nose-throat and lung malignancies are common in elderly transplant candidates with active or prior history of smoking. Most transplant centers require a tumor-free interval of 1 to 5 years for LT candidacy, except for some cancers that have curative expected survival that exceeds post-LT survival (eg, a few histologic variants of renal cell carcinoma) that have curative expected survival that exceeds post-LT survival.[27,28] No defined screening protocols are in place for elderly LT candidates; however, it is prudent to screen for EHCs based on the risk factors.

Nutritional and functional status

Pre-LT evaluation must include evaluation of candidates' functional and nutritional status. Sarcopenia, defined as a loss of skeletal muscles, is commonly seen in elderly patients,[29] as is malnutrition. Other markers of functional and nutrition status are also notably impaired in the elderly. Elderly patients more than 65 years old have more functional impairment and lower Short Physical Performance Battery (SPPB) scores than their younger counterparts. SPPB score less than 9 in elderly LT candidates was associated with higher waiting-list mortality compared with younger, not impaired patients with SPPB score more than 9.[30] Taking the intrinsic vulnerabilities and increased health burden from the comorbid conditions into consideration, the pre-transplant evaluation of elderly transplant candidates should be more inclusive and multidisciplinary than for the general population.[5]

Intraoperative Morbidity

Intraoperative hemorrhage, volume status, ascites, and cardiomyopathy can cause serious alterations in cardiac output, especially in the elderly.[31] However, operative time does not seem to be affected by recipient age.[6,10,32] Higher requirement for fluid resuscitation and transfusions, packed red blood cells (PRBCs), platelets, and fresh frozen plasma among the elderly had been reported in older studies,[32] but recent studies have reported no differences.[6,10] Cardiovascular events are responsible for 40% of early post-LT mortality (within 30 days) and is more frequent in the elderly, especially in those with NASH, DM, hypertension, and chronic obstructive pulmonary disease (COPD). Older age, DM, and COPD have been associated with higher rate of cardiac arrest.[33] Patients older than 50 years have a higher cardiac event rate of 7.5% (compared with 5.1% in younger patients) and a mortality of 0.8% to 1.2%.[33,34] Intraoperative complications could be higher than the reported rates because the data are possibly biased by the strict selection and may not apply to all elderly transplant candidates. Nonetheless, advanced age and NASH seem to have a negative impact on the early post-LT survival because of higher rates of cardiovascular events.

Posttransplant Complications

Graft survival

In general, acute cellular rejection is less frequent in elderly solid organ transplant recipients. A combination of factors, such as reduction in the proportion of naive T cells, dysfunction of memory cells, and age-related altered metabolism of immunosuppressant, are implicated as plausible mechanisms for the low rates of rejection in elderly LT recipients.[35] Aging also reduces the tolerance of foreign antigens and self-antigens (autoimmunity).[35] According to the OPTN database, early graft survival rates were similar among younger recipients and recipients older than 65 years of age, but the survival rate diminishes in the elderly in subsequent years. Graft survival at 1, 3, and 5 years is 89.1%, 79.8%, and 71% in the younger recipients, whereas it is 86.6%, 75.2%, and 65.9% in elderly recipients (**Fig. 2**). Graft survival at 10 years post-LT in the elderly more than 70 years old is 41.7% compared with 60.9% in younger recipients.[6] According to the OPTN database, early graft survival rates were comparable among younger and older recipients but the survival rate diminishes in the elderly in subsequent years. Data regarding immunosuppressive regimens in the elderly are scarce and have been limited to single-center experiences. It is common practice in

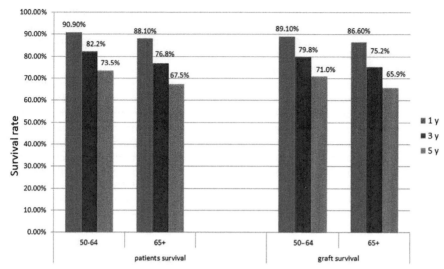

Fig. 2. Patient and graft survival rates for transplant from 2008 to 2015 in United States (based on OPTN database as of June 12, 2020).

most centers to administer lower doses of immunosuppression in most elderly transplant recipients because they are generally at high risk for DM, hypertension, CVD, and renal impairment.[36] Immunosenescence and immunosuppression may play a role in HCC recurrence in elderly recipients. Biliary complications account for 9.6% of graft failures and have similar incidences in younger and elderly LT recipients.[37]

Patient survival
Elderly patients with chronic liver disease are at higher risk of other comorbidities, such as malignant neoplasms, CVD (hypertension, ischemic heart disease, arrhythmias, cardiomyopathies, aortic dissection), respiratory illnesses, diabetes, dyslipidemia, gout, hypothyroidism, cerebrovascular disease, and renal failure.[38] The presence of these comorbidities, as well as other characteristics inherent to the elderly, in particular an impaired immune system, increases the likelihood of opportunistic infections and other complications, such as erectile dysfunction, osteoporosis, malignancy, and depression.[11] The utility and benefit of LT in this population have been evaluated since the 1990s, reporting what were initially contradictory and variable posttransplant survival rates ranging from 35% to 83% at 3 years.[39,40] Most of the early evidence showed that selected elderly (adults >60 years of age) had variable outcomes and survival compared with younger adults.[41–48] In 1991, a single-center retrospective analysis of 156 LT patients more than the age of 60 years found that the 3-year survival rate in the elderly population was comparable with the younger recipients, concluding that advanced age was not a contraindication to LT.[43] In another prospective trial including 735 LT recipients between 1990 and 1994, recipients older than 60 years had longer hospital/intensive care unit (ICU) stay and lower 1-year post-LT survival rate compared with the younger recipients: 81% versus 90% respectively.[47] The excess mortality among the older recipients was attributable to infections, cardiac events, or neurologic events.[47] Advances in immunosuppression and management of chronic comorbidities have improved outcomes in more recent years across all ages and in the elderly.

A single-center analysis from the Mayo Clinic included all LTs performed between 1998 and 2004, reporting that mortalities at 1, 3, and 5 years after transplant for elderly recipients were 10%, 14%, and 27% respectively, compared with those of younger patients, which in turn were 12%, 21%, and 24%.[32] An analysis of 46,772 LTs performed from 1994 to 2005 in the United Network for Organ Sharing (UNOS)/OPTN database found that 17% of the recipients were older than 60 years. Out of the 5 strongest factors that would predict poor patient survival, 4 of those elements were inherent to the recipients, such as the need for mechanical ventilation, history of DM, positive HCV serology, and creatinine levels of 1.6 mg/dL or higher. The fifth factor was a combined recipient and donor age of 120 years or more. Taking these variables into account, an older recipient prognostic score (ORPS) was created, with each variable accounting for 1 point. ORPS groups ranged from 1 to 5, and patients in ORPS group 1 experienced 1-year, 3-year, and 5-year survival rates of 85%, 77%, and 69%, whereas those in ORPS group 5 had 1-year, 3-year, and 5-year survival rates of 73%, 48%, and 41% respectively. In this patient population, data from this study found that the Model for End-stage Liver Disease (MELD) score was a poor posttransplant prognostic indicator.[49]

A retrospective study that analyzed LT recipients from the UNOS/OPTN registry between 2002 and 2012 reported an overall 5-year survival of 59% in elderly (>70 years old) HCC recipients and 68.6% in younger HCC recipients. In those without HCC, the 5-year survival rate was 61.2% versus 74.2% in elderly and younger patients, respectively. Similar trends were noted in those with or without HCV, 5-year survival in HCV-positive elderly versus younger patients was 60.7% and 69%, and in HCV-negative elderly versus younger patients was 62.6% and 78.5% respectively.[50]

Another retrospective analysis of 3104 recipients from a single-center database in the United States, transplanted from 1998 through December 2016, aimed to determine other factors that were related to decreased overall patient survival, identifying those in the pretransplant, peritransplant, and posttransplant settings. In terms of the recipients, they found that advanced age, HCC history, the need for hospitalization before LT, and increasing PRBC requirement were significant. Around the time of transplant, a longer total operating time, the cold ischemia time (CIT), and the warm ischemia time all correlated negatively with survival. Posttransplant events such as hospital length of stay, need for ICU management, and donor characteristics (University of California, Los Angeles, extended criteria donors [ECD] score equal or higher than ≥2 and cerebrovascular/stroke as the cause of death) were significantly associated with decreased overall patient survival.[6]

Another study used information from a national database in Korea that included all adult patients who underwent LT from 2007 to 2016, totaling 9614. Of these, a cohort of 84 LT patients more than 70 years of age was evaluated; elderly patients had increased in-hospital mortality and hospitalization costs.[51] Despite this and other data supporting worse transplant survival in the elderly, some investigators argue that, without transplant, these patients would also have a lower survival than younger patients at any MELD score, and therefore support transplant, finding that these patients do have a survival benefit derived from it.[4] **Table 1** summarizes results of studies evaluating outcomes after LTs in elderly patients since 2002 (post-MELD era). In the postoperative period, the care of elderly recipients poses a few characteristic challenges compared with younger patients, in order to avoid complications that could negatively affect posttransplant morbidity and mortality, such as decline of bone health, worsening of CVD, and development of malignancies.[39]

Table 1
Reported data for patients and graft survival in literature

Study, Year	Area	Donor Type	Sample Size (n)	Age at LT (y)	Patients Survival
Goldberg et al,[80] 2020	United States UNOS 2002–2018 SLK	NA	93	≥70	5 y: 68.8% (without CKD) 5 y: 57.8% (with CKD)
Mousa et al,[6] 2019	United States Single center	DDLT	162	≥70	5 y: 70.8% 10 y: 43.6%
Cullaro et al,[7] 2020	United States UNOS 2003–2017	LDLT-DDLT	11,775	≥65	HCC: 1 y: 90% 5 y: 79% No HCC: 1 y: 87% 5 y: 78.5%
Kollmann et al,[102] 2018	European Union (Austria) Single center	NA	76	≥65	1 y: 71% (73% MELD era) 5 y: 48% (60% MELD era)
Sharma et al,[50] 2017	United States UNOS/OPTN 2002–2012	DDLT	1514	≥70	5 y: 60%
Su et al,[4] 2016	United States UNOS 2002–2014	LDLT-DDLT	1666	≥70	5 y: 62%
Sonny et al,[9] 2015	United States Single center 2004–2010	NA	223	≥60	5 y: 75.8%
Wilson et al,[8] 2014	United States SRTR/UHC	DDLT	323	≥70	1 y: 85% 5 y: 64%
Malinis et al,[37] 2014	United States UNOS 2002–2011	LDLT-DDLT	4254 1265	60–69 ≥70	5 y: 65% 5 y: 57.5%
Schwartz et al,[103] 2012	United States UNOS 2010	DDLT 1 LDLT	480	≥70	5 y: 55%
Taner et al,[104] 2012	United States Single center	DDLT	13	≥75	5 y: 54%
Aloia et al,[49] 2010	United States UNOS 1994–2005	NA	631	≥70	5 y: 56%
Aduen et al,[32] 2009	United States Single center	DDLT	42	≥70	5 y: 63%
Lipshutz et al,[105] 2007	United States Single center	DDLT	62	≥70	1 y: 73.3% 3 y: 65.8% 5 y: 47.1% 10 y: 39.7%
Safdar et al,[11] 2004	United States Single center	DDLT	33	≥70	1 y: 78.79% 3 y: 71.43%,
Zetterman et al,[47] 1998	Multiple centers	NA	135	≥60 y od	1 y: 81%
Rudich & Busuttil,[45] 1999	United States Single center	DDLT	33	≥70	1 y: 60%

Abbreviations: CKD, chronic kidney disease; DDLT, deceased donor LT; LDLT, living donor LT; NA, not available; SLK, simultaneous liver-kidney transplant; SRTR, Scientific Registry of Transplant Recipients; UHC, University HealthSystem Consortium.
    Data from Refs.[4,6–9,11,32,37,45,47,49,50,80,102–105]

Bone health in post–liver transplant setting

Bone loss accelerates in the first 6 months after LT, regardless of the pretransplant bone mineral density, and it is associated with increased risk of fractures, which in turn causes significant morbidity and reduced quality of life; 6 to 12 months after LT, bone loss reverses and there is a gain in bone density.[52] Osteoporosis is reported in up to 36% of elderly LT candidates compared with 5% in age-matched healthy peers regardless of gender.[53] There is a substantial risk of decline in bone health and an increase in pathologic fractures of up to 35% in the immediate posttransplant period.[54] Of the 360 LT recipients with cholestatic liver disease transplanted at the Mayo, 20% had a fracture in the pre-LT period. There was a sharp increase in fracturing, with a 30% cumulative incidence of fractures at 1 year post-LT, and the strongest risk factors were pretransplant fractures, severity of osteopenia, and glucocorticoid use.[55] Limiting the exposure to corticosteroids is generally possible because of the decreased requirement for immunosuppressants in the elderly. Single-center studies have found a lower incidence of rejection and higher rates of infection and cancer in the elderly.[11,32,43] The changes of the immune system in the elderly seem to confer a protective effect against rejection, because most cell-mediated and humoral immune responses decline with advancing age. Both T-cell and B-cell activation, transit through the cell cycle, and subsequent differentiation are significantly diminished in the elderly.[56]

Cardiovascular diseases

Cardiovascular health can significantly affect the perioperative period, as well as posttransplant outcomes. In the past, evidence suggested that patients with angiographically proven CAD had an overall mortality of 50% over a follow-up period of 1 to 3 years.[57] Physiologic changes in this age group, such as increased left ventricular mass, increased arterial stiffness, coronary atherosclerosis, and altered vascular regulation, can be responsible for their limited reserve. Data from a multicenter study that evaluated the outcomes of 630 patients who had undergone coronary angiography as part of their pretransplant evaluation, comparing the 151 patients who had CAD with the rest, were published in 2013. Despite the presence of several cardiovascular risk factors, revascularization and medical therapies used before LT were shown to be effective did not affect survival post-LT; patients with a history of severe CAD who underwent preoperative coronary intervention were able to safely undergo LT without being at a higher risk for short-term mortality.[58]

Malignancies

De novo malignancies represent another leading cause of mortality in the elderly after LT[59–61] and are mostly triggered by the immune dysregulation caused by immunosuppressive agents and opportunistic infections with carcinogenic viruses (Epstein-Barr virus, human papilloma virus), primary sclerosing cholangitis, smoking, and alcohol abuse.[52] In a registry that included 175,732 solid organ transplant recipients (21.6% for liver) in the United States, incidence of overall cancers was 1375 per 100,000 person years, with the most common malignancies being non-Hodgkin lymphoma and cancers of the lung, liver, and kidney.[62] An analysis of the National Institute of Diabetes and Digestive and Kidney Diseases (NIDDK) Liver Transplantation Database, including liver recipients from 3 clinical centers, showed that 22% of transplanted patients developed a de novo malignancy during the 12.6-year study period. The incidences of de novo malignancy within 1, 5, and 10 years were 3.5%, 11.9%, and 21.7%, respectively, with highest risk of solid organ malignancies (hazard ratio [HR], 1.26) and skin malignancies (HR, 1.81) in the elderly recipients.[59,63,64]

Does donor age matter in elderly liver transplant recipients?

With increasing demand for organs, transplant centers have used several donor pool expansion strategies, such as the use of living donors, cadaveric split livers, and ECDs. ECDs have underlying factors associated with poor graft function and increased risk of graft failure, such as hypernatremia, prolonged warm ischemia time, pressor requirement, donation after cardiac death, and advanced donor age.[65] Older liver grafts could have unfavorable age-related attributes, such as fibrosis, steatosis, atherosclerosis, and increased activation of proinflammatory and apoptotic genes, which can result in higher risk of injury during ischemia-reperfusion.[66] Grafts from older donors also carry a higher susceptibility to CIT,[67,68] primary nonfunction, and delayed graft function[69] and is independently associated with poor 5-year graft survival.[37] A single-center, retrospective analysis of LT from 1990 to 2007 that included 91 older donors (>60 years old) and 650 younger donors reported that neither patient survival rates nor graft survival rates had any disadvantage.[70] In 2016, Barbier and colleagues[71] compared 253 recipients of younger grafts with 157 recipients of older grafts (>75 years old) and reported no significant differences in primary nonfunction, hepatic artery thrombosis, biliary complications, graft survival, or retransplant rates among both cohorts. A very small, single-center study had also reported favorable outcomes with donors older than 80 years, using morphologic appearance of the liver at time of harvesting and presence of steatosis as factors that determined the use of these organs.[72] A larger cohort study from Italy also found comparable 1-year, 3-year, and 5-year survival rates in recipients of grafts from octogenarian and younger donors. However, the study pointed out that increased donor age may portend worse outcome if the donor had increased transaminase levels and if the graft was used in sicker recipients (HCV positive, higher MELD scores).[73] Since 2006, the donor risk index, a model based on quantified surrogates of donor quality, has been used to differentiate between lower-risk and high-risk donors, with higher scores correlating with decreased survival.[74] Evidence from the analysis of 8070 liver recipients aged 60 years or older, transplanted from 1994 to 2005, suggested that the strongest prognostic factor for LT recipients 60 years old or older was the allocation of a liver allograft from an older donor that created a recipient and donor age combination equal to or greater than 120 years, because in those cases there was a 20% reduction in postoperative survival.[49] In an age-matched LT study, older recipients were at higher risk of death posttransplant, independent of age matching, and the predictors of poor prognosis were high MELD scores, retransplant, and prolonged CIT.[75] Elderly donors did not affect patient survival, and, even though the recipient's age independently increased the risk of death, matching older donors to older recipients did not confer an additional risk. The optimal recipients of older donor grafts are first-time recipients, those with body mass index less than 35, non–status 1, low biological MELD score, and CIT of less than 8 hours. Resulting evidence therefore supports the use of older livers in older recipients, as long as other risk factors are minimized.[75] Grafts from donors older than 70 years of age are still underused in some parts of the United States, with a discard rate of approximately 26%, but the use of older donor organs could be optimized by adjusting for aforementioned recipient-specific factors. Current UNOS/OPTN allocation for livers does not follow age matching, but transplant centers assign the livers from elderly donors in the appropriately selected patient populations in whom the strategy was proved to be safe.[76,77]

LIVING DONOR LIVER TRANSPLANT IN THE ELDERLY

Scarce data mostly derived from single-center non-US transplant centers is available with regard to living donor LT (LDLT) in the elderly. Ethics discussion for LDLT in the elderly is even more difficult and needs to balance the operative risks of the younger donor to be justified by recipient gain of life years and quality of life. Japanese and Korean studies reported no survival differences in the elderly and the younger LDLT recipients.[61,78] Moreover, a significantly lower incidence of graft failure in recipients older than 65 years was observed.[61] In US studies, Su and colleagues[4] reported 3% of LDLT in recipients older than 70 years, but the post-LT survival rate for this subgroup was not reported. LDLT in elderly recipient seems to be feasible and confers a reasonably good survival rate in high-volume LDLT centers. However, the existing data are limited and the impact of LDLT in the elderly needs to be evaluated in a more systematic fashion.

SIMULTANEOUS LIVER-KIDNEY TRANSPLANT IN ELDERLY

Current data with regard to simultaneous liver-kidney transplant (SLK) in the elderly are limited. An age cutoff of 65 or 70 years has been proposed because of previous reports of unfavorable outcomes in SLK recipients.[79] A recent study analyzing the UNOS database of SLK recipients from 2002 to 2018 reported a constant increase of older recipients with chronic kidney disease. Among the total SLK recipients, 17% were older than 65 years of age and 3% were older than 70 years. The latter age group showed a statistically significant increased mortality risk after SLK compared with all other age groups. Comparison between young nondiabetic recipients and older recipients (independent of DM status) showed survival rate differences of 10.3%, 25%, and 31% at 1, 5, and 10 years. Among all age groups, the elderly cohort (>70 years old) experienced a 5-year survival less than 60%.[80] Therefore, in the SLK setting, a chronologic age of 70 years seems to be a reasonable cutoff, at least until more systematic data become available in the future.

ETHICS

In 1984, the National Organ Transplant Act (NOTA) established the OPTN and the initial policies regarding an equitable organ allocation system.[81] In 1998, the OPTN Final Rule was adopted by Congress, with the goal of establishing the regulatory requirements for the OPTN and improving the effectiveness and equity of the transplant system, furthering the objectives established in NOTA.[82] However, this document was not meant to be an ethical guide, enumerating only the minimal legal and governmental policy requirements that must be included in a just allocation policy. A report adopted in 1992 by the OPTN Ethics Committee, then revised in 2010, describes the ethical principles that should be applied in the allocation of organs. These principles include:

- Utility, which is described as maximizing the benefits of available resources
- Justice, which ensures the fair distribution of these benefits
- Respect for persons or autonomy,[83] in a background of equity as described by NOTA when referring to desired outcomes of organ allocation[81]

The liver allocation system based on the MELD follows a justice system that prioritizes patients with the highest risk of waiting-list mortality. An ideal allocation system would consider the principle of utility and parameters such as predicted graft survival and predicted years of life added after transplant. These parameters are some of the standardized measures used to determine the strategies for organ allocation and are balanced with the potential negative consequences of transplant, such as mortality, postoperative complications, and long-term outcomes.[83] In this setting, the recipient age unequivocally becomes a major determinant because transplant of an elderly patient would be expected to result in a time-limited benefit (fewer years added after transplant compared with nonelderly recipients). Several guiding principles have been endorsed to overcome this age paradox; some contend that all patients in liver failure have equal worth and, as such, the sickest should have an equal chance at getting an organ, regardless of their age.[84]

Others argue in favor of intergenerational equity, or the principle of fair innings, claiming that everyone is entitled to a normal lifespan, and that anyone who is deprived of that is at a disadvantage. Therefore, prolonging the lives of those who had achieved an older age with transplant and taking away the organ from the nonelderly recipient should not be the priority.[85] In 2012, Ross and colleagues[86] evaluated the role that age can play in the allocation of deceased donor kidneys, based on a model that they called Equal Opportunity Supplemented by Fair Innings. This principle allows allocation of kidneys based on 2 strategies: the first was that all waiting-list candidates had an equal chance of getting a deceased donor kidney transplant, regardless of age. Second, this was supplemented by the principle of fair innings, which prioritized patients developing end-stage renal disease at a younger age as being worse off than those who developed it later in life. Hence, the proposed allocation of higher-quality organs (using donor age as proxy for quality) to younger patients (a young-to-young allocation) provides them with a higher probability of achieving a full lifespan.[86,87] A few years later, a group of Italian investigators published the results of a study that evaluated how recipient and donor ages affected allocation and therefore affected the life expectancy of LT recipients. The study analyzed 2476 candidates and 1371 grafts and the effect of fair innings, age matching, and age mapping. Age mapping defends that all candidates have an equal chance of getting a liver, good-quality organs (typically from younger donors) being offered to the sickest. Such liver allocation based on age mapping resulted in a significant reduction (33%) in the gap between years of life lost between youngest and oldest candidates, and showed improved equity and efficiency compared with those observed in prognostic models.[84]

UNOS provides age-specific risk adjustment that is capped at a recipient age of 65 years and is potentially discouraging to the centers toward transplant in the elderly population, because their increased mortality risk is not adjusted for.[88] Based on the most recent data reports from UNOS, a total of 20,810 patients more than the age of 65 years have been transplanted from 1988 to date; more than 60% of these patients were transplanted after 2010, with cases almost doubling every year since 2016, indicating more frequent transplants in this population. In 2020, there are 3496 candidates more than 65 years of age wait-listed for an LT in the UNOS database.[89] In a study of 122,606 adults listed for transplant and 60,820 that underwent liver transplant from 2002 to 2014, the proportion of registrants aged more than 60 years increased from 19% to 41%; those more than 65 years old increased from 8.1% to 17% and those more than 70 years old increased from 1.4% to 3.1%. Increased age was significantly associated with increased waiting-list mortality and also increased posttransplant mortality. However, older age did not affect the transplant-related survival benefit.[4] Similar results had also been described by Wilson and colleagues,[8] who analyzed the Scientific Registry of Transplant Recipients (SRTR) and the University HealthSystem Consortium databases of 12,445 patients who underwent LT from 2007 to 2011. Whether or not current policies should be modified to include the age of the recipient as part of the allocation algorithm for LT, akin to the kidney allocation system, remains a topic of discussion.[88]

CORONAVIRUS DISEASE-19 AND TRANSPLANT IN ELDERLY

Severe acute respiratory syndrome–coronavirus-2 (SARS-CoV-2) virus and its related disease COVID-19 (coronavirus disease 2019) continue to spread worldwide, affecting 6,713,881 persons globally with 393,709 deaths as of June 5, 2020.[90] In the early half of 2020, COVID-19 has dramatically changed the medical world and the approach to managing chronic diseases. The rapid spread of COVID-19 has affected the most vulnerable first: older patients and those with comorbidities such as DM, HTN, and CAD. The overall impact of the COVID-19 pandemic on the elderly population has been devastating people who have the highest risk of mortality.[91,92] A report from China on the elderly population affected by SARS-CoV-2 showed that age older than 60 years was associated with more severe disease than the general population.[91] Recent data from an Italian LT unit in Milan reported 3 deaths among long-term LT recipients in a short time frame of 3 weeks. Interestingly, the fatalities occurred in patients older than 65 years with multiple comorbidities (HTN, DM, hyperlipidemia, overweight), who underwent LT longer than 10 years previously and were on minimal immunosuppressive regimen.[93] A report from the Italian epicenter of the pandemic, Bergamo, concluded that immunosuppression does not constitute a risk factor in solid organ recipients.[94] Data from Spain on 18 solid organ tumor recipients reported a median age of 71 years, among which 6 were LT recipients. The study reported severe disease presentation and course in most the patients, with a case-fatality rate of 27.8%.[95] Contradictory results in terms of mortality in solid organ recipients infected with SARS-CoV-2 have been published so far in the United States. Data from the New York area showed an overall mortality of 18% in solid organ recipients positive for SARS-CoV-2. Recipient age older than 65 years was associated with a 60% rate of severe disease presentation.[96] A different cancer center reported data from 21 solid organ transplant recipients with only 5 patients older than 65 years. In this cohort, 67% of patients were hospitalized and half of them required ICU care, with only 1 deceased patient (mortality 4.8%) reported.[97] Liver transplant practices have also changed because of the COVID-19 pandemic, which mandates aggressive screening of donors and recipients for SARS-CoV-2. Wait-listed patients with acute SARS-CoV-2 infection are ineligible for LT. The high rates of false-negative results and accuracy of the assays at various phases of the COVID-19 infection have to be taken into consideration for appropriate patient selection.[98] Polymerase chain reaction on bronchoalveolar lavage testing for SARS-CoV-2 has been proposed as a better screening test, with a sensitivity of 93%, than nasopharyngeal swabs.[99,100] LT candidates who test positive for SARS-CoV-2 can be considered for transplant after 14 to 21 days of symptom resolution and after 2 negative tests for SARS-CoV-2.[98] Immunosuppression in itself would likely prolong the viral shredding rather than increase the severity of the infection.[94] Current consensus does not recommend empiric reduction of immunosuppression in LT recipients, even in the elderly.[98] More robust data are needed for a better understanding of the disease and its implications in immunosuppressed patients.

SUMMARY

Advances in medicine and population behavior led to increased life expectancy in developed countries until the COVID-19 pandemic, which has been significantly deleterious in the elderly. Effective antiviral therapies for HCV and HBV and improved management of cirrhosis complications and hepatocellular carcinoma have led to an increased prevalence of elderly patients with ESLD who need LT. Current epidemiologic trends show decreasing prevalence of chronic HCV and progressively increasing prevalence of NASH, alcoholic liver disease, and hepatocellular carcinoma as indications for LT in the elderly population. Recent evidence suggests that elderly LT recipients are generally healthier and have comparable functional status with their younger counterparts. According to the UNOS database, the oldest transplant recipient is 88 years old and there is a steady surge in the transplant volume in those older than 70 years of age.[101] The volume of LTs performed in patients older than 65 years increased from 716 in 2010 to 1920 in 2019 (see **Fig. 1**). Posttransplant survival and graft outcomes in patients older than 70 years have also reportedly been similar to younger patients, which provides a favorable argument for advocating that chronologic age should not be considered as an absolute contraindication for LT. However, elderly transplant candidates are carefully selected with stringent pre-LT screening, which could explain the favorable outcomes and survival data observed in the cohort. Specific algorithms for elderly patient selection for LT are not well established; however, consensus agreement is that elderly LT candidates need a more rigorous selection process. Presence of comorbidities such as CVD, obesity, DM, and HTN have a negative impact on early post-LT survival, especially in the growing NASH population. In conclusion, there is no specific upper age cutoff for liver transplant. Elderly patient selection for transplant must be individualized and strategies from high-volume centers that transplant the elderly need to be validated in future studies to assess how far clinicians can "push the envelope" in this aging cohort.

CLINICS CARE POINTS

- Increased life expectancy and aging population has led to a trend of increasing LT volume in the elderly.
- Elderly LT candidates typically have an age-associated burden of comorbid conditions that can pose several clinical challenges during the selection/evaluation process for LT.
- Cardiovascular complications and de novo malignancies are the most common causes of post-LT mortality in elderly LT recipients.
- Although the early survival rate after LT is comparable with the younger recipients, the delayed patient and graft survival rates are lower in the elderly recipients. However, the number of years gained in elderly patients after LT is significant and, therefore, there is no strict chronologic age cutoff for LT.
- A thorough individualized evaluation is the current strategy, but development of rigorous transplant protocols geared to improving outcomes in the elderly cohort are necessary in the future.

DISCLOSURE

C. Cottone and N.P. Polanco have nothing to disclose. K.R. Bhamidimarri receives research grants from Allergan, Gilead, Genfit, Mallinckrodt, Viking therapies, and Hepquant; participates in scientific advisory boards for Gilead, Abbvie, Mallinckrodt, and Intercept, and receives speaker honoraria from Alexion and Intercept.

REFERENCES

1. Beard JR, Officer A, de Carvalho IA, et al. The World report on ageing and health: a policy framework for healthy ageing. Lancet 2016;387(10033): 2145–54.
2. Department of economics and social affairs of the UN: world population prospects 2019 revision. Data Booklet (ST/ESA/SER.A/424).

3. Kwong A, Kim WR, Lake JR, et al. OPTN/SRTR 2018 annual data report: liver. Am J Transplant 2020;20(s1):193–299.

4. Su F, Yu L, Berry K, et al. Aging of liver transplant registrants and recipients: trends and impact on waitlist outcomes, post-transplantation outcomes, and transplant-related survival benefit. Gastroenterology 2016;150(2):441–53.e6 [quiz: e416].

5. Martin P, DiMartini A, Feng S, et al. Evaluation for liver transplantation in adults: 2013 practice guideline by the American association for the study of liver diseases and the american society of transplantation. Hepatology 2014;59(3): 1144–65.

6. Mousa OY, Nguyen JH, Ma Y, et al. Evolving role of liver transplantation in elderly recipients. Liver Transplant 2019;25(9):1363–74.

7. Cullaro G, Rubin JB, Mehta N, et al. Differential impact of age among liver transplant candidates with and without hepatocellular carcinoma. Liver Transpl 2020; 26(3):349–58.

8. Wilson GC, Quillin RC 3rd, Wima K, et al. Is liver transplantation safe and effective in elderly (>/=70 years) recipients? A case-controlled analysis. HPB(Oxford) 2014;16(12):1088–94.

9. Sonny A, Kelly D, Hammel JP, et al. Predictors of poor outcome among older liver transplant recipients. Clin Transplant 2015;29(3):197–203.

10. Li HY, Wei YG, Yan LN, et al. Outcomes between elderly and young hepatocellular carcinoma living donor liver transplantation recipients: a single-center experience. Medicine 2016;95(5):e2499.

11. Safdar K, Neff GW, Montalbano M, et al. Liver transplant for the septuagenarians: importance of patient selection. Transplant Proc 2004;36(5):1445–8.

12. Samji NS, Heda R, Satapathy SK. Peri-transplant management of nonalcoholic fatty liver disease in liver transplant candidates . Transl Gastroenterol Hepatol 2020;5:10.

13. Malik SM, DeVera ME, Fontes P, et al. Outcome after liver transplantation for NASH cirrhosis. Am J Transplant 2009;9(4):782–93.

14. Carey WD, Dumot JA, Pimentel RR, et al. The prevalence of coronary artery disease in liver transplant candidates over age 50. Transplantation 1995;59(6): 859–64.

15. Liu H, Jayakumar S, Traboulsi M, et al. Cirrhotic cardiomyopathy: implications for liver transplantation. Liver Transpl 2017;23(6):826–35.

16. Bargehr J, Trejo-Gutierrez JF, Patel T, et al. Preexisting atrial fibrillation and cardiac complications after liver transplantation. Liver Transpl 2015;21(3):314–20.

17. Le Pavec J, Souza R, Herve P, et al. Portopulmonary hypertension: survival and prognostic factors. Am J Respir Crit Care Med 2008;178(6):637–43.

18. Krowka MJ, Miller DP, Barst RJ, et al. Portopulmonary hypertension: a report from the US-based REVEAL registry. Chest 2012;141(4):906–15.

19. Choi JM, Kong Y-G, Kang J-W, et al. Coronary computed tomography angiography in combination with coronary artery calcium scoring for the preoperative cardiac evaluation of liver transplant recipients. Biomed Res Int 2017;2017: 4081525.

20. Kemmer N, Safdar K, Kaiser TE, et al. Liver transplantation trends for older recipients: regional and ethnic variations. Transplantation 2008;86(1):104–7.

21. Kong YG, Kang JW, Kim YK, et al. Preoperative coronary calcium score is predictive of early postoperative cardiovascular complications in liver transplant recipients. Br J Anaesth 2015;114(3):437–43.

22. Lentine KL, Costa SP, Weir MR, et al. Cardiac disease evaluation and management among kidney and liver transplantation candidates: a scientific statement from the American heart association and the american college of cardiology foundation: endorsed by the American society of transplant surgeons, American society of transplantation, and national kidney foundation. Circulation 2012; 126(5):617–63.

23. Snipelisky DF, McRee C, Seeger K, et al. Coronary interventions before liver transplantation might not avert postoperative cardiovascular events. Tex Heart Inst J 2015;42(5):438–42.

24. Kim D, Adejumo AC, Yoo ER, et al. Trends in mortality from extrahepatic complications in patients with chronic liver disease, from 2007 through 2017. Gastroenterology 2019;157(4):1055–66.e11.

25. Allen AM, Hicks SB, Mara KC, et al. The risk of incident extrahepatic cancers is higher in non-alcoholic fatty liver disease than obesity - a longitudinal cohort study. J Hepatol 2019;71(6):1229–36.

26. Allaire M, Nahon P, Layese R, et al. Extrahepatic cancers are the leading cause of death in patients achieving hepatitis B virus control or hepatitis C virus eradication. Hepatology 2018;68(4):1245–59.

27. Fayek S, Moore D, Bortecen KH, et al. Liver transplantation in the setting of extra-hepatic malignancy: two case reports. Transplant Proc 2007;39(10): 3512–4.

28. Falkensammer CE, Bonatti H, Falkensammer J, et al. Combined liver transplantation together with partial/total nephrectomy in patients with renal cell cancer and nonalcoholic steatohepatitis. Transpl Int 2007;20(5):471–2.

29. Englesbe MJ, Patel SP, He K, et al. Sarcopenia and mortality after liver transplantation. J Am Coll Surg 2010;211(2):271–8.

30. Wang CW, Covinsky KE, Feng S, et al. Functional impairment in older liver transplantation candidates: from the functional assessment in liver transplantation study. Liver Transpl 2015;21(12):1465–70.

31. Therapondos G, Flapan AD, Plevris JN, et al. Cardiac morbidity and mortality related to orthotopic liver transplantation. Liver Transpl 2004;10(12):1441–53.

32. Aduen JF, Sujay B, Dickson RC, et al. Outcomes after liver transplant in patients aged 70 years or older compared with those younger than 60 years. Mayo Clin Proc 2009;84(11):973–8.

33. VanWagner LB, Lapin B, Levitsky J, et al. High early cardiovascular mortality after liver transplantation. Liver Transpl 2014;20(11):1306–16.

34. Eleid MF, Hurst RT, Vargas HE, et al. Short-term cardiac and noncardiac mortality following liver transplantation. J Transplant 2010;2010:910165.

35. Martins PN, Tullius SG, Markmann JF. Immunosenescence and immune response in organ transplantation. Int Rev Immunol 2014;33(3):162–73.

36. Krenzien F, El Hajj S, Tullius SG, et al. Immunosenescence and immunosuppressive drugs in the elderly. In: Fulop T, Franceschi C, Hirokawa K, et al, editors. Handbook of immunosenescence: basic understanding and clinical implications. Cham (Switzerland): Springer International Publishing; 2019. p. 2147–67.

37. Malinis MF, Chen S, Allore HG, et al. Outcomes among older adult liver transplantation recipients in the model of end stage liver disease (MELD) era. Ann Transplant 2014;19:478–87.

38. Hoshida Y, Ikeda K, Kobayashi M, et al. Chronic liver disease in the extremely elderly of 80 years or more: clinical characteristics, prognosis and patient survival analysis. J Hepatol 1999;31(5):860–6.

39. Keswani RN, Ahmed A, Keeffe EB. Older age and liver transplantation: a review. Liver Transpl 2004;10(8):957–67.
40. Filipponi F, Roncella M, Boggi U, et al. Liver transplantation in recipients over 60. Transplant Proc 2001;33(1–2):1465–6.
41. Pirsch JD, Kalayoglu M, D'Alessandro AM, et al. Orthotopic liver transplantation in patients 60 years of age and older. Transplantation 1991;51(2):431–3.
42. Emre S, Mor E, Schwartz ME, et al. Liver transplantation in patients beyond age 60. Transplant Proc 1993;25(1 Pt 2):1075–6.
43. Stieber AC, Gordon RD, Todo S, et al. Liver transplantation in patients over sixty years of age. Transplantation 1991;51(1):271–3.
44. Bromley PN, Hilmi I, Tan KC, et al. Orthotopic liver transplantation in patients over 60 years old. Transplantation 1994;58(7):800–3.
45. Rudich S, Busuttil R. Similar outcomes, morbidity, and mortality for orthotopic liver transplantation between the very elderly and the young. Transplant Proc 1999;31(1–2):523–5.
46. Collins BH, Pirsch JD, Becker YT, et al. Long-term results of liver transplantation in older patients 60 years of age and older. Transplantation 2000;70(5):780–3.
47. Zetterman RK, Belle SH, Hoofnagle JH, et al. Age and liver transplantation: a report of the Liver transplantation database. Transplantation 1998;66(4):500–6.
48. Levy MF, Somasundar PS, Jennings LW, et al. The elderly liver transplant recipient: a call for caution. Ann Surg 2001;233(1):107–13.
49. Aloia TA, Knight R, Gaber AO, et al. Analysis of liver transplant outcomes for United Network for Organ Sharing recipients 60 years old or older identifies multiple model for end-stage liver disease-independent prognostic factors. Liver Transpl 2010;16(8):950–9.
50. Sharma M, Ahmed A, Wong RJ. Significantly higher mortality following liver transplantation among patients aged 70 years and older. Prog Transplant 2017;27(3):225–31.
51. Gil E, Kim JM, Jeon K, et al. Recipient age and mortality after liver transplantation: a population-based cohort study. Transplantation 2018;102(12):2025–32.
52. EASL Clinical Practice Guidelines. Liver transplantation. J Hepatol 2016;64(2):433–85.
53. Ninkovic M, Love SA, Tom B, et al. High prevalence of osteoporosis in patients with chronic liver disease prior to liver transplantation. Calcif Tissue Int 2001;69(6):321–6.
54. Jeong HM, Kim DJ. Bone diseases in patients with chronic liver disease. Int J Mol Sci 2019;20(17):4270.
55. Guichelaar MM, Schmoll J, Malinchoc M, et al. Fractures and avascular necrosis before and after orthotopic liver transplantation: long-term follow-up and predictive factors. Hepatology 2007;46(4):1198–207.
56. Weigle WO. Effects of aging on the immune system. Hosp Pract (Off ed) 1989;24(12):112–9.
57. Plotkin JS, Scott VL, Pinna A, et al. Morbidity and mortality in patients with coronary artery disease undergoing orthotopic liver transplantation. Liver Transpl Surg 1996;2(6):426–30.
58. Wray C, Scovotti JC, Tobis J, et al. Liver transplantation outcome in patients with angiographically proven coronary artery disease: a multi-institutional study. Am J Transplant 2013;13(1):184–91.
59. Watt KD, Pedersen RA, Kremers WK, et al. Long-term probability of and mortality from de novo malignancy after liver transplantation. Gastroenterology 2009;137(6):2010–7.

60. Cross TJ, Antoniades CG, Muiesan P, et al. Liver transplantation in patients over 60 and 65 years: an evaluation of long-term outcomes and survival. Liver Transpl 2007;13(10):1382–8.

61. Ikegami T, Bekki Y, Imai D, et al. Clinical outcomes of living donor liver transplantation for patients 65 years old or older with preserved performance status. Liver Transplant 2014;20(4):408–15.

62. Engels EA, Pfeiffer RM, Fraumeni JF Jr, et al. Spectrum of cancer risk among US solid organ transplant recipients. JAMA 2011;306(17):1891–901.

63. Herrero JI, Lucena JF, Quiroga J, et al. Liver transplant recipients older than 60 years have lower survival and higher incidence of malignancy. Am J Transplant 2003;3(11):1407–12.

64. Herrero JI, España A, Quiroga J, et al. Nonmelanoma skin cancer after liver transplantation. Study of risk factors. Liver Transpl 2005;11(9):1100–6.

65. Gordon Burroughs S, Busuttil RW. Optimal utilization of extended hepatic grafts. Surg Today 2009;39(9):746–51.

66. Kireev RA, Cuesta S, Ibarrola C, et al. Age-related differences in hepatic ischemia/reperfusion: gene activation, liver injury, and protective effect of melatonin. J Surg Res 2012;178(2):922–34.

67. Chela H, Yousef MH, Albarrak AA, et al. Elderly donor graft for liver transplantation: never too late. World J Transplant 2017;7(6):324–8.

68. Colvin MM, Smith CA, Tullius SG, et al. Aging and the immune response to organ transplantation. J Clin Invest 2017;127(7):2523–9.

69. Ploeg RJ, D'Alessandro AM, Knechtle SJ, et al. Risk factors for primary dysfunction after liver transplantation–a multivariate analysis. Transplantation 1993; 55(4):807–13.

70. Anderson CD, Vachharajani N, Doyle M, et al. Advanced donor age alone does not affect patient or graft survival after liver transplantation. J Am Coll Surg 2008; 207(6):847–52.

71. Barbier L, Cesaretti M, Dondero F, et al. Liver transplantation with older donors: a comparison with younger donors in a context of organ shortage. Transplantation 2016;100(11):2410–5.

72. Zapletal C, Faust D, Wullstein C, et al. Does the liver ever age? Results of liver transplantation with donors above 80 years of age. Transplant Proc 2005;37(2): 1182–5.

73. Ghinolfi D, Marti J, De Simone P, et al. Use of octogenarian donors for liver transplantation: a survival analysis. Am J Transplant 2014;14(9):2062–71.

74. Flores A, Asrani SK. The donor risk index: a decade of experience. Liver Transpl 2017;23(9):1216–25.

75. Gilbo N, Jochmans I, Sainz-Barriga M, et al. Age matching of elderly liver grafts with elderly recipients does not have a synergistic effect on long-term outcomes when both are carefully selected. Transplant direct 2019;5(4):e342.

76. Segev DL, Maley WR, Simpkins CE, et al. Minimizing risk associated with elderly liver donors by matching to preferred recipients. Hepatology 2007;46(6): 1907–18.

77. Durand F, Levitsky J, Cauchy F, et al. Age and liver transplantation. J Hepatol 2019;70(4):745–58.

78. Kwon JH, Yoon YI, Song GW, et al. Living donor liver transplantation for patients older than age 70 years: a single-center experience. Am J Transplant 2017; 17(11):2890–900.

79. Eason JD, Gonwa TA, Davis CL, et al. Proceedings of consensus conference on simultaneous liver kidney transplantation (SLK). Am J Transplant 2008;8(11): 2243–51.

80. Goldberg DS, Vianna RM, Martin EF, et al. Simultaneous liver kidney transplant in elderly patients with chronic kidney disease: is there an appropriate upper age cutoff? Transplantation 2020. Online First.

81. US National organ transplant act (NOTA), Pub L 98-507. 1984.

82. Organ Procurement and Transplantation Network–HRSA. Final rule with comment period. Fed Regist 1998;63(63):16296–338.

83. Ethical principles in the allocation of human organs. 2015. Available at: https://optn.transplant.hrsa.gov/resources/ethics/ethical-principles-in-the-allocation-of-human-organs/. Accessed May 13, 2020.

84. Cucchetti A, Ross LF, Thistlethwaite JR Jr, et al. Age and equity in liver transplantation: an organ allocation model. Liver Transpl 2015;21(10):1241–9.

85. Williams A. Intergenerational equity: an exploration of the 'fair innings' argument. Health Econ 1997;6(2):117–32.

86. Ross LF, Thistlethwaite JR Jr. Age should not be considered in the allocation of deceased donor kidneys. Semin Dial 2012;25(6):675–81.

87. Ross LF, Parker W, Veatch RM, et al. Equal opportunity supplemented by fair innings: equity and efficiency in allocating deceased donor kidneys. Am J Transplant 2012;12(8):2115–24.

88. Goldberg DS, Charlton M. Usefulness of liver transplantation in the elderly: the converging impact of risk and benefit. Gastroenterology 2016;150(2):306–9.

89. Network OPaT. Organ by age. current U.S. waiting list. Available at: https://optn.transplant.hrsa.gov/data/view-data-reports/national-data/#. Accessed May 19, 2020.

90. Johns Hopkins Coronavirus Resource Center. 2020. Available at: https://coronavirus.jhu.edu/map.html. Accessed June 5, 2020.

91. Liu K, Chen Y, Lin R, et al. Clinical features of COVID-19 in elderly patients: a comparison with young and middle-aged patients. J Infect 2020;80(6):e14–8.

92. Abbatecola AM, Antonelli-Incalzi R. Editorial: COVID-19 spiraling of frailty in older Italian patients. J Nutr Health Aging 2020;24(5):453–5.

93. Bhoori S, Rossi RE, Citterio D, et al. COVID-19 in long-term liver transplant patients: preliminary experience from an Italian transplant centre in Lombardy. Lancet Gastroenterol Hepatol 2020;5(6):532–3.

94. D'Antiga L. Coronaviruses and immunosuppressed patients: the facts during the third epidemic. Liver Transpl 2020;26(6):832–4.

95. Fernández-Ruiz M, Andrés A, Loinaz C, et al. COVID-19 in solid organ transplant recipients: a single-center case series from Spain. Am J Transplant 2020;20(7):1849–58.

96. Pereira MR, Mohan S, Cohen DJ, et al. COVID-19 in solid organ transplant recipients: initial report from the US epicenter. Am J Transplant 2020;20(7): 1800–8.

97. Yi SG, Rogers AW, Saharia A, et al. Early experience with COVID-19 and solid organ transplantation at a US high-volume transplant center. Transplantation 2020. https://doi.org/10.1097/TP.0000000000003339.

98. Fix OK, Hameed B, Fontana RJ, et al. Clinical best practice advice for hepatology and liver transplant providers during the COVID-19 pandemic: AASLD expert panel consensus statement. Baltimore, (Md): Hepatology; 2020.

99. Umberto M, Luciano C, Daniel Y, et al. The impact of the COVID-19 outbreak on liver transplantation programs in Northern Italy. Am J Transplant 2020;20(7): 1840–8.
100. Wang W, Xu Y, Gao R, et al. Detection of SARS-CoV-2 in different types of clinical specimens. JAMA 2020;323(18):1843–4.
101. OPTN Ethics Committee Minutes. Available at: https://optn.transplant.hrsa.gov/media/2772/20181029_ethics_committee_minutes.pdf.
102. Kollmann D, Maschke S, Rasoul-Rockenschaub S, et al. Outcome after liver transplantation in elderly recipients (>65 years) - a single-center retrospective analysis. Dig Liver Dis 2018;50(10):1049–55.
103. Schwartz JJ, Pappas L, Thiesset HF, et al. Liver transplantation in septuagenarians receiving model for end-stage liver disease exception points for hepatocellular carcinoma: the national experience. Liver Transpl 2012;18(4):423–33.
104. Taner CB, Ung RL, Rosser BG, et al. Age is not a contraindication for orthotopic liver transplantation: a single institution experience with recipients older than 75 years. Hepatol Int 2012;6(1):403–7.
105. Lipshutz GS, Hiatt J, Ghobrial RM, et al. Outcome of liver transplantation in septuagenarians: a single-center experience. Arch Surg 2007;142(8):775–81 [discussion: 781–74].

Transplants for Acute Alcoholic Hepatitis
Controversies and Early Successes

Jessica Hause, MD, John P. Rice, MD*

KEYWORDS

- Alcohol • Hepatitis • Liver • Transplant • Controversy

KEY POINTS

- Liver transplant for medically refractory, severe acute alcohol-associated hepatitis offers a survival benefit compared with medical therapy.
- Alcohol relapse rates in published studies of liver transplant recipients for alcohol-associated hepatitis are comparable with liver transplant recipients with alcohol-associated cirrhosis.
- Optimal patient selection for liver transplant in alcohol-associated hepatitis is challenging and remains a primary source of controversy in the transplant community.
- Concerns regarding objectivity in the selection process are well founded but not necessarily unique to alcohol-associated hepatitis.

HISTORY OF LIVER TRANSPLANT, ALCOHOL-ASSOCIATED LIVER DISEASE, AND THE 6-MONTH RULE

Alcohol-associated liver disease (ALD) is currently the leading indication for liver transplant (LT) in the United States.[1] This increase in LT for ALD is thought to be in part explained by a decline in hepatitis C virus as an indication for LT but also by an absolute increase in patients with ALD undergoing LT.[2] This emergence of ALD as the leading indication for LT has occurred despite early skepticism that ALD would be a frequent indication for LT. In 1983, the National Institutes of Health (NIH) Consensus Conference declared LT a modality deserving of broader application for end-stage liver disease (ESLD).[3,4] In reference to ALD, the NIH recommended LT be considered in "patients judged likely to abstain from alcohol," but that "only a small proportion of alcoholic patients with liver disease would be expected to meet these rigorous criteria."[4]

Disclosures: Drs J. Hause and J.P. Rice have no commercial or financial conflicts of interest to disclose.
Division of Gastroenterology and Hepatology, Department of Medicine, University of Wisconsin School of Medicine and Public Health, 4th Floor MFCB, 1685 Highland Avenue, Madison, WI 53705, USA
* Corresponding author.
E-mail address: jrice@medicine.wisc.edu

Clin Liver Dis 25 (2021) 229–252
https://doi.org/10.1016/j.cld.2020.08.010
1089-3261/21/© 2020 Elsevier Inc. All rights reserved.

Subsequently, the early experiences in LT for ALD were generally positive. In 1988, Starzl and colleagues[5] published an early experience in performing LT for ALD. They did not mandate a fixed "dry" period before consideration of LT, arguing that, although abstinence was considered to be a favorable factor, a "dry" period of specific duration was not required because this would have invited systematic falsification of the medical history and because death often would have been the price of a significant wait. In addition to acceptable 1-year post-LT survival in the postcyclosporine era, the investigators observed that alcohol relapse was uncommon, occurring in only 1 of the 30 patients that survived 6 months in the postcyclosporine era. The investigators opined that, "the imposition of an arbitrary period of abstinence before going forward with transplantation would seem medically unsound or even inhumane."[5]

Over the next 2 decades, LT for ALD rapidly expanded across the globe and ALD became a leading indication for LT. Encouragingly, LT outcomes in ALD seemed comparable with other indications and further reinforced LT as an acceptable treatment of ALD leading to ESLD and hepatocellular carcinoma.[6,7] As more follow-up data became available, it became clear that, contrary to the early experience of Starzl and colleagues,[5] LT was not "the ultimate sobering experience." Numerous studies have attempted to determine alcohol use after LT. Many of the studies were retrospective and thus limited in terms of standardization of alcohol use assessments and quantification of amount of alcohol consumed. In addition, the definition of alcohol relapse was not standardized and suffered from a lack of discrimination of moderate from harmful use and sustained alcohol use versus self-limited "slips." In addition, the lack of available alcohol biomarkers made detecting subclinical or surreptitious alcohol use difficult. Acknowledging these limitations, these studies estimated rates of alcohol use after LT for ALD from approximately 10% to 50%.[8–12] The best study in post-LT alcohol use remains the prospective longitudinal study from DiMartini and colleagues,[10] at the University of Pittsburgh. They followed 208 patients that underwent LT for ALD over 10 years and found that slightly less than half (46%) drank some alcohol after LT. Although most drank alcohol infrequently, 19% drank in a potentially harmful manner. They identified 5 distinct patterns of alcohol use after LT (none, infrequent, early onset accelerating to moderate use, late onset accelerating to heavy use, and early onset accelerating use). Thus, despite Starzl and colleagues'[5] early observation, post-LT alcohol use is common. However, context is important. Alcohol relapse seems to be much less common in LT recipients than in patients completing community alcohol treatment programs.[13]

Initially, there was uncertainty whether alcohol relapse negatively affected post-LT outcomes.[14] However, as data regarding alcohol use after LT accumulated over time, it became clear that harmful drinking after LT was clearly associated with allograft damage and inferior post-LT outcomes. In the DiMartini and colleagues[10] study, a few patients with heavy alcohol use developed steatohepatitis on liver biopsy and 5 patients did succumb to recurrent ALD.[10] Other retrospective studies have consistently shown the association between alcohol use after LT, allograft damage, and inferior graft and survival outcomes.[8,9,11,12] Thus, absolute alcohol abstinence after LT should be the recommendation for every LT recipient. In addition, it should be the goal of every LT program to select patients for LT with a favorable prognosis for long-term abstinence.

The origins of the 6-month rule are not clear; however, as ALD emerged as an indication for LT, the practice of enforcing mandatory intervals of sobriety before consideration of LT became widespread. A survey of LT programs in 1998 revealed that 85% of LT programs in the United States enforced some sobriety interval rule before LT eligibility.[15] There is sound medical logic for monitored sobriety. With time and alcohol abstinence, liver failure and complications of portal hypertension can improve and thus remove the need for LT.[16] However, in practice, the use of a fixed sobriety interval was adopted as a tool for relapse prevention after LT. The scientific evidence for such a practice is weak. Although length of sobriety pre-LT is associated with decreased risk of alcohol relapse, 6 months of sobriety has not been consistently shown to decrease risk of post-LT relapse.[10,17,18] In longitudinal studies of non-LT patients, relapse is common and sustained sobriety achieved only after 5 years of abstinence, an interval rarely achieved before LT.[19] Therefore, in accordance with the original opinion of Starzl and colleagues,[5] the enforcement of fixed sobriety intervals before evaluation for a lifesaving LT is likely ethically unsound.

ALCOHOL-ASSOCIATED HEPATITIS AND LIVER TRANSPLANT

Alcohol-associated hepatitis (AH) is a clinical syndrome manifested as the development of jaundice in the setting of heavy antecedent alcohol use. The severity of AH is highly variable. Although mild AH may be largely asymptomatic, severe AH is a life-threatening illness complicated by severe liver failure and complications of portal hypertension. When refractory to medical therapy, severe AH carries a poor short-term prognosis, with mortalities of 25% to 45% at 1 month.[20–22]

The NIH has created consensus criteria for diagnosing suspected AH (**Table 1**).[23] Essential to the diagnosis of AH is a history of heavy antecedent alcohol use. This threshold has been set at 4 standard drinks ($\sim$50–60 g) per day for men and 3 standard drinks (40 g) per day for women. This level of drinking should have occurred for at least 6 months and jaundice should have been noted within 60 days of the last drink. In practice, most patients with AH greatly exceed this minimum threshold for diagnosis.

The most common histopathologic finding in AH is alcoholic steatohepatitis (ASH).[24] The pathologic hallmarks of ASH are macrovesicular hepatic steatosis; hepatocellular injury manifested as swollen hepatocytes, termed ballooning; neutrophil-predominant inflammation; and the presence of Mallory-Denk hyaline. Although the features of steatohepatitis can be seen in other diagnoses, such a nonalcoholic steatohepatitis (NASH) and drug injury, the combination of clinical AH and ASH on biopsy confirms the diagnosis. In the United States, a diagnosis of AH is usually made by clinical judgment, and liver biopsy is rarely performed.

Occasionally, patients with a clinical AH diagnosis do not have concomitant histopathologic ASH but have cirrhosis without associated steatohepatitis. In turn, most patients with clinical AH and histologic ASH have concomitant cirrhosis.[24] Thus, there may be considerable overlap between AH and acute-on-chronic liver failure (ACLF), defined as the acute deterioration of liver function associated with a high short-term mortality. In studies of ACLF, alcohol use is a common precipitant of ACLF.[25–27] Therefore, there is no consensus that AH and ACLF with recent heavy alcohol use are distinct clinical syndromes. Although therapeutics designed to treat ASH may make the histopathologic distinction important, for patients with recent harmful alcohol use and severe liver failure being considered for LT, the presence or absence of histopathologic ASH is likely inconsequential.

The mainstay of treatment of AH is abstinence from alcohol and nutritional support (**Fig. 1**). Most patients with AH have significant protein calorie malnutrition and may have refeeding syndrome. Although a randomized trial of intensive enteral nutrition did not show a mortality benefit compared with conventional nutritional support, the study did find a significantly increased mortality in patients with severe AH consuming less than 21.5 kcal/kg/d[28] For patients that cannot reach that threshold by conventional diet, consideration of a feeding tube and enteral supplementation should be

Table 1	
National Institute on Alcohol Abuse and Alcoholism consensus definitions in the diagnosis of alcoholic hepatitis	
Minimum criteria for a diagnosis of alcoholic hepatitis: • Serum bilirubin level >3.0 mg/dL • Drinking more than 3 standard drinks (40 g) per day for women and 4 drinks (50–60 g) per day for men • Minimum criteria drinking for >6 mo • <60 d from last drink to the development of jaundice • AST>50 IU/L but AST/ALT<400 IU/L • AST/ALT ratio of >1.5	Definite alcoholic hepatitis: clinical AH and biopsy-proven ASH Probable alcoholic hepatitis: meets minimum criteria for AH without confounding factors: • Negative immune markers (ANA<1:160, ASMA<1:80 dilution) • Absence of sepsis, shock, cocaine use, or drug use at risk of DILI within 30 d • Biopsy not required for diagnosis Possible alcoholic hepatitis: does not meet minimum criteria or potential confounders • Inconsistent alcohol history • Atypical laboratory studies (AST<50 IU/L, ALT/AST>400 IU/L, or AST/ALT ratio<1.5) • Recent shock (hemorrhagic or septic) • Positive immune markers (ANA>1:160 or ASMA>1:80) • Suspicion of DILI • Biopsy recommended to confirm diagnosis

Abbreviations: ALT, alanine aminotransferase; ANA, antinuclear antibody; ASH, alcoholic steatohepatitis; ASMA, anti–smooth muscle antibody; AST, aspartate aminotransferase; DILI, drug induced liver injury.

Data from Crabb DW, Bataller R, Chalasani NP, et al. Standard Definitions and Common Data Elements for Clinical Trials in Patients With Alcoholic Hepatitis: Recommendation From the NIAAA Alcoholic Hepatitis Consortia. Gastroenterology. 2016;150(4):785-790.

considered.[28] With time and abstinence, liver function and complications from portal hypertension may dramatically improve, even at the point of cirrhosis. Improvement, when it does occur, typically does so over a span of weeks to a few months, but can be delayed as much as 12 months.

For patients with severe AH, consideration should be made for pharmacotherapy in addition to abstinence and nutritional support. Severe AH can be defined by several scoring systems using widely available laboratory variables (**Table 2**). Corticosteroids, typically prednisolone 40 mg daily, remain the first-line therapy for severe AH as recommended by guidelines from the major liver disease societies.[29–31] Studies of corticosteroids in severe AH have yielded conflicting results, but the totality of the evidence suggests some benefit.[20,22] However, corticosteroids should not be initiated in patients with uncontrolled infection or gastrointestinal hemorrhage. In addition, the use of corticosteroids increases the risk of subsequent infection, a major cause of morbidity and mortality in severe AH.[32,33] For that reason, once initiated, an assessment of corticosteroid response is essential. The Lille model is a validated score to determine corticosteroid response at 7 days at a cutoff of 0.45.[21] A Lille model greater than 0.45 at day 7 indicates nonresponse and a poor prognosis, and corticosteroids should be discontinued. A Lille model less than 0.45 indicates a good prognosis and is an indication to continue corticosteroids for 28 days and then taper off. One study suggested a 4-day Lille model performed as well as the 7-day Lille model.[34] In addition, a declining bilirubin level or Model for End-stage Liver Disease (MELD) score also signals recovery and can be used as a surrogate for the Lille model.[35,36]

Patients with severe AH that are either nonresponders or ineligible for corticosteroids generally have a poor short-term prognosis, although outcomes have varied

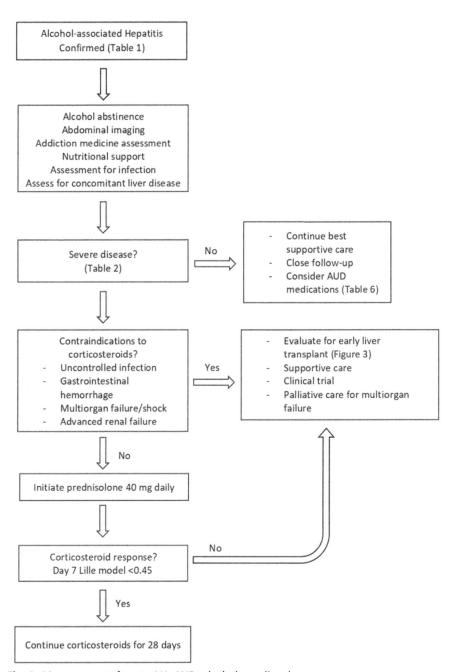

Fig. 1. Management of acute AH. AUD, alcohol use disorder.

substantially in different studies. In the Lille model cohort, corticosteroid nonresponse carried a 6-month mortality of ~75%.[21] In the randomized controlled Steroids or Pentoxyfylline for Alcoholic Hepatitis (STOPAH) trial, 28-day mortality was less than 20% in all study arms.[22] Multiple risk factors have been associated with

Table 2
Scoring systems for determining severity in alcohol associated hepatitis

	Discriminant Function	MELD	GAHS	Age, Bilirubin, INR, Creatinine	Lille Model[a]
Variables Collected	• Serum total bilirubin • Prothrombin time • Control prothrombin time	• Serum total bilirubin • INR • Serum creatinine	• Age • WBC • Blood urea nitrogen • Prothrombin time • Control prothrombin time	• Age • Serum total bilirubin • INR • Serum creatinine	• Age • Serum albumin at day 0 • Serum creatinine at day 0 • Prothrombin time at day 0 • Serum total bilirubin at day 0 • Serum total bilirubin at day 4 or 7
Interpretation at Diagnosis	Severe AH: MDF ≥32	Severe AH: undefined values >20–25 considered high mortality risk	Poor prognosis: ≥9	High mortality risk: >9 Intermediate risk: 6.71–9.00 Low risk: <6.71	NA
Corticosteroid Threshold	MDF>32	Unknown	GAHS ≥9	Unknown	NA
Interpretation After 7 d of Corticosteroid Treatment	NA	Favorable prognosis: MELD decline by ≥2.6 points	NA	NA	Favorable prognosis: Lille model <0.45 Poor prognosis: Lille>0.45

Abbreviations: GAHS, Glasgow Alcoholic Hepatitis Score; INR, International Normalized Ratio; MDF, Maddrey's Discriminant Function; MELD, Model for End-stage Liver Disease; NA, not available; WBC, white blood cell count.

[a] The Lille model is calculated from serum data on the date of corticosteroid initiation (day 0) and at day 4 or 7 of corticosteroid therapy.

a poor outcome, including older age, degree of leukocytosis, amount of alcohol consumed, renal failure, and the development of multiple organ failure.[27,37] At the present time, no additional medical treatments have been proved to improve outcomes in severe AH.

As a result, LT is a potential lifesaving option for patients with severe AH refractory to medical therapy. However, the widespread enforcement of fixed sobriety intervals almost exclusively excluded AH from consideration of LT. In addition, the idea of offering LT to patients with untreated alcohol use disorder (AUD) and limited sobriety was considered anathema to the LT community. European transplant centers were the first to question, and study, early (before 6 months of abstinence) LT for severe AH refractory to medical care. The landmark Franco-Belgian study was a prospective, multicenter study performed from 2005 to 2010 and showing that early LT in severe, refractory AH had superior 6-month survival compared with controls treated with best medical care (77% vs 23%, P<.001).[38] The selection process was rigorous. Patients considered for early LT needed to commit to lifelong abstinence, have strong social support, and no previous episodes of decompensation from ALD. Complete consensus of the LT selection committee was required for approval. Most medical nonresponders were not selected (France 19.4%, Belgium 26.1% approval rates, respectively). Of the entire cohort of severe AH, including medical responders, less than 2% ultimately underwent LT, accounting for 2.9% of allografts used during the study period. Alcohol relapse was infrequent, occurring in only 10% of patients.[38] This study successfully challenged the 6-month dogma and set the stage for expansion of LT for severe AH across the globe.

Subsequently, LT for severe AH moved across the Atlantic as 2 pilot studies were published in the United States. The first study, by Im and colleagues,[39] reported the results of a single-center pilot study from 2012 to 2015 at Mount Sinai Hospital in New York City. Out of 111 patients with severe AH refractory to medical therapy, 9 (8.1%) ultimately underwent LT, with 8 (89%) surviving 6 months. One LT recipient did relapse to harmful alcohol use post-LT.[39] Subsequent, another single-center study from Johns Hopkins published their experience in AH and ALD, in general.[40,41] Between 2012 and 2017, 46 patients underwent LT for AH compared with 34 for alcohol-associated cirrhosis (AC). One-year graft survival (89% vs 93%, P = .7), any alcohol use (24% vs 28%, P = .8), and harmful alcohol use (12% vs 17%, P = .5) were no different in AC versus AH despite comparable follow-up times (678 days vs 484 days, P = .2), respectively.[41] More recently, an additional single-center study of 10 patients that underwent LT with recent drinking showed excellent 1-year survival and only 1 patient (10%) returned to drinking.[42]

The largest US experience in LT for AH was a retrospective, multicenter study (including Mount Sinai and Johns Hopkins data) of LT for clinical AH from 2006 to 2017.[43] Among 147 patients that underwent LT for severe AH, cumulative patient survival after LT was 94% at 1 year and 84% at 3 years, a significant survival benefit compared with previous studies of medically refractory severe AH. Harmful alcohol use was infrequent, with the cumulative incidence of sustained alcohol use of 10% at 1 year and 17% at 3 years. However, sustained alcohol use after LT was associated with increased mortality and ultimately, among the 9 deaths to occur after the first year, 7 were alcohol related.[43] Patient selection in this study was more heterogeneous but generally followed the framework put forth by the Franco-Belgian study. Nine of the 12 centers could provide selection data and 35.9% of patients were waitlisted. Patients included in this study had no prior diagnosis of decompensated liver disease or episodes of AH and endured comprehensive psychosocial assessments as part of the selection process.[43]

LIVER TRANSPLANT FOR ALCOHOL-ASSOCIATED HEPATITIS: THE DEBATE

The practice of rescue LT in medically refractory severe AH may be the most controversial current topic in LT (**Table 3**). Many providers in the field, whether they be surgeons, hepatologists, transplant coordinators, social workers, or addiction specialists, have strong feelings about the practice, one way or the other.

Arguments Supporting Early Liver Transplant for Severe Alcohol-Associated Hepatitis

For proponents of LT in AH, the debate centers on the lifesaving nature of LT for AH. Given the poor survival of medically refractory AH, early LT offers lifesaving treatment and a survival benefit.[38,43] One-year survival outcomes have generally been good and likely comparable with other indications for transplant. In addition, the rates of alcohol relapse have not significantly differed from the published rates of alcohol relapse in AC. Most LT recipients have remained abstinent from alcohol and thus show that a fixed interval of sobriety before LT is neither necessary nor sufficient for some patients to achieve long-term abstinence and a good LT outcome. Even in the worst-case scenario of refractory harmful alcohol relapse post-LT, modeling has suggested that the mortality benefit of early LT would be preserved.[44] Given the lifesaving nature of early LT in AH and the lack of evidence that AH portends a significantly higher risk of alcohol relapse or graft loss, proponents of LT for AH believe strongly that there is no ethical basis to deny LT candidacy in AH based on fixed-sobriety rules.

In addition, proponents argue that fixed-interval sobriety rules subject patients with AUD to a bias not found in other so-called lifestyle liver diseases, such as obesity-induced NASH or in intentional overdose leading to acute liver failure (ALF). Most LT programs do not mandate weight loss before consideration of LT, nor do they mandate mental health treatment before considering LT in all cases of suicide attempt. These candidates undergo a thorough medical and psychosocial assessment to determine LT suitability and are not subject to inflexible mandates. Thus, subjecting patients with AUD to a different standard is likewise unethical.

Table 3
Arguments for and against early liver transplant for severe alcohol-associated hepatitis

Arguments for early LT for severe AH	Arguments against early LT for severe AH
• Improved survival compared with medical therapy	• Lack of long-term outcome data to show acceptable outcomes
• Weak evidence that mandatory sobriety intervals improve LT outcome	• Concerns regarding early graft loss from recurrent ALD
• Alcohol relapse rates comparable with AC with fixed-interval sobriety	• Subjectivity in selection process
• Denial of early LT is a result of bias not enforced in other lifestyle-related liver diseases (eg, NASH, ALF secondary to intentional overdose)	• Lack of program transparency in selection process
	• Lack of oversight of programs performing early LT for AH
	• Lack of LT program resources to adequately assess and monitor patients undergoing early LT for AH
	• Workload on LT team
	• Potential for spontaneous hepatic recovery obviating need for transplant
	• Worsening organ shortage
	• Disparity in access to early transplant
	• Negative public perception

Public perception of the practice of LT has always been a critical focus of the transplant community. Deceased donor LT remains the dominant modality of LT in the United States and Europe. Because LT depends on the generosity of the public in terms of organ donation, public confidence in the process of LT selection and performance is understandably and appropriately of the utmost importance. Critics are concerned that expanding LT to patients with ALD without significant pre-LT sobriety will be rejected by the public and risk organ donation. Proponents of LT for AH believe that, if the selection process for LT is transparent, rigorous, and backed by scientific evidence, the public will accept opening LT to patients with limited sobriety and high short-term mortality. Surveys of public opinion suggest that the public, at this point, is at least neutral to the practice.[45]

Arguments Against Early Liver Transplant in Severe Alcohol-Associated Hepatitis

Critics of LT for AH think that the existing scientific literature is insufficient to show acceptable post-LT outcomes in AH, both in terms of survival and alcohol relapse. As stewards of organ transplantation, transplant providers should prove acceptable outcomes for a given indication before widespread adoption. The United States experience in LT for AH consists of a few, small, single-center experiences and a multicenter retrospective analysis that included data from the 2 initial single-center published experiences.[39,41–43] Concerns regarding patient survival are driven by the 77% 1-year survival reported in the Franco-Belgian study.[38] However, in the American Consortium of Early Liver Transplantation for Alcoholic Hepatitis (ACCELERATE-AH) multicenter retrospective study, survival was an excellent 94% at 1 year and 84% at 3 years[43] Of greater concern is the risk of alcohol relapse potentially leading to consequences of AUD and adverse graft outcomes. In the Franco-Belgian study, only 3 patients relapsed to alcohol. However, in ACCELERATE, 34% of patients had some alcohol use by 3 years and sustained use was present in 17%.[38,43] Sustained alcohol use was associated with graft loss. In addition, although post-LT survival in ACCELERATE-AH was excellent and alcohol relapse not significantly greater than published experiences in cirrhosis, the median follow-up was only 1.8 years, and thus follow-up is likely not sufficient to truly capture the impact of relapse post-LT. In addition, studies of AH survivors, with or without LT, show that severe alcohol relapse is common and associated with poor outcomes.[46–48] Thus, critics argue that data on LT for AH lack sufficient quality, and longer-term follow-up is needed to show acceptable outcomes before the widespread adoption of the practice. In addition, graft loss is only 1 potential consequence of alcohol relapse. Medical nonadherence, other alcohol-related medical complications, and social or legal consequences of harmful drinking are also potential consequences of relapse. Critics argue that, even in the absence of graft loss, alcohol relapse damages LT program morale and may negatively affect public perception of LT.[40]

A second critique of the practice of LT for AH focuses on lack of clearly defined criteria and transparency in patient selection. At present, although published experiences in LT for AH have noted stringent selection criteria, specifics are frequently lacking. Although numerous scoring systems (**Table 4**) are available to help provide a risk estimate for future alcohol use, no scoring system predicts alcohol relapse sufficiently to be used as the sole arbiter of LT candidacy.[49–51] In addition, although multiple factors may portend prognosis in AUD, the natural history is unpredictable. Thus, critics note that LT selection may be increasingly subjective and therefore subject to bias and external influences. Providers may lose objectivity in the evaluation process and feel compelled to advocate for an unacceptably high-risk candidate

Table 4
Prediction tools for post–liver transplant alcohol relapse

Prediction Tool	Variables Assessed	Study Population	Interpretation	Outcome of Interest
MAPS[71]	1. Acceptance of AUD 2. Substitute activities 3. Behavioral consequences 4. Source of hope/self-esteem 5. Social relationship 6. Steady job 7. Stable residence 8. Does not live alone 9. Stable marriage	LT recipients for ALD	Scored 5–20 with higher numbers favorable	Alcohol relapse after LT. MAPS not predictive on 1 retrospective study[72]
ARRA[50]	10. Absence of hepatocellular carcinoma 11. Tobacco use 12. Continued use despite liver disease 13. Low motivation for AUD treatment 14. Poor stress management skills 15. Lack of a rehabilitation relationship 16. Limited social support 17. Lacks nonmedical behavioral consequences 18. Engagement in social activities where alcohol is present	138 LT recipients with a history of alcohol abuse or dependence Single center	Single point per variable ARRA I (0 points): 0% ARRA II (1–3 points): 8% ARRA III (4–6 points): 57% ARRA IV (7–9 points): 75%	Return to any alcohol consumption

Score	Components	Study population	Scoring	Outcome
HRAR [49]	1. Duration of heavy drinking 2. Daily drinks 3. Prior alcohol inpatient treatments	387 LT recipients for alcohol-related cirrhosis; Two centers	Variables scored 0–2 points; HRAR>3 significantly associated with outcome	40 g of alcohol consumption daily
Stanford Integrated Psychosocial Assessment for Transplantation [73]	Psychosocial domains assessed: 1. Patient readiness level and illness management 2. Social support system level of readiness 3. Psychological stability and mental disorder 4. Lifestyle and effect of substance use	102 solid organ transplant recipients, including 52 LT recipients; Single center	Scored 0–86 based on the 4 domains; Higher scores indicated greater psychosocial risk	Higher scores correlated with higher rates of rejection, medical hospitalization, infection rate, psychiatric decompensations, support system failure [74]
HPSS [40,41]	1. Self-admission to the hospital 2. Drinks per day 3. Insight 4. Marital status 5. Abstinence duration 6. Psychiatric comorbidity 7. History of other substance abuse 8. History of failed rehabilitation attempt 9. Family history of AUD 10. Employment 11. Legal history	80 patients that underwent LT for ALD, including 46 with AH; Single center	Variables scored −2 to +2; HPSS ≤ 0 associated with alcohol relapse	Any alcohol use after LT
Sustained Alcohol Use after Liver Transplant [51]	1. >10 drinks per day 2. Multiple failed rehabilitation attempts 3. Alcohol-related legal trouble 4. Other substance use	134 patients that underwent LT for clinical alcohol abuse diagnosis; Multicenter	Scored 0–11; Scores <5 had a 95% negative predictive value for sustained alcohol use after LT	Sustained use defined as alcohol use for a minimum of 100 d

Abbreviations: ARRA, Alcohol Relapse Risk Assessment; HPSS, Hopkins Psychosocial Scale; HRAR, High Risk for Alcohol Relapse; MAPS, Michigan Alcohol Prognosis Score.

Data from Refs. [40,41,49–51,71–74]

secondary to personal feelings or pressure from the patient support system. The propensity to bias in the selection process increases in importance in the setting of MELD-based organ allocation and wider geographic sharing of organs. Programs under pressure to grow transplant volume are at risk for relaxing selection standards in pursuit of transplant volume.

Many critics of LT for AH are concerned that widespread adoption of LT for AH could overwhelm an LT program and worsen the organ shortage. Epidemiologic data show that deaths from ALD are increasing in the United States.[52,53] ALD is now the leading indication for LT in the United States.[1] Although epidemiologic data on AH are more difficult to fully discern, severe AH is clearly a frequent cause of inpatient liver-related hospital admissions and medical failures are likewise common. A recent study of International Classification of Diseases coded AH hospital admissions in 4 US states showed that the incidence of AH admissions had increased across all age groups over time, with the greatest increase in the demographic aged 20 to 39 years.[54] The incidence of AH admissions was highest among non-Hispanic white people. Offering LT for AH will add considerable workload to an LT program and potentially overwhelm existing program resources.[55] Thus, critics fear that expanding LT to AH will dramatically increase the number of LT evaluations performed, yield few acceptable candidates, and increase the risk of burnout in the program. In addition, analyses of the United Network for Organ Sharing (UNOS) database suggest that LT for AH is already occurring more frequently than is reported and many LT programs are now accepting AH as an indication for LT in selected patients.[2,56,57] In addition to increasing the workload for an LT program, increasing the pool of transplant candidates in the absence of increased organ availability will worsen this disparity between LT candidates and availability given that the transplant community faces a permanent scarcity of donor organs.

Disparity is also a concern in patient selection and availability of rescue LT for AH. Payer acceptance of early LT in AH is variable and an audit of state Medicaid requirements shows continued adherence to fixed intervals for ALD before LT consideration in many states.[58] In addition, given that a minority of patients with AH are ultimately selected for LT, there is concern that early LT for AH will favor patients who have the financial means to access multiple programs in pursuit of LT listing.

In addition, critics note that the natural history of medically refractory, severe AH is still unpredictable. In the Franco-Belgian trial, 6-month survival in a matched nontransplanted cohort was 30%.[38] This 6-month survival is similar to previous studies of corticosteroids in AH.[20,21] However, some studies have shown higher short-term prognosis in corticosteroid nonresponders.[22] Thus, the potential exists that premature LT in medically refractory severe AH may subject patients with severe AH that would have recovered to life-altering operations and deplete the donor pool.

PATIENT SELECTION

At the heart of the controversy surrounding LT for AH is patient selection (**Fig. 2**). Severe AH presents several unique challenges in the transplant selection process. The severity of liver failure, compressed time frame, and the LT evaluation process create an unfavorable environment for a comprehensive assessment of AUD. AUD is itself a complex medical problem and often coexistent with psychiatric comorbidities. On an individual basis, the unpredictable natural history of AUD means no 1 factor or combination of risk factors can guarantee alcohol abstinence or relapse after LT. Ultimately, LT programs are forced to assess AUD prognosis despite the limitations noted earlier. Consistency and uniformity in the selection process are essential to

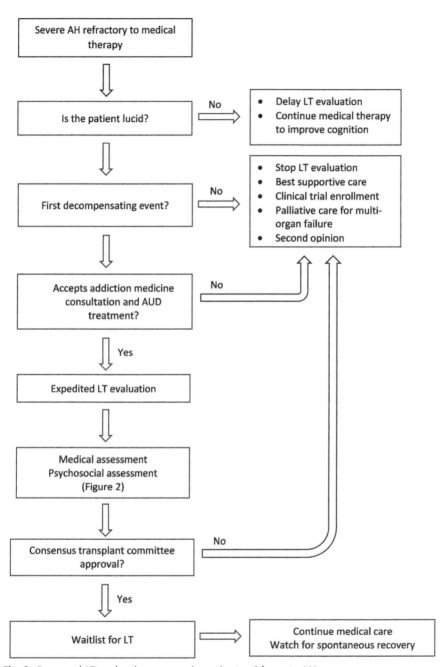

Fig. 2. Proposed LT evaluation process in patients with acute AH.

justice in the transplant selection process, ethical distribution of allografts, and to ensure a sense of integrity for a transplant team.

Recognition of AUD as a separate diagnosis from AH and ALD is essential to beginning an objective transplant evaluation, regardless of sobriety length. Rather than a moral failing or a failure of willpower, AUD is a complex biopsychosocial disease with its own treatment and prognosis. As such, any LT program performing LT for ALD, regardless of AH, should have dedicated personnel with experience in the assessment and management of addictive disorders. The addiction medicine and social work teams should become involved while the patient with AH is lucid and ideally before the initiation of the transplant discussion. The presence of impaired cognitive function, secondary to either hepatic encephalopathy (HE) or another medical condition, should ideally postpone the addiction assessment until patient lucidity can be established. This requirement presents a unique challenge in severe AH because patients frequently have at least minimal HE, thus making a detailed interview difficult.[59] If the patient cannot participate in the addiction assessment because of persistent mental status change, LT evaluation should only proceed under extreme caution. The patient interview is the most critical diagnostic tool in the AUD assessment and is severely limited if the patient cannot participate. Not surprisingly, HE at the time of evaluation is associated with post-LT harmful alcohol use.[43]

Corroborative information and interviews with close patient family and friends are important.[60,61] First, in gathering information from third parties, the interviewer may discover confirmation or discrepancy in the history provided by the patient. A fuller picture of AUD severity may develop. Second, interviewing close family or friends helps establish the presence or absence of social support necessary for the LT process. Because AUD can be an isolating disease, the interviewer may find third-party reservations about the patient as an LT candidate and reluctance to serve as a support system after LT. In addition, pathologic alcohol use may be shared between patients and their support partners. The interviewer should take an alcohol use history and consider screening individuals for harmful drinking if identified as support in the LT process.

There is no standard evaluation of AUD for the ALD population being evaluated for LT. The Diagnostic and Statistical Manual of Mental Disorders (DSM-V) combined the previous DSM-IV diagnoses of alcohol abuse and alcohol dependence into the diagnosis of AUD (https://dsm.psychiatryonline.org/doi/book/10.1176/appi.books. 9780890425596).[62] A diagnosis of AUD is made if 2 of the 11 criteria for AUD are met. The severity of AUD is graded as mild, moderate, or severe depending on the number of criteria met. An assessment of AUD severity is important as an objective measure of severity of illness. In addition to an assessment of AUD severity, the assessment should include a detailed history of alcohol use and other substance use, prior history of substance use treatment, previous periods of sobriety, and a history of use despite negative substance-related health, and legal and social consequences. A history of childhood upbringing and adverse childhood experiences, including a family history of substance use disorders, is important to establish both a developmental and biological basis for substance abuse.[63] A detailed psychiatric history should be taken, including a history of mental health diagnoses and treatment, including the exploration of untreated symptoms of anxiety or depression. In addition, and most importantly, patients should be assessed as to their level of insight into their AUD diagnoses and willingness to seek AUD treatment as their health allows.

The goal of the addiction medicine and social work assessment is to provide the LT program selection committee an estimation of prognosis regarding AUD and risk of harmful alcohol use after LT. As mentioned previously, no 1 factor has reliably been shown to predict prognosis in AUD; however, numerous factors have been shown to predict risk for and protection from future harmful drinking.[40,46,49–51,60,64] Prognostic tools (see **Table 4**) can assist in the selection process but should be used as an adjunct rather than as a sole arbiter of transplant candidacy. In the absence of a

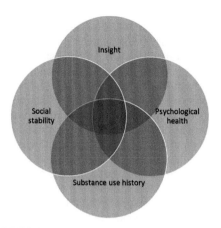

Protective Factors	Risk Factors
Insight	
• Acceptance of AUD diagnosis • Willingness to seek AUD treatment	• Ambivalence or denial of AUD diagnosis • Ambivalence or refusal of AUD treatment • Acceptance of AUD treatment only as mandatory for LT candidacy
Psychological Health	
• Absence of personality disorder • Absence of untreated or poorly treated mental health disorder • Normal childhood • Source of hope/self-esteem	• Personality disorder • Untreated/poorly treated mental health disorder • Deprived childhood • Impaired cognition
Social stability	
• Strong sober support/rehabilitation relationship • Structured time • Employment • Negative behavioral reinforcer	• Social isolation • Substance use disorder in partner
Substance use history	
• Longer sobriety length • Older age • Alcohol use only • Lower daily alcohol consumption • Shorter duration of drinking • Mild or moderate AUD diagnosis[a]	• Shorter sobriety length • Younger age • Polysubstance use disorder • Higher daily alcohol consumption • Longer duration of drinking • Severe AUD diagnosis[a] • Previous failed AUD treatment • Alcohol-related legal trouble

Fig. 3. Protective factors and risk factors for alcohol relapse in patients with AUD. [a]AUD has replaced alcohol abuse and alcohol dependence in the DSM-V. Alcohol dependence was previous thought to be a risk factor for harmful drinking after LT. The category of severe AUD is used as a substitute for alcohol dependence. AUD severity has not been well studied in the LT population.

validated process by which to evaluate and select prospective LT candidates with ALD, a 4-domain assessment model, derived from work by Beresford and Lucey,[60,65] can provide a nuanced and comprehensive assessment of risk (**Fig. 3**).[3,60,65] These 4 domains encompass patient insight and acceptance of the drinking problem, social stability, psychological health, and AUD history. Each domain contains several protective and risk factors for relapse to harmful alcohol use. Insight and acknowledgment of problematic alcohol use, particularly in the setting of LT evaluation, is of critical importance. Ambivalence toward drinking or an unwillingness to seek dedicated AUD treatment, particularly in the setting of AH, should be viewed as a major risk factor for harmful post-LT relapse and ideally these patients should undergo a prolonged period of monitoring before consideration of LT.[60,61] Social stability has been described as the "foundation upon which ongoing medical adherence and favorable prognosis are built."[60] For patients attempting to rehabilitate from LT and AUD, having a strong, supportive, and sober social network is paramount for success. Likewise, structured time was identified by Vaillant[19] as a factor that predicted sobriety. This structured time can include employment, Alcoholics Anonymous meetings, or any activity that provides value to the patient and fills idle time. Mental illness and AUD are frequently comorbid. Although mental illness is a risk factor for harmful alcohol use, harmful alcohol use itself can precipitate many of the symptoms common to mental illness. Severe or poorly controlled mental illness, particularly personality disorders, should be considered a major risk factor for relapse. In addition, a comprehensive assessment of any LT candidate with AUD should include a detailed alcohol history. Multiple risk factors for relapse can be identified in a detailed history. Risk factors that have been associated with relapse include younger age at presentation, shorter duration of sobriety, greater amounts of daily drinking and duration of heavy drinking, polysubstance use, failed rehabilitation attempts, alcohol-related legal difficulties, and AUD severity.[46,49–51] As mentioned previously, these patient factors have been used to create numerical risk estimates for post-LT risk (see **Table 4**). Specifically, in the early LT for AH population, more than 10 drinks per day, multiple failed rehabilitation attempts, alcohol-related legal difficulties, and prior illicit substance abuse were associated with harmful alcohol use after transplant and were used to create a predictive model.[51] This model, named the Sustained Alcohol Use Post–Liver Transplant (SALT) score is a numerical score based on the aforementioned criteria. Patients that scored less than 5 on the SALT score had a 95% negative predictive value for harmful drinking after LT. It has not been externally validated.

At transplant selection, for most patients with AH under consideration for LT, discussion centers on the comprehensive psychosocial assessment. The transplant selection committee should strive to review the medical and psychosocial report objectively and make an unbiased assessment of transplant candidacy. However, objectivity may be difficult in practice. A previous study of transplant selection by Volk and colleagues[66] showed that committees had difficulty maintaining objectivity in making life-and-death decisions. External influences affected decision making and members found the lack of written policies a barrier to effective group decision making. For this reason, despite the lack of reliable predictors of future relapse, many centers have published specific selection criteria for rescue LT in AH. Although inherently imperfect, such policies may permit easier decision making and equality in the transplant evaluation process and decision.

DELIVERING BAD NEWS

Informing patients and their loved ones that they were not selected for rescue LT is difficult. The difficulty stems primarily from 2 factors. First and foremost, the patient and family recognize that, without LT, the patient is likely to die soon. Second, unlike medical contraindications to LT, the rationale for LT denial is typically a belief by the LT selection committee that the patient's AUD is of such severity that sobriety is unlikely after LT. This subjective assessment often runs contrary to a sincere belief by the patient and loved ones that the patient will maintain sobriety. This belief in future abstinence may be strong despite a long history of harmful alcohol use and relapses despite extensive consequences and attempts at treatment.

When delivering the transplant selection committee outcome, it is important for the LT team to decide who will deliver the bad news and answer questions. The patient and family should view the decision as a committee decision and not the arbitrary decision of 1 individual or a select few individuals. For that reason, in some situations, it may be desirable for multiple specialties from the LT selection committee to be present at the delivery of bad news. If a program has a written policy used in candidate selection, reference to those criteria may be helpful in explaining the rationale for LT denial. The timing and location of bad news delivery should be at the discretion of the patient and family. Providers should be seated and deliver the committee decision directly and without ambiguity. Providers should empathize with patient and family emotions and frustration with the decision and answer any questions they might have about the selection process and plan going forward. For patients with multiorgan failure, the prognosis is extremely poor. It is appropriate to discuss palliative care and hospice. However, given the shock of the selection committee decision, palliative care discussions may need to be deferred until the patient and family have processed the transplant decision. For patients without multiorgan failure, some patients with severe AH may recover or eventually be an LT candidate with AUD treatment and monitored sobriety. Although the time frame for LT candidacy may not be realistic, it is important to outline a specific pathway to LT candidacy, when possible. It is also important for the patient and family to know that the patient will still receive high-quality, longitudinal care for the liver disease despite lack of LT candidacy. In addition, some patients or families may request a second opinion regarding LT from another program. Providers should attempt to facilitate this request whenever possible. It is important for providers to communicate that approval for a second opinion does imply selection for LT.

FUTURE DIRECTIONS

LT for AH remains among the most controversial and contentious topics in transplantation. For many transplant professionals, the lifting of mandatory sobriety intervals before LT consideration in ALD is akin to lifting the lid on Pandora's box. Many factors in LT for AH seem ripe for unintended consequences. The volume of patients with AH is considerable and expanding LT consideration may strain the resources allocated to an LT program and health system. Many programs lack the addiction medicine expertise to effectively evaluate and manage a high-risk population. The lack of strong predictors to guide selection puts the onus on a subjective process that struggles with objectivity even with less contentious diagnoses. Recent changes in organ distribution coupled with MELD-based allocation could incentivize a program to lax selection standards in AH in pursuit of transplant volume. In addition, the excellent 1-year survival seen in the ACCLERATE study means excessive risk in patient selection is unlikely to be captured in the Scientific Registry of Transplant Recipients (SRTR) program-specific reporting. Based on these concerns, critics' fear of the so-called race to the bottom seems valid.

However, although these concerns are valid, there is no question that LT saves lives in the setting of severe AH refractory to medical therapy. In addition, mandatory sobriety intervals do not sufficiently predict future relapse and LT outcomes such that they should exclude a candidate with a favorable psychosocial assessment for AUD rehabilitation. Mandatory sobriety intervals are frankly unethical as the sole arbiter of LT candidacy.

So, how should the LT community move forward in making LT for AH a success story rather than a race to the bottom? First, more data are needed, ideally prospective, but certainly longer term. The availability of alcohol biomarkers such as ethyl glucuronide and phosphatidylethanol grant LT programs specific tools to detect potential harmful drinking after LT.[67,68] These tools can be used to better document and understand alcohol use after LT for patients with all forms of ALD and non-ALD indications for LT. With enhanced monitoring biomarkers, alcohol use and relapse definitions need to be used consistently. In the past, studies involving relapse after LT have defined any use as relapse. This lack of nuance does not distinguish nonharmful alcohol consumption or self-limited slips/relapses from refractory AUD relapse, the latter most commonly leading to poor outcomes. Thus, the LT community needs to move away from merely equating any alcohol use with a poor outcome. Similarly, there is a significant need for evidence-based relapse prevention interventions for LT recipients. Trials of relapse prevention medications and strategies to minimize risk of relapse and reestablish sobriety are critical to long-term LT success, regardless of sobriety length. In addition, the UNOS database should revise the transplant candidate registration worksheet to more accurately define ALD. At present, UNOS has diagnosis listing codes for alcoholic cirrhosis and alcoholic hepatitis. The distinction between AH and AC is not always clear; frequently overlaps; and, for the purposes of early LT, is likely irrelevant. This lack of clarity has limited the UNOS database as a source for accurate, nuanced research in ALD.[57] UNOS should begin collecting the date of last alcohol use before listing, rather than asking for a distinction between AH and AC. In addition, modifying the UNOS adult LT recipient follow-up reporting worksheet to include data points on alcohol use post-LT and recurrent ALD as a cause of, or contributing to, graft failure would facilitate mapping of geographic trends in LT for ALD and a more nuanced analysis of long-term outcomes.

Second, programs need to create comprehensive programs for AUD assessment and treatment as well as implement protocols for relapse prevention, monitoring, and treatment. This process starts with adequate human resources. Programs should have adequate addiction medicine and mental health resources to provide a thorough LT candidate assessment and recommendations for AUD rehabilitation. Programs should be resourced for frequent monitoring of LT recipients for relapse, especially in the first year after LT when relapse risk seems the highest.[10,43] With the increasing availability of biomarkers, programs should strongly consider implementing biomarkers in monitoring protocols. Patients should be informed in the LT evaluation process that they will undergo biomarker surveillance and the rationale for monitoring. In addition, candor should be encouraged should relapse occur. Patients need to be reassured that relapse will not be met with scorn or resentment from the transplant team. Instead, patients should be reassured that relapse will be treated compassionately with a goal of assisting the patient in regaining sustained sobriety and ensuring a good LT outcome. In the early post-LT period, programs should consider multidisciplinary visits with addiction medicine specialists and transplant surgery/hepatology.[69] Traditionally, most LT visits focus on the allograft and immunosuppression management. Addiction specialists are better trained to detect alcohol relapse and monitor progress of addiction recovery. In addition, LT programs should consider more widespread use of medication therapy for AUD (**Table 5**). Such treatments are not frequently used in patients with liver disease, but may assist in preventing relapse, particularly in highly vulnerable periods such as in the first year after LT.[70]

In addition, transparency and oversight are essential to ensure successful and ethical LT for AH. Programs should publish their selection processes and criteria for LT in AH/ALD. Detailed data elements from the psychosocial assessment should be recorded and periodically reviewed to determine whether selection guidelines are being adhered to and whether updates to the process and criteria are needed. Posttransplant, published protocols should be put into place detailing processes for alcohol

Table 5
Relapse prevention medications for consideration in alcohol-associated liver disease

Medication	Dosage	Mechanism of Action	Studied in ALD	Concerns
Acamprosate[a]	666 mg by mouth 3 times per day	NMDA receptor antagonist	No	Contraindicated for creatinine clearance <30 mL/min
Naltrexone[a]	50 mg by mouth daily or 380 mg subcutaneously monthly	Opioid receptor antagonist	No	Potential hepatotoxicity
Gabapentin	600–1800 mg by mouth daily	Modulates GABA activity	No	Needs dose reduction for renal impairment
Baclofen	30–60 mg/d	GABA-B receptor agonist	Single RCT suggested benefit	—
Topiramate	75–400 mg/d	GABA action augmentation	No	—

Abbreviations: GABA, gamma-aminobutyric acid; NMDA, N-methyl-ᴅ-aspartate; RCT, randomized controlled trial.
[a] Denotes US Food and Drug Administration approval.
Data from Crabb, DW et al. Diagnosis and Treatment of Alcohol-Related Liver Diseases: 2019 Practice Guidance from the American Association for the Study of Liver Diseases. In. Hepatology. 2019

relapse prevention, monitoring, and intervention should alcohol relapse occur. Similarly, programs should have a systematic process for recording relevant post-LT outcomes such as relapse and graft loss. These documents should be available for audit by regulators to ensure adherence to published selection standards.

LT for AH creates several challenges in oversight. First, the unpredictable natural history of AUD, potential for reviewer bias, and relative urgency of LT for severe AH render external review by the UNOS National Liver Review Board potentially unfavorable. Nevertheless, external review may be a viable strategy for oversight and objectivity in LT selection. Second, 1-year LT outcomes do not adequately capture psychosocial risk in most circumstances. Even in the case of early, severe refractory alcohol relapse, allograft loss within 1 year would be considered exceptional. Whether use of 3-year graft and patient outcomes from the SRTR program-specific report in determination of Centers for Medicare and Medicaid Services (CMS) Conditions of Participation or private payer Center of Excellence status would adequately capture risk in ALD selection is unknown. However, with longer follow-up, confounding factors leading to allograft loss may render 3-year outcomes nonspecific for determining risk in AH selection.

SUMMARY

In the absence of better medical therapy for severe AH, salvage LT remains the only hope for survival for many patients with severe AH that are refractory to, or ineligible for, corticosteroids. Clearly, well-selected patients with favorable psychosocial profiles for AUD rehabilitation can do well after LT with excellent survival and a low risk for sustained alcohol relapse. At the heart of the debate surrounding LT for AH is the selection process. This process is made difficult by the volume of patients with severe AH, unpredictable natural history of AUD, lack of specific criteria to reliably predict outcomes, and the potential for loss of objectivity in the selection process. For LT for severe AH to be successful, programs need to be adequately resourced for AUD assessment, monitoring, and treatment; transparent in their selection processes; and subject to appropriate regulatory oversight. More longitudinal data are needed to better capture long-term outcomes after LT for AH and UNOS data recording elements modified to reflect the reality that the 6-month rule is increasingly being abandoned in the United States. It is up to the LT community to ensure that LT for AH is being performed in a manner that upholds utility and justice in the process.

CLINICS CARE POINTS

- Liver Transplantation can be performed successfully with a significant survival benefit in severe alcohol-associated hepatitis unresponsive to medical therapy.
- Liver Transplantation for alcohol-associated hepatitis should be reserved for patients with a favorable prognosis for rehabilitation from alcohol use disorder.
- Numerous risk factors help predict risk for harmful alcohol use after liver transplantation, however no one factor nor combinations of factors can reliably predict outcome for an individual patient.
- Liver Transplant programs performing early liver transplantation for alcohol-associated hepatitis should be transparent in the selection process.

REFERENCES

1. Cholankeril G, Ahmed A. Alcoholic liver disease replaces hepatitis C virus infection as the leading indication for liver transplantation in the United States. Clin Gastroenterol Hepatol 2018;16(8):1356–8.

2. Lee BP, Vittinghoff E, Dodge JL, et al. National trends and long-term outcomes of liver transplant for alcohol-associated liver disease in the United States. JAMA Intern Med 2019;179(3):340–8.
3. Im GY, Cameron AM, Lucey MR. Liver transplantation for alcoholic hepatitis. J Hepatol 2019;70(2):328–34.
4. National Institutes of health consensus development conference statement: liver transplantation–june 20-23, 1983. Hepatology 1984;4(1 Suppl):107S–10S.
5. Starzl TE, Van Thiel D, Tzakis AG, et al. Orthotopic liver transplantation for alcoholic cirrhosis. JAMA 1988;260(17):2542–4.
6. Lucey MR, Schaubel DE, Guidinger MK, et al. Effect of alcoholic liver disease and hepatitis C infection on waiting list and posttransplant mortality and transplant survival benefit. Hepatology 2009;50(2):400–6.
7. Burra P, Senzolo M, Adam R, et al. Liver transplantation for alcoholic liver disease in Europe: a study from the ELTR (European Liver Transplant Registry). Am J Transplant 2010;10(1):138–48.
8. Pfitzmann R, Schwenzer J, Rayes N, et al. Long-term survival and predictors of relapse after orthotopic liver transplantation for alcoholic liver disease. Liver Transpl 2007;13(2):197–205.
9. Rice JP, Eickhoff J, Agni R, et al. Abusive drinking after liver transplantation is associated with allograft loss and advanced allograft fibrosis. Liver Transpl 2013;19(12):1377–86.
10. DiMartini A, Dew MA, Day N, et al. Trajectories of alcohol consumption following liver transplantation. Am J Transplant 2010;10(10):2305–12.
11. Cuadrado A, Fábrega E, Casafont F, et al. Alcohol recidivism impairs long-term patient survival after orthotopic liver transplantation for alcoholic liver disease. Liver Transpl 2005;11(4):420–6.
12. Erard-Poinsot D, Guillaud O, Hervieu V, et al. Severe alcoholic relapse after liver transplantation: what consequences on the graft? A study based on liver biopsies analysis. Liver Transpl 2016;22(6):773–84.
13. Vaillant GE. The natural history of alcoholism and its relationship to liver transplantation. Liver Transpl Surg 1997;3(3):304–10.
14. Bellamy CO, DiMartini AM, Ruppert K, et al. Liver transplantation for alcoholic cirrhosis: long term follow-up and impact of disease recurrence. Transplantation 2001;72(4):619–26.
15. Everhart JE, Beresford TP. Liver transplantation for alcoholic liver disease: a survey of transplantation programs in the United States. Liver Transpl Surg 1997; 3(3):220–6.
16. Lucey MR, Brown KA, Everson GT, et al. Minimal criteria for placement of adults on the liver transplant waiting list: a report of a national conference organized by the American Society of Transplant Physicians and the American Association for the Study of Liver Diseases. Transplantation 1998;66(7):956–62.
17. Jauhar S, Talwalkar JA, Schneekloth T, et al. Analysis of factors that predict alcohol relapse following liver transplantation. Liver Transpl 2004;10(3):408–11.
18. Egawa H, Nishimura K, Teramukai S, et al. Risk factors for alcohol relapse after liver transplantation for alcoholic cirrhosis in Japan. Liver Transpl 2014;20(3): 298–310.
19. Vaillant GE. A 60-year follow-up of alcoholic men. Addiction 2003;98(8):1043–51.
20. Mathurin P, O'Grady J, Carithers RL, et al. Corticosteroids improve short-term survival in patients with severe alcoholic hepatitis: meta-analysis of individual patient data. Gut 2011;60(2):255–60.

21. Louvet A, Naveau S, Abdelnour M, et al. The Lille model: a new tool for therapeutic strategy in patients with severe alcoholic hepatitis treated with steroids. Hepatology 2007;45(6):1348–54.
22. Thursz MR, Richardson P, Allison M, et al. Prednisolone or pentoxifylline for alcoholic hepatitis. N Engl J Med 2015;372(17):1619–28.
23. Crabb DW, Bataller R, Chalasani NP, et al. Standard definitions and common data elements for clinical trials in patients with alcoholic hepatitis: recommendation from the NIAAA Alcoholic Hepatitis Consortia. Gastroenterology 2016;150(4):785–90.
24. Roth NC, Qin J. Histopathology of alcohol-related liver diseases. Clin Liver Dis 2019;23(1):11–23.
25. Moreau R, Jalan R, Gines P, et al. Acute-on-chronic liver failure is a distinct syndrome that develops in patients with acute decompensation of cirrhosis. Gastroenterology 2013;144(7):1426–37, 1437.e1-9.
26. Gustot T, Jalan R. Acute-on-chronic liver failure in patients with alcohol-related liver disease. J Hepatol 2019;70(2):319–27.
27. Sersté T, Cornillie A, Njimi H, et al. The prognostic value of acute-on-chronic liver failure during the course of severe alcoholic hepatitis. J Hepatol 2018;69(2):318–24.
28. Moreno C, Deltenre P, Senterre C, et al. Intensive enteral nutrition is ineffective for patients with severe alcoholic hepatitis treated with corticosteroids. Gastroenterology 2016;150(4):903–10.e8.
29. Crabb DW, Im GY, Szabo G, et al. Diagnosis and treatment of alcohol-related liver diseases: 2019 practice guidance from the American association for the study of liver diseases. Hepatology 2020;71(1):306–33.
30. easloffice@easloffice.eu EAftSotLEa, Liver EAftSot. EASL clinical practice guidelines: management of alcohol-related liver disease. J Hepatol 2018;69(1):154–81.
31. Arab JP, Roblero JP, Altamirano J, et al. Alcohol-related liver disease: clinical practice guidelines by the Latin American association for the study of the liver (ALEH). Ann Hepatol 2019;18(3):518–35.
32. Vergis N, Atkinson SR, Knapp S, et al. In patients with severe alcoholic hepatitis, prednisolone increases susceptibility to infection and infection-related mortality, and is associated with high circulating levels of bacterial DNA. Gastroenterology 2017;152(5):1068–77.e4.
33. Louvet A, Wartel F, Castel H, et al. Infection in patients with severe alcoholic hepatitis treated with steroids: early response to therapy is the key factor. Gastroenterology 2009;137(2):541–8.
34. Garcia-Saenz-de-Sicilia M, Duvoor C, Altamirano J, et al. Corrigendum: a day-4 lille model predicts response to corticosteroids and mortality in severe alcoholic hepatitis. Am J Gastroenterol 2017;112(4):666.
35. Mathurin P, Abdelnour M, Ramond MJ, et al. Early change in bilirubin levels is an important prognostic factor in severe alcoholic hepatitis treated with prednisolone. Hepatology 2003;38(6):1363–9.
36. Forrest EH, Atkinson SR, Richardson P, et al. Application of prognostic scores in the STOPAH trial: discriminant function is no longer the optimal scoring system in alcoholic hepatitis. J Hepatol 2018;68(3):511–8.
37. Lucey MR, Mathurin P, Morgan TR. Alcoholic hepatitis. N Engl J Med 2009;360(26):2758–69.
38. Mathurin P, Moreno C, Samuel D, et al. Early liver transplantation for severe alcoholic hepatitis. N Engl J Med 2011;365(19):1790–800.

39. Im GY, Kim-Schluger L, Shenoy A, et al. Early liver transplantation for severe alcoholic hepatitis in the United States–a single-center experience. Am J Transplant 2016;16(3):841–9.
40. Lee BP, Chen PH, Haugen C, et al. Three-year results of a pilot program in early liver transplantation for severe alcoholic hepatitis. Ann Surg 2017;265(1):20–9.
41. Weeks SR, Sun Z, McCaul ME, et al. Liver transplantation for severe alcoholic hepatitis, updated lessons from the world's largest series. J Am Coll Surg 2018;226(4):549–57.
42. Sundaram V, Wu T, Klein AS, et al. Liver transplantation for severe alcoholic hepatitis: report of a single center pilot program. Transplant Proc 2018;50(10): 3527–32.
43. Lee BP, Mehta N, Platt L, et al. Outcomes of early liver transplantation for patients with severe alcoholic hepatitis. Gastroenterology 2018;155(2):422–30.e1.
44. Lee BP, Samur S, Dalgic OO, et al. Model to calculate harms and benefits of early vs delayed liver transplantation for patients with alcohol-associated hepatitis. Gastroenterology 2019;157(2):472–80.e5.
45. Stroh G, Rosell T, Dong F, et al. Early liver transplantation for patients with acute alcoholic hepatitis: public views and the effects on organ donation. Am J Transplant 2015;15(6):1598–604.
46. Altamirano J, López-Pelayo H, Michelena J, et al. Alcohol abstinence in patients surviving an episode of alcoholic hepatitis: prediction and impact on long-term survival. Hepatology 2017;66(6):1842–53.
47. Degré D, Stauber RE, Englebert G, et al. Long-term outcomes in patients with decompensated alcohol-related liver disease, steatohepatitis and Maddrey's discriminant function <32. J Hepatol 2020;72(4):636–42.
48. Louvet A, Labreuche J, Artru F, et al. Main drivers of outcome differ between short term and long term in severe alcoholic hepatitis: a prospective study. Hepatology 2017;66(5):1464–73.
49. De Gottardi A, Spahr L, Gelez P, et al. A simple score for predicting alcohol relapse after liver transplantation: results from 387 patients over 15 years. Arch Intern Med 2007;167(11):1183–8.
50. Rodrigue JR, Hanto DW, Curry MP. The Alcohol Relapse Risk Assessment: a scoring system to predict the risk of relapse to any alcohol use after liver transplant. Prog Transplant 2013;23(4):310–8.
51. Lee BP, Vittinghoff E, Hsu C, et al. Predicting low risk for sustained alcohol use after early liver transplant for acute alcoholic hepatitis: the sustained alcohol use post-liver transplant score. Hepatology 2019;69(4):1477–87.
52. Tapper EB, Parikh ND. Mortality due to cirrhosis and liver cancer in the United States, 1999-2016: observational study. BMJ 2018;362:k2817.
53. Moon AM, Yang JY, Barritt AS, et al. Rising mortality from alcohol-associated liver disease in the United States in the 21st century. Am J Gastroenterol 2020;115(1): 79–87.
54. Doshi SD, Stotts MJ, Hubbard RA, et al. The changing burden of alcoholic hepatitis: rising incidence and associations with age, gender, race, and geography. Dig Dis Sci 2020. https://doi.org/10.1007/s10620-020-06346-8.
55. Vogel A, Nahas J, Shenoy A, et al. Center level impact of early liver transplantation for alcoholic hepatitis. Hepatology 2017;66(S1):88.
56. Bangaru S, Pedersen MR, MacConmara MP, et al. Survey of liver transplantation practices for severe acute alcoholic hepatitis. Liver Transpl 2018;24(10):1357–62.
57. Lee BP, Im GY, Rice JP, et al. Underestimation of liver transplantation for alcoholic hepatitis in the national transplant database. Liver Transpl 2019;25(5):706–11.

58. Lee BP, Vittinghoff E, Pletcher MJ, et al. Medicaid policy and liver transplant for alcohol-associated liver disease. Hepatology 2020;72(1):130–9.
59. Louvet A, Thursz MR, Kim DJ, et al. Corticosteroids reduce risk of death within 28 days for patients with severe alcoholic hepatitis, compared with pentoxifylline or placebo-a meta-analysis of individual data from controlled trials. Gastroenterology 2018;155(2):458–68.e8.
60. Beresford TP, Lucey MR. Towards standardizing the alcoholism evaluation of potential liver transplant recipients. Alcohol Alcohol 2018;53(2):135–44.
61. Asrani SK, Trotter J, Lake J, et al. Meeting report: the dallas consensus conference on liver transplantation for alcohol associated hepatitis. Liver Transpl 2020;26(1):127–40.
62. American Psychiatric Association. American Psychiatric Association. DSM-5 Task Force. Diagnostic and statistical manual of mental disorders: DSM-5. 5th edition. Washington, DC: American Psychiatric Association; 2013.
63. Jung J, Rosoff DB, Muench C, et al. Adverse childhood experiences are associated with high-intensity binge drinking behavior in adulthood and mediated by psychiatric disorders. Alcohol Alcohol 2020;55(2):204–14.
64. Vaillant GE. The natural history of alcoholism revisited. Cambridge (MA): Harvard University Press; 1995.
65. Beresford TP, Lucey MR. Alcoholics and liver transplantation: facts, biases, and the future. Addiction 1994;89(9):1043–8.
66. Volk ML, Biggins SW, Huang MA, et al. Decision making in liver transplant selection committees: a multicenter study. Ann Intern Med 2011;155(8):503–8.
67. Beckmann M, Paslakis G, Böttcher M, et al. Integration of clinical examination, self-report, and hair ethyl glucuronide analysis for evaluation of patients with alcoholic liver disease prior to liver transplantation. Prog Transplant 2016;26(1):40–6.
68. Fleming MF, Smith MJ, Oslakovic E, et al. Phosphatidylethanol detects moderate-to-heavy alcohol use in liver transplant recipients. Alcohol Clin Exp Res 2017; 41(4):857–62.
69. Magistri P, Marzi L, Guerzoni S, et al. Impact of a multidisciplinary team on alcohol recidivism and survival after liver transplant for alcoholic disease. Transplant Proc 2019;51(1):187–9.
70. Rogal S, Youk A, Zhang H, et al. Impact of alcohol use disorder treatment on clinical outcomes among patients with cirrhosis. Hepatology 2020;71(6):2080–92.
71. Beresford T. Alcoholism prognosis scale for major organ transplant candidates. In: Craven J, Rodin GM, editors. Psychiatric aspects of organ transplantation. New York: Oxford University Press; 1992. p. 31–2.
72. Lucey MR, Carr K, Beresford TP, et al. Alcohol use after liver transplantation in alcoholics: a clinical cohort follow-up study. Hepatology 1997;25(5):1223–7.
73. Maldonado JR, Dubois HC, David EE, et al. The Stanford Integrated Psychosocial Assessment for Transplantation (SIPAT): a new tool for the psychosocial evaluation of pre-transplant candidates. Psychosomatics 2012;53(2):123–32.
74. Maldonado JR, Sher Y, Lolak S, et al. The stanford integrated psychosocial assessment for transplantation: a prospective study of medical and psychosocial outcomes. Psychosom Med 2015;77(9):1018–30.

Moving?

Make sure your subscription moves with you!

To notify us of your new address, find your **Clinics Account Number** (located on your mailing label above your name), and contact customer service at:

Email: journalscustomerservice-usa@elsevier.com

800-654-2452 (subscribers in the U.S. & Canada)
314-447-8871 (subscribers outside of the U.S. & Canada)

Fax number: 314-447-8029

Elsevier Health Sciences Division
Subscription Customer Service
3251 Riverport Lane
Maryland Heights, MO 63043

*To ensure uninterrupted delivery of your subscription, please notify us at least 4 weeks in advance of move.

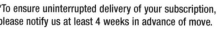

ELSEVIER

Moving?

Make sure your subscription moves with you!

To notify us of your new address, find your Clinics Account number (located on your mailing label above your name), and contact customer service at:

Email: journalscustomerservice-usa@elsevier.com

800-654-2452 (subscribers in the U.S. & Canada)
314-447-8871 (subscribers outside of the U.S. & Canada)

Fax number: 314-447-8029

Elsevier Health Sciences Division
Subscription Customer Service
3251 Riverport Lane
Maryland Heights, MO 63043

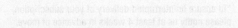